AF885256

# CPC Study Guide

# 2025-2026

***Complete Review + 500 Questions and Detailed Answer Explanations for the Certified Professional Coder Exam (5 Full-Length Exams + Medical Coding Review)***

# Table of Contents

# Chapter 1: Tips for the AAPC Certification Exam

## Why AAPC Certification?

The American Academy of Professional Coders (AAPC) certification examination is vital for a career as a certified professional coder. The test is advantageous for coders who are just starting or already working in the industry. AAPC certification provides evidence of acquired skills and understanding of healthcare intricacies.

Passing the test gives a coder credibility as a professional, improves job prospects, and allows them to command more value in the highly competitive profession. This translates to an uptick in expected monetary remuneration. It is a commitment to a blooming career as a certified professional coder.

## Where to Start?

**Relax**. Maintain a calm state while studying. Breathe in, hold, breathe out, hold, and repeat for a few minutes. Candidates need to be relaxed under examination pressure on their test day, hence the need to practice relaxation techniques.

**Start early**. Begin preparing for this exam as soon as possible to be well-rounded. Preparation is a marathon and requires careful planning and diligent dedication.

**Not starting early?** This book will guide candidates through the requisite sections and knowledge base. However, they will need to spend more time daily and be more locked in than ever.

## Break Large Goals into Smaller Targets

Little drops of water make a mighty ocean, and a thousand-mile journey comprises many tiny steps. Set an overarching goal of exceptional performance for the exam. Achieving this goal depends on a candidate's ability to recall the details of the material and review their skills every day. Break a study goal into months, weeks, days, and hours. Choose an accountability partner to help keep on track.

## Draw an Information Map

An information map overviews all the concepts a candidate must learn for this exam. An outline of this book is a good start, as it closely mirrors the official test outline. Write down the chapter titles, then visualize them and group the concepts based on their relationship. Put those that can be studied together in the same group.

During this process, identify the vocabularies specific to each of these sections and list them. This step is handy when studying these sections later, as it makes an easy-to-reference glossary. Keep this list close and update it regularly. This book also helps in this regard. Chapters are arranged and discussed sequentially, and most have a glossary subsection.

## Have a Schedule and Timeline

After creating an information map, make a strategy that covers the timeline for each section. Although the plan may be broad, keep it simple. *Create achievable, clear targets for each day.* Deadlines and measurable goals clarify what needs to be done and when it needs to be finished.

Also, studying a small section per day helps retain learned material and concepts. It also reduces the chance of becoming overwhelmed. Building this practice of regular, deliberate study goals and routines is an integral step on the journey to success.

## Study Environment Is Everything

The environment has a massive impact on the effectiveness of studying. This includes the candidate's physical location and the people surrounding them during this period. Although, in theory, study can be done anywhere, a study location should ideally be away from distractions.

During the preparation period for this exam, a candidate should have a team of other test takers. Being in a study group can help one develop a study plan. Study groups make reviewing concepts less stressful, as the members can devise a plan to examine critical points at predetermined intervals. These meetings could include drills and quizzes.

## Study Techniques

Everyone has a preferred learning style. Identify which study technique works best. This helps maximize study time regarding concept understanding, retention of studied materials, and recall. Some options include visualization, listening, and discussing.

Candidates who learn best with visualization could draw flowcharts for the main concepts, the key points, and their details. Also, they could color-code their study materials, make representative illustrations and symbols, and mentally attach specific ideas to them.

Alternatively, if a candidate learns more by hearing or discussing the topics, they can make a voice recording of the subjects and associated concepts. The recorded notes can become a way to review at a later date. Another effective method is to get a study partner to discuss the topics being studied. Planning group discussions ensures that most of the time is dedicated to studying rather than other distractions.

Irrespective of the chosen technique, flashcards are a helpful addition. Mnemonics encode study materials to make storage and later recall easier. Using mnemonics is another viable option to explore as a study tool. In reality, candidates usually use a combination of most of these techniques. The key is to find the best variety and timing and stick with it religiously.

## Practice Review Questions

Practice questions are an effective way to see how prepared a candidate is for the examination. It is a reliable approach to studying actively. It also helps calibrate speed and accuracy. The approach below can help channel one's attention to benefit maximally from answering questions.

Start practicing questions without time constraints and using an open-book approach. This will give a candidate a feel for the test, and they can focus on answering the questions correctly. Next, practice the questions within a set time and with a closed-book approach. This may be difficult initially, but it will become easier with repetition.

**Review the questions that were answered incorrectly.** These questions highlight incomplete understanding. Reexamine the relevant sections of your study materials. Make sure to understand why these questions were wrong.

**Pay attention to the questions that were difficult or required extra time to solve.** This helps identify places where a candidate has some knowledge but a weak understanding of concepts. Candidates may also need to unravel the gist of particularly wordy questions.

Many practice questions include answers and explanations. This only provides a superficial knowledge of why the supplied answer is correct. Be sure to study the concept and any other related details properly to gain a thorough understanding. Simply relying on the given explanation does not guarantee a solid grasp of the concept.

Ultimately, the goal should be to answer all the questions in each section with enough time to review. This means that if the total time for a section with 100 questions is sixty minutes, the expected time for each question is estimated to be thirty seconds. Endeavor to spend less time than this for each question, perhaps twenty-three to twenty-five seconds on average. This strategy builds in time to review answers. Aim for about eighty-five to ninety percent correct answers in the practice sessions.

## Approach to Answering Questions

- **Code manual use:** Code manuals are allowed for the examination, one each for the CPT Professional, HCPCS Level II, and ICD-10-CM. The use of a medical dictionary is prohibited for this examination.

- **Read the instructions carefully:** It is essential to read the questions carefully to ensure correct answers. It would be terrible to miss questions simply because of misread instructions.

- **Take note of questions that use absolute terms:** These are frequently false as they leave no room for other possibilities. Examiners often add them as trick questions. The words used in these questions are definitive and include always and exactly, in contrast to words like usually, mostly, may, and sometimes.

- **Identify re-orienting words within the question:** These words indicate a switch in the flow or direction of the question and may be the key to the correct answer. Examples include: however, but, on the other hand, although, despite, and regardless. Be sensitive to these clues.

- **Do not be in a hurry:** Rushing through questions increases the chances of mistakes. Candidates should find a pace that allows them to be confident in their choices. Sometimes, a few more seconds are needed to discern distracting information examiners add to the questions. These additional seconds could have a significant impact on the overall score.

- **Leave enough time to review:** Candidates should ensure they have not made any costly omissions or errors in their answers. If possible, give all answers a second look.

  Now that the basics have been sorted, it is time to prepare for a successful CPC Examination.

# Chapter 2: Introduction to Medical Coding

## Introduction

The proper assignment of standardized documentation is vital for the clinical and business components of healthcare. Medical coding creates a common language for data collection and delivery of quality care. It also helps determine billing and appropriate reimbursement. A physician or a professional coder can code. When the physician does the coding, an external auditor verifies the consistency of the medical documentation and the code. The auditor also ensures that the medical record is both accurate and complete. This is because if the documentation is incorrect or incomplete, it will be translated poorly into code.

## Different Coder Settings

Coding can be done in either outpatient or inpatient settings. Physician professional services and outpatient facility codes are the primary concerns of coding in the outpatient context. Regardless of the environment, coders must continue self-education and stay updated with industry changes. There could be updates to code sets or insurance payment policies at different cycles.

## Different Payer Types

When patients come to the hospital and incur medical expenses, most use insurance coverage rather than paying out of pocket. A patient who seeks insurance can choose a plan from two types:

**Private Plans:** Companies provide insurance with varying coverage levels for individuals and groups based on the package purchased and medical procedure type.

**Government Plans:** This is the largest insurer, the most significant part of which is Medicare. This federal health insurance scheme covers citizens over sixty-five, individuals with certain disabilities, and those with End-Stage Renal Disease (ESRD). The Centers for Medicare and Medicaid Services (CMS) oversees government-based insurance. The CMS is responsible for the coding parameters for public healthcare programs and other payer systems. The Medicare Program comprises various components, which include:

- **Medicare Part A** mainly serves hospital-based treatment. This involves residential care, hospitalization, specialized nursing care, and palliative care. Part A is designed to assist beneficiaries with the costs associated with inpatient care.

- **Medicare Part B** complements Part A and covers outpatient care and medically necessary services provided by physicians. This includes doctor visits, preventive care, ambulance services, and certain outpatient hospital services.
- **Medicare Part C**, also known as Medicare Advantage, integrates the benefits of Medicare Part A and Part B and includes Medicare Part D for prescription drugs. Unlike Original Medicare, Part C plans are offered by Medicare-approved private insurers. Medicare Advantage plans may offer additional benefits not found in Original Medicare, and the costs for premiums, deductibles, and coinsurance can vary by plan.
- **Medicare Part D** is managed by Medicare-approved private organizations. It is designed specifically to cover drugs that are prescription-only. All Medicare enrollees can access it. Part D helps individuals afford the costs of prescription medications. Beneficiaries can choose from various Part D plans provided by private insurers, each with its own formulary and cost-sharing structure.

Another government-funded insurance program is Medicaid, which is designed to assist low-income individuals and families. While Medicaid places significant priority on pregnant women and children, it also serves the elderly, disabled, and other eligible low-income adults. Both state and federal governments sponsor it with strict guidelines.

## Resource-Based Relative Value Scale (RBRVS)

A method to estimate the value of a service performed and the implied compensation is necessary for Medicare payments to be authorized. This must be stratified so that every service does not just pull figures out of thin air. A relative value scale based on resources is employed to achieve this. This standardized payment system for medical providers determines the amount to be paid for tiered services. It is based on the cost of resources for providing different services.

The resource cost is divided into physician work, practice expense, and professional liability insurance.

- **Physician Work**: This is the most important element of the RBRVS. It represents around half of the relative worth of a technique. The time needed to complete the service and the stress of possible risk to patients are often utilized to evaluate a doctor's work. Additionally, it considers the technical, physical, and mental effort, as well as the professional judgment required.

- **Practice Expense**: This refers to the expense of services provided at different locations and the relative availability of resources at these locations. This may include office space, staff, and equipment costs. As a result, even when identical treatments are provided in both settings, e.g., the hospital and the doctor's office, different costs (values) may be associated with the same service. Approximately forty-four percent of the entire relative value of each service is made up of practice expenses.

- **Professional Liability Insurance**: This insurance policy protects healthcare professionals against claims from possible negligence, malpractice, or misrepresentation. It reflects the cost of purchasing malpractice insurance. It represents around four percent of the total relative value.

Every year, the Physician Fee Schedule (PFS) and the formula used to determine the amount of PFS payment are published on the CMS website. The formula is as given below:

**Non-Facility Pricing Amount** = [(Work RVU × Work GPCI) + (Non-Facility PE RVU × PE GPCI) + (MP RVU × MP GPCI)] × (CF).

**Facility Pricing Amount** = [(Work RVU × Work GPCI) + (Facility PE RVU × PE GPCI) + (MP RVU × MP GPCI)] × (CF).

PE = Physician Expense.

MP = Malpractice.

CF = Conversion Factor (a preset dollar rate, predetermined by the CMS, to convert RVU into payable charges).

GCPI = Geographical practice cost index (compares each element of a region's resource cost to its national average).

RVU = Relative Value Unit.

However, the Conversion Factor and Relative Value Unit may change from one year to another. Hence, a coder must routinely check the CMS website to stay updated.

## Medical Necessity

Medical necessity refers to the suitability of a treatment or technique provided to a patient in a specific scenario. A procedure or service is considered a medical necessity if it is the most straightforward procedure or service that successfully treats a patient's condition or meets their medical need.

To ensure standardization of these services, the CMS developed a framework for medical necessities based on statutory regulations in the Social Security Act. For a service to be termed as a medical necessity, it should be:

- Essential for the diagnosis, treatment, or relief of a health condition, injury, disease, or its attendant symptoms. Exceptions include services not covered under the policy, such as those deemed experimental or cosmetic, unless specifically allowed under certain conditions.

- Necessary to diagnose, treat, or cure the disease, injury, or symptoms or relieve a health condition.

- Within the standard of care that is generally accepted in the medical community.

It should not be for the sole purpose of the convenience of the patient, the relatives of the patient, or the healthcare service provider.

For this reason, when a doctor performs these treatments for a Medicare-eligible patient, the doctor only bills for services deemed "reasonable and necessary" for the patient's diagnosis and course of treatment.

Each Medicare Administrative Contractor (MAC) translates federal guidelines into local directives known as Local Coverage Determinations (LCD). This document outlines what is considered essential or necessary. The LCD also outlines what services are included, the limitations of their coverage, and the CPT and ICD-10-CM codes that are appropriate for medical necessity reporting for the service or procedure.

Other non-Medicare commercial insurers can develop separate medical policies that may not be in accordance with the Medicare guidelines. However, these policies are private. Thus, the contract terms are defined between the payer and the healthcare service provider.

## The Need for Safety and Confidentiality

The career path of medical coding involves access to sensitive information about peoples' private lives and clinical conditions. The Health Insurance Portability and Accountability Act (HIPAA) ensures federal protection for private health information stored by and accessible to a covered entity. According to the guidelines of this act, covered entities may be:

- **Health Care Providers**: Who transmit any health information in electronic form in connection with a transaction for which the Department of Health and Human Services has adopted a standard. This encompasses physicians, healthcare facilities, care homes, and pharmacies.

- **Health Plans**: This includes private health insurance providers, health maintenance organizations (HMOs), Medicare, Medicaid, and the Veteran Healthcare Program.

- **Health Care Clearinghouses**: These processing companies convert non-standard health information that they have received from another company or establishment into a standard format. Their role could also be in the opposite direction–conversion of standardized health information to an unstandardized one.

HIPAA provision has a *minimum necessary* requirement. This requirement states that only the minimum necessary protected health information (PHI) should be shared for a particular purpose. This means that such information should be withheld if the information is not essential or is surplus to the requirements for a specific purpose.

Under the Privacy Rule, however, there are exceptions to applying the minimum necessary PHI. These include:

- Disclosures made to a healthcare provider for treatment.
- Requests for treatment made by a healthcare professional.
- Disclosure of information to the individual for whom it is intended.
- Disclosure or usage that is necessary for adherence to HIPAA Administrative Simplification Rules.
- Disclosure or usage that follows the individual's authorization.
- Disclosure to the United States Department of Health and Human Services (HHS) in the event that the disclosed information is needed for enforcement reasons under the Privacy Rule.
- Uses or disclosures mandated under other laws.

The duty lies on covered entities to develop and implement in-house policies to meet HIPAA requirements. Also, access to PHI should be restricted to individuals whose job description requires it.

## HITECH and Its Impact on HIPAA

The Health Information Technology for Economic and Clinical Health Act (HITECH) was drafted to facilitate the use of Electronic Health Records (EHRs). It has sections that fortify HIPAA regulations as it addresses confidentiality and integrity concerns connected to the electronic transmission of health information.

Thanks to HITECH, patients have the right to receive an accounting of certain disclosures of their health information made through an electronic health record, including for treatment, payment, and health care operations, for the three years prior to the request. A person must also be informed if and when their health information is used without authorization, in accordance with HITECH regulations.

## Fraud and Abuse

The Office of Inspector General (OIG) is obligated by law to engage in activities that test the efficiency of government programs. The OIG investigates suspected fraud and abuse in healthcare programs, an activity aggressively pursued by the government.

Abuse consists of the payment for items or services billed in error by the providers and should not be reimbursed by Medicare. Fraud occurs when services are billed for but not given or when a higher reimbursement is billed for a service than the one provided. Fraud requires intent, meaning an individual must knowingly submit false claims or representations to be considered engaging in fraud. Similarly, an individual is not required to know about the violation for it to be considered an offense.

## Compliance Rules and Audits

Every healthcare facility, including physician offices, must have a protocol for complying with the many rules, regulations, and policies. The compliance plan is a set of guidelines that describes how to code and submit accurate claims and what to do if discrepancies are discovered.

Reimbursement payments for claims and billings are usually the source of fraud and abuse. These payments and claims have recently been the focus of government regulations, scrutiny, and sanctions. The use of a compliance plan by companies might help them improve the accuracy of their coding and claim payments. It also significantly reduces the chances of violating policies and statutes.

The increased accuracy of physician documentation, which results from a compliance program, can assist with improved patient care. It shows the commitment of the healthcare facility or medical practice to submit accurate claims in good faith. It also serves as a cue to others on the importance of compliance and that erroneous and fraudulent reporting is not condoned.

# Chapter 3: Coding Guidelines

## Introduction

Different coding conventions, with their respective peculiarities, are guided by different rules for the system of code in question. The techniques and intricacies of these concepts and contexts cannot be fully explored in this chapter, but an overview of some will be included. This chapter also serves as a summarized digest for concepts that will be continually applied in future chapters and a medical coding career.

## ICD-10-CM Official Guidelines

The ICD-10-CM coding system translates the medical terms for a multitude of diseases and procedures into numerical code. The United States publishes it to classify clinical diagnoses in all healthcare settings during patient visits. It has a rich history dating back to the seventeenth century and has evolved over the years into its current iteration.

The ICD-10-CM is maintained by the National Center for Health Statistics, which is a part of the Centers for Disease Control and Prevention, and is based on the ICD-10. The ICD-10 is a systematic classification of medical illnesses by the World Health Organization (WHO). The ICD-10-CM guidebook has many abbreviations and symbols to provide sufficiently rich information in as little space as possible. The knowledge of these particulars is integral to coding in different diagnostic scenarios.

### General Guidelines

There are some general guidelines when coding with the ICD-10-CM to accurately, quickly, and effectively report different diagnoses. These should always be followed when writing ICD-10-CM codes.

- Only confirmed conditions or diseases are to be coded in outpatient settings. This means that a condition considered only a suspected case will not be reported with this code. Though this usually holds in an inpatient situation, the suspected diagnosis may be reported if an individual's diagnosis remains unclear until discharge.

- The code should support the necessity of the treatment strictly on medical grounds. This should be based solely on available facts and has no place for speculation.

- The utmost amount of detail possible should be used while coding. This means a general code should not be chosen if a more precise code is available.

- Each unique code is to be reported once in each encounter. Repeating code for a diagnosis or procedure in the same encounter is prohibited. This also applies to bilateral conditions where there is no specific code to indicate if it affects one or both sides.

- When coding ICD-10-CM conditions that show lateralization, use the corresponding code. Record the code for the right or left sides individually if the condition lacks a bilateral code.

- The code should be ordered to put the primary concern of the patient encounter first.

- If a doctor reports a borderline (somewhat uncertain) diagnosis when a patient is ready for discharge, the diagnosis is classified as confirmed.

## Common Coding Conventions

The usual coding conventions in ICD-10-CM are rules used for classification and are independent of their respective guidelines.

<table>
<tr><th>Item</th><th colspan="2">Use Case</th></tr>
<tr><td>INCLUDES</td><td colspan="2">Conditions or other content written after this are used to explain further or define the code it follows.</td></tr>
<tr><td>EXCLUDES 1</td><td colspan="2">The code written after this should never be used simultaneously with the ones preceding it.</td></tr>
<tr><td>EXCLUDES 2</td><td colspan="2">This signifies that the conditions (code) written after it are not part of the condition represented by the preceding code, but they may coexist, so both can be coded if applicable in the patient’s case.</td></tr>
<tr><th colspan="3">ABBREVIATIONS</th></tr>
<tr><td>-</td><td></td><td>Signifies there are other characters associated with the code.</td></tr>
<tr><td>( )</td><td>Parentheses</td><td>Used to enclose supplementary words for the disease or procedure in both the Supplementary List and Alphabetic Index. They are alternatively known as non-essential modifiers.</td></tr>
<tr><td>[ ]</td><td>Brackets</td><td>Used to include additional synonyms or alternative terms in the Tabular List. This covers the explanations as well.</td></tr>
<tr><td>NEC</td><td>Not elsewhere classifiable</td><td>Used to signify that there is no existing code available for the condition.</td></tr>
<tr><td>NOS</td><td>Not otherwise classified</td><td>Used to represent that the condition is unspecified.</td></tr>
<tr><td>X</td><td>Placeholder “X”</td><td>Used to signify the possibility for future code expansion to include other conditions. When there are placeholders in a code, they must always be included when writing it.</td></tr>
</table>

## Coding Signs and Symptoms

A symptom is any sensation or change in bodily function associated with a particular disease experienced by a patient. Signs, on the other hand, are those features of a disease that are elicited by a clinician. Although some indications and manifestations could be more frequently linked to a certain ailment, they do not directly result in a diagnosis. It is acceptable to code this for reporting when the diagnosis for the condition has not yet been established.

## Coding Sequela

Sequela refers to the after-effects or residual symptoms that develop following treatment for a disease or injury. A sequela may be specific to that disease type or not. Sequelae have no defined time limit. They can occur within days or many years after the initial disease, condition, or injury. Examples can include scarring following burn injury and infertility following pelvic inflammatory diseases.

## Coding HIV

A list of guidelines is stipulated in the specific section of ICD-10-CM for coding HIV infections. This includes its interaction with other related conditions.

- Only use this code for HIV infections that have been conclusively verified. The medical professional's confirmed diagnosis of a positive HIV infection will be enough in this instance.
- If a patient's present illness is linked to HIV, the HIV code (B20) should be used as the initial diagnosis, and any related codes should come after that.
- The primary diagnosis for an unrelated ailment should come first, followed by the HIV code when an HIV-positive patient seeks treatment.
- An individual who has been identified as *HIV-positive* or *known HIV* but does not currently exhibit any symptoms should be given the Asymptomatic Human Immunodeficiency Virus code Z21.
- The inconclusive HIV serology code R75 should be applied to a patient who has an inconclusive HIV serology result but no clinical manifestation of the illness.
- O98.7 should be the primary diagnosis in cases where a patient presents or is hospitalized with an HIV-related illness during labor, pregnancy, or the postpartum period.

## Coding COVID-19

There are some stipulated guidelines in the specific section of ICD-10-CM for coding COVID-19 infection. This is a relatively novel infection caused by a strain in the coronavirus family, Severe Acute Respiratory Syndrome Coronavirus 2 (SARS-COV-2). It includes coding for the infection and common manifestations:

- Only code when the patient's COVID-19 illness has been confirmed, either by test results or provider documentation. Use the code U07.1 in these situations.
- If COVID-19 is suspected but not confirmed, do not use code U07.1 for COVID-19. Instead, code the symptoms that the patient exhibits.
- Should a patient's present state be linked to COVID-19, the primary diagnosis should be the code for COVID-19, which is then followed by the codes for the respective manifestation of the disease.
- For an asymptomatic person who has had exposure (either actual or suspected) to COVID-19 but without a definitive diagnosis or an inconclusive test result, Z20.828 should be used in cases when exposure to other viral infectious illnesses is suspected or confirmed.

## Sequencing Neoplasm Code

Determining whether a tumor is benign, in-situ, malignant, or has an unclear histologic character is essential to code for neoplasms accurately. If it is a malignant tumor, secondary locations must also be verified. The respective codes for various neoplasms are mainly seen in the specific body system section of the ICD-10-CM. However, common guidelines for code sequencing include the following:

- When a patient receives treatment for a malignancy, the code for the principal diagnosis (the malignancy) should be listed first. This is then followed by the care given. This does not apply to patients admitted for radiation, immunotherapy, or chemotherapy. For that situation, code the procedure first, followed by the primary condition.
- When a patient is hospitalized for treatment of a cancer that has spread to other areas of their body, the original site should be coded first, followed by the secondary locations.
- Even when there is a primary tumor present, the secondary site neoplasm should be identified as the primary diagnosis if the patient is being admitted only to treat a secondary site neoplasm (such as pathologic femoral shaft fracture).
- If a patient's visit or admission is due to malignancy-associated anemia, code for the primary malignancy followed by the appropriate code for anemia.
- When a patient is hospitalized due to anemia following radiation therapy for their initial cancer, the anemia should be coded first. The neoplasm is coded next, followed by Y84.2, which represents the radiologic relationship of the complication that necessitates admission/encounter.

## Coding for Diabetes

Diabetes mellitus (DM) is the most prevalent endocrine system disorder. The ICD-10-DM codes for DM are standard guidelines for coding for the disease. These coding guidelines are as follows:

- Code E11 for type II diabetes mellitus should be used if the operation note or medical record does not specify the type of diabetes.
- Use the code for type II diabetes mellitus (E11) if the procedure notes or medical record mentions using insulin but does not specify the type of diabetes. Additional codes for long-term insulin or other hypoglycemic medication use can be assigned from category Z79.
- Use the code E89.1 for diabetes mellitus that develops following the surgical excision of some segments or all of the pancreas (post-pancreatectomy diabetes mellitus).
- If the diagnosis is gestational diabetes occurring in pregnancy, the code should be from subcategory O24.4 rather than the standard diabetes code.

## Coding for Hypertensive Heart and Chronic Kidney Disease

Before assigning a patient's disease a code, the coder must recognize that the patient has a combination of diseases. Thus, designate a code that falls within the combination category I13. If heart failure is detected, indicate the kind of heart failure with a supplementary code from I50.

## Coding External Cause of Morbidity

The ICD-10-CM usually uses the phrase *external cause of morbidity* to signify an injury or disease that occurs due to external forces. This may include falls, auto crashes, tornadoes, tsunamis, or fire outbreaks. Further details on the circumstances that preceded this condition can be provided with these codes. This covers the incident's location, the status of the patient (civilian or military), and the motive (deliberate or accidental).

When coding for external cause for morbidity, it is best to use as many codes to denote the cause as necessary to explicitly represent the patient's condition as documented in the procedure notes. The external cause of morbidity is not to be sequenced first. Instead, it should be coded as an add-on to other ranges when there is mention of an external cause.

### Screening Codes

Screening codes are used for patient encounters where testing is done in otherwise healthy individuals for early detection and subsequent treatment of any condition identified. The codes for screening tests are in section Z of the Tabular List in ICD-10-CM. They are in sections Z11 through Z13, and Z36. When the encounter is coded solely because of the screening, the screening code should be sequenced. Any condition found during this screening should be coded separately after the screening code.

## CPT Coding Guidelines

### Common Conventions for CPT Codes

The CPT codebook is a compilation that uses different symbols and formatting to allow anyone to understand the information presented to them quickly. However, to understand and properly use these codes, there is a need to know the basic conventions for coding in CPT. This includes:

- **Indentation**: The use of a code indentation signifies a modification of the non-indented code above it. This means that whatever the preceding code identifies still generally applies, but it is a noteworthy variation. For example, code 25100 reads *Arthrotomy, wrist joint; with biopsy*. Code 25105 reads *with synovectomy*. Since the part before the indentation is considered a part of the code, the full description is *25105 Arthrotomy, wrist joint, with synovectomy.*
- **The plus (+) sign**: The inclusion of the plus symbol with a code indicates an extension code. This means it should not be reported alone but in addition to the primary code. The only exception to this is the critical care add-on code +99292.
- **Red text**: In the CPT codebook, when a code is written in red, this signifies that there has been a change to the code from the previous year, such as a modification or revision.

### Criteria for Code Categories

The American Medical Association has categorized the CPT codes into three groups. These categories are determined by whether they meet general and specific criteria within each group. This includes a stipulation that the descriptor for the code must be unique, well-defined, and identifiable from existing procedures and services. It must meet the requirements stipulated by the appropriate oversight bodies and the leveled financial implication of the procedure or service.

CPT codes are grouped into Categories I, II, and III.

- **Category I**: This category is for procedures or services that have received FDA approval. The procedures must be performed at a frequency commensurate with their intended clinical usefulness by doctors and other authorized healthcare providers. For example, procedures and services for common conditions should be done frequently, and procedures for rare diseases should be rarely done. There must also be documented evidence of its efficacy in medical literature. This category of five-digit codes constitutes the majority of CPT codes.

- **Category II**: This category is for procedures and services commonly included in E/M services but not associated with usual fees. These services have evidence-based measurements that state their relationship to health outcomes. It also addresses high-risk, high-cost, or high-prevalence clinical conditions. Other criteria for a category II code which are mandatory include:

    - A definition of a measure consistent with the intended use.
    - The physician or other healthcare professional must have a significant impact on the aspect of care that is being measured.
    - It must lessen the workload of gathering data for doctors and other medical professionals.
    - It must be detailed enough to be useful for multiple purposes.

- **Category III**: This category codes for services and procedures only recently performed in humans. Additionally, these circumstances must fulfill at least one of the following requirements:
    - At least one CPT or HCPAC adviser who represents practitioners who might use the procedure or service has endorsed the application.
    - The potential or actual clinical effectiveness of the procedure or service has been reported in a peer-reviewed publication.
    - The following information is required: a study protocol of the procedure or service that an Institutional Review Board has approved, a description of an ongoing trial in the United States that demonstrates the effectiveness of the procedure or service, and additional evidence of clinical utilization changes.

## The Healthcare Common Procedure Coding System (HCPCS)

### Common Coding Symbols and Conventions

The HCPCS uses various symbols and conventions to clearly provide information as needed for coding Medicare procedures in as little space as possible. The knowledge of these conventions helps coders understand HCPCS coding for medical procedures and services. Some of the common conventions include:

- **Colored text** is used to signify indicators in some coding manuals. The use of color in coding manuals can vary by publisher, and coders should refer to the specific manual's legend or introduction for the meaning of colored text.
- **Letters in block form** are used to signify circumstances that affect payment. C is for carrier judgment, D is for special coverage instructions, M is for noncovered by Medicare, and S is for noncovered by Medicare statute.
- **MIPS** is a light blue box with text that indicates the code is within the purview of the merit-based incentive payment system (MIPS).

## Different Code Types

- **Permanent national codes** describe the products and services permanently. They provide a standardized way to identify and bill for established healthcare offerings. Examples include CPT (Current Procedural Terminology) codes and HCPCS (Healthcare Common Procedure Coding System) Level II codes.
- **Temporary national codes** represent services without permanent codes. They are used to meet operational requirements within a short time. They can subsequently be converted into a permanent national code.
- **Miscellaneous codes** allow suppliers to submit billing for a product or service with no permanent national code. These codes are helpful in situations where a unique or infrequent service needs to be documented and billed.

# Chapter 4: Medical Terminology and Human Anatomy

## Introduction to Medical Terminology

Medical terminology refers to specialized language or vocabulary used in medical practice. These terms describe, diagnose, treat, and communicate information about the human body, medical conditions, treatments, and procedures. Medical terminologies are well structured and comprise word roots, prefixes, suffixes, and combining forms.

These fundamental parts are systematically combined to create terms that convey precise meanings. A structured system for medical communication in the form of medical terminologies is essential in medical practice. It has many significant purposes, some of which are highlighted below.

- **Precision and Clarity**
  Medical terminology ensures that healthcare professionals can communicate precisely. It gives standardized, unambiguous terms to describe symptoms, diagnoses, and treatments, which reduces the risk of miscommunication or misunderstanding.

- **Efficient Communication**
  Healthcare is often a fast-paced environment where quick and accurate communication is critical. Medical terminology allows professionals to convey complex medical information efficiently, which saves time and, potentially, lives.

- **Accurate Documentation**
  In healthcare, meticulous record-keeping is essential. Accurate medical terminology is used in patient records, charts, and reports. This ensures that the patient's medical history and condition are documented consistently and clearly.

- **Global Standard**
  Medical terminology is a universal language in the medical field. Regardless of where they are in the world, healthcare professionals can understand and use the same terminology, which facilitates collaboration and knowledge sharing.

- **Diagnostic Precision**
  Medical terminology is essential for diagnosing medical conditions. It enables healthcare providers to describe symptoms and conditions accurately. This helps identify diseases and develop treatment plans.

- **Treatment Planning**
  Medical professionals use specific terminology to plan and execute medical procedures, surgeries, and treatments. Planning is critical to the success of these interventions.

- **Patient Empowerment**
  Patients benefit from medical terminology as it allows healthcare providers to explain their conditions and treatment options in a way they can comprehend. Informed patients can actively participate in their healthcare decisions.

- **Adaptation to Medical Advancements**
  As medical science evolves, new terminology is constantly introduced to describe emerging diseases, treatments, and technologies. Keeping up with these developments is vital for staying at the forefront of healthcare.

- **Legal and Ethical Considerations**
  Legal and ethical standards in healthcare require accurate terminology in medical records, reports, and informed consent documents.

Medical terminology is of utmost significance in healthcare because it underpins effective and precise communication, accurate diagnosis and treatment, and the global standardization of medical language, ultimately contributing to delivering high-quality healthcare services.

## Roots, Prefixes, and Suffixes

Medical terminology often uses word roots, prefixes, and suffixes to create complex medical terms. Below are some common examples.

**Word roots** in medical terminology are the foundation of medical words and provide the basic meaning of a term. Some common word roots used in medical terminology are as follows:

| Root | Meaning | Example |
|---|---|---|
| Angi | Vessel, usually blood vessel | Angiogram, i.e., X-ray of blood vessels |
| Athr | Joint | Arthritis, i.e., inflammation of joint |
| Cardi | Heart | Cardiology, i.e., study of the heart |
| Cerebr | Brain | Cerebral, i.e., related to the brain |
| Cholecyst | Gallbladder | Cholecystectomy, i.e., surgical removal of the gallbladder |
| Chondr | Cartilage | Chondrocyte, i.e., cartilage cell |
| Cran | Skull | Craniotomy, i.e., surgical opening of the skull |
| Cyt | Cell | Cytology, i.e., study of cells |
| Dactyl | Finger, toe | Polydactyly, i.e., having more than the normal number of digits |
| Dent | Tooth | Dentistry, i.e., study and treatment of teeth |
| Derm | Skin | Dermatology, i.e., study of skin |
| Gastr | Stomach | Gastroenterology, i.e., study of the stomach and intestines |
| Glyc | Sugar | Glycemia, i.e., presence of sugar in the blood |
| Gynec | Woman, female | Gynecology, i.e., study of the female reproductive system |
| Hemat | Blood | Hematology, i.e., study of blood |
| Hepat | Liver | Hepatitis, i.e., inflammation of the liver |
| Hyster | Uterus | Hysterectomy, i.e., surgical removal of the uterus |
| Laryng | Voice box, throat | Laryngitis, i.e., inflammation of the voice box |
| Myo | Muscle | Myocardium, i.e., muscular tissue of the heart wall |
| Nas | Nose | Nasogastric, i.e., pertaining to the nose and stomach |
| Nephro | Kidney | Nephritis, i.e., inflammation of the kidney |
| Neur | Nerve | Neurology, i.e., study of neural networks |
| Onc | Tumor, mass | Oncology, i.e., study of tumors or cancer |
| Ophthalm | Eye | Ophthalmology, i.e., study of the eye |
| Orth | Straight, correct | Orthodontics, i.e., straightening of teeth |
| Oste | Bone | Osteoporosis, i.e., condition of porous bones |
| Pneum | Lung | Pneumonia, i.e., inflammation of the lungs |
| Pod | Foot | Podiatry, i.e., study and treatment of foot disorders |
| Psych | Mind, mental | Psychology, i.e., study of mind and behavior |
| Pulm | Lung | Pulmonary, i.e., related to the lungs |
| Ren | Kidney | Renal, i.e., related to the kidneys |
| Rhin | Nose | Rhinoplasty, i.e., surgical repair of the nose |
| Splen | Spleen | Splenomegaly, i.e., enlargement of the spleen |
| Thromb | Clot | Thrombolysis, i.e., dissolution of a blood clot |
| Ureter | Ureter | Ureteroplasty, i.e., surgical repair of the ureter |
| Vas | Vessel, duct | Vasectomy, i.e., surgical cutting or sealing of the vas deferens |

**Prefixes** are placed at the beginning of a word root to adjust its meaning. These prefixes give the medical term a more precise meaning. This enables medical practitioners to characterize body parts, locations, and connections. Some common prefixes used in medical terminology are as follows:

| Prefix | Meaning | Example |
|---|---|---|
| A-, an- | Without, lack of | Apathy, i.e., lack of interest or enthusiasm |
| Anti- | Against | Antibiotic, i.e., against bacteria |
| Bi- | Two | Bifocal, i.e., having two focal lengths |
| Brady- | Slow | Bradycardia, i.e., abnormally slow heartbeat |
| Circum- | Around | Circumference, i.e., distance around a circular object |
| Dia- | Through, across | Diarrhea, i.e., passage of water stools |
| Dys- | Abnormal, difficult, painful | Dysfunction, i.e., impaired function |
| Endo- | Within, inner | Endoscopy, i.e., examination inside the body |
| Eu- | Good, normal | Euphoria, i.e., feeling of well-being or happiness |
| Hyper- | Excessive, above | Hyperactivity, i.e., excessively active |
| Hypo- | Deficient, below | Hypothyroidism, i.e., underactive thyroid |
| Intra- | Within | Intravenous, i.e., within a vein |
| Iso- | Equal | Isometric, i.e., having equal measure or length |
| Leuko- | White | Leukocyt, i.e., white blood cell |
| Macro- | Large, long | Macrocephaly, i.e., abnormally large head |
| Mal- | Bad, abnormal | Malnutrition, i.e., poor nutrition |
| Micro- | Small | Microorganism, i.e., tiny living organisms like bacteria and viruses |
| Neo- | New | Neoplasm, i.e., new growth or tumor |
| Pan- | All, entire | Pancreas, i.e., organ with both endocrine and exocrine functions |
| Peri- | Around | Pericardium, i.e., membrane around the heart |
| Poly- | Many | Polyneuropathy, i.e., dysfunction of multiple nerves |
| Post- | After, behind | Postoperative, i.e., after surgery |
| Pre- | Before, in front of | Prenatal, i.e., before birth |
| Quadri- | Four | Quadriplegia, i.e., paralysis of all four limbs |
| Retro- | Behind, backward | Retrograde, i.e., moving backward |
| Sub- | Below, under | Subcutaneous, i.e., under the skin |
| Tachy- | Fast | Tachycardia, i.e., abnormally fast heartbeat |
| Trans- | Across, through | Transdermal, i.e., through the skin |

**Suffixes** in medical terminology are added to the end of a word root to adjust its meaning. Suffixes help to indicate the nature of a medical condition, procedure, or diagnostic test. This provides valuable information to healthcare professionals. Some common suffixes used in medical terminology are below.

| Suffix | Meaning | Example |
|---|---|---|
| -algia | Pain | Neuralgia, i.e., nerve pain |
| -centesis | Surgical puncture | Arthrocentesis, i.e., surgical puncture of a joint |
| -cyte | Cell | Leukocyte, i.e., white blood cell |
| -ectomy | Surgical removal | Appendectomy, i.e., surgical removal of the appendix |
| -emia | Blood condition | Anemia, i.e., lack of red blood cells |
| -genesis | Formation, origin | Carcinogenesis, i.e., formation of cancer |
| -graphy | Process of recording | Mammography, i.e., imaging of the breast |
| -ia | Condition | Hypoxia, i.e., condition of low oxygen |
| -ic | Pertaining to | Cardiac, i.e., pertaining to the heart |
| -ism | State of | Hyperthyroidism, i.e., state of excessive thyroid activity |
| -itis | Inflammation | Dermatitis, i.e., inflammation of the skin |
| -logy | Study of | Cardiology, i.e., study of the heart |
| -oma | Tumor, mass | Lipoma, i.e., fatty tumor |
| -osis | Abnormal condition | Osteoporosis, i.e., condition of porous bone |
| -pathy | Disease | Neuropathy, i.e., nerve disease |
| -plasia | Development, formation | Hyperplasia, i.e., excessive development of cells |
| -plasty | Surgical repair | Rhinoplasty, i.e., surgical repair of nose |
| -rrhea | Flow, discharge | Diarrhea, i.e., discharge of watery stool |
| -rrhage | Bursting forth | Hemorage, i.e., excessive bleeding |
| -scopy | Examination, inspection | Endoscopy, i.e., examination inside the body |

## How Medical Terms are Formed

Word roots, prefixes, and suffixes are combined to generate medical terminology systematically. Here are some common examples:

| Term | Prefix | Root | Suffix |
|---|---|---|---|
| Antibiotic | Anti- (against) | Bio (life) | -tic (pertaining to) |
| Arthritis | | Arthr (joint) | -itis (inflammation) |
| Cardiology | | Cardio (heart) | -logy (study of) |
| Cerebral | | Cerebr (brain) | -al (pertaining to) |
| Cytology | | Cyt (cell) | -logy (study of) |
| Dermatitis | | Derma (skin) | -itis (inflammation) |
| Gastroenteritis | | Gastro (stomach) Enter (small intestine) | -itis (inflammation) |
| Gynecology | | Gynec (woman, female) | -logy (study of) |
| Hematology | | Hema (blood) | -logy (study of) |
| Hepatitis | | Hepat (liver) | -itis (inflammation) |
| Hysterectomy | | Hyster (uterus) | -ectomy (surgical removal) |
| Hypothyroidism | Hypo- (deficient, below) | Thyroid (thyroid gland) | -ism (state of) |
| Myocardium | | Myo (muscle Cardi (heart) | -um (structure) |
| Nephritis | | Nephro (kidney) | -itis (inflammation) |
| Neurology | | Neuro (nerve) | -logy (study of) |
| Oncology | | Onc (tumor) | -logy (study of) |
| Ophthalmology | | Ophthalm (eye) | -logy (study of) |
| Osteoporosis | | Osteo (bone) | -osis (abnormal condition) |
| Podiatry | | Pod (foot) | -iatry (medical specialty) |
| Polydactyly | Poly- (many) | Dactyl (finger or toe) | -y (condition, process) |
| Psychology | | Psych (mind, mental) | -logy (study of) |
| Rhinoplasty | | Rhin (nose) | -plasty (surgical repair) |

## Introduction to Human Anatomy

The study of human anatomy focuses on the composition and general arrangement of the human body. It is a fundamental science and forms the basis of medical practice. Understanding human anatomy is essential for healthcare professionals. It provides insights into the body's function and the relationships between various organs and body systems. Understanding human anatomy is required to diagnose and treat medical conditions.

The human body is a complex structure comprised of various types of cells, tissues, organs, and other systems that work in harmony. Anatomy is broadly subdivided into two main branches: Macroscopic anatomy, which includes gross anatomy and the study of visible body structures, and microscopic anatomy, which examines cells and tissues at a cellular level.

### Major Body Systems

The human body is an intricate and complex biological masterpiece with numerous interconnected systems with unique functions and roles. These systems work together in synchrony to maintain homeostasis. The following sections discuss the major bodily systems.

**The skeletal system** supports the body's structure, shields essential organs, and aids in red blood cell synthesis and movement. Its components include the following:

- **Bones**: There are 206 bones in the human body. This comprises flat bones (cranium, scapula), short bones (tarsals, carpals), long bones (tibia, fibula), and irregular bones (vertebrae).
- **Joints**: Joints are the point of articulation between two or more bones. This allows for movement.
- **Cartilage**: Cartilage covers the ends of bones at the joints, which reduces friction.
- **Ligaments**: Connective tissue bands known as ligaments function to hold bones in place where they come together at joints.

**The muscular system:** The muscular system maintains posture, produces heat, and controls movement and stability. There are three types of muscles:

- **Skeletal muscles** are used for movement and are controlled voluntarily.
- **Smooth muscles** are the involuntary muscles found in the digestive system and other visceral organs.

- **Cardiac muscles** are the involuntary muscles of the heart that contract to pump blood throughout the body.

**The circulatory system** is also called the cardiovascular system. It transports oxygen, nutrients, and hormones to body cells. It also removes waste products from the body. Components include:

- **Heart**: The heart is a muscular organ with four chambers (atria and ventricles) that pump blood throughout the body.
- **Blood vessels**: Arteries transport oxygen-rich blood from the heart to body organs. Veins transport oxygen-depleted blood back to the heart. Capillaries facilitate the exchange of substances with body tissues.
- **Blood**: Red blood cells supply oxygen, white blood cells serve immunological functions, platelets facilitate clotting, and plasma is the fluid part of blood.

**The nervous system** controls and coordinates body functions, which enables rapid communication and responses to internal and external stimuli. Components include:

- **The central nervous system (CNS)** comprises the brain and spinal cord, processes information, and controls body functions.
- **The peripheral nervous system (PNS)** comprises nerves that extend from the CNS to transmit information. It is further divided into the somatic (voluntary) and autonomic (involuntary) nervous systems.
- **Neurons** are central to the nervous system and transmit electrical signals to communicate information.

**The respiratory system** facilitates the exchange of gases (oxygen and carbon dioxide) between the blood and the environment. Components include:

- **Lungs**: The lungs are the primary respiratory organs, where oxygen is absorbed into the bloodstream, and carbon dioxide is expelled.
- **Trachea and bronchi**: The trachea, or windpipe, branches into the bronchi. They carry air to and from the lungs.
- **Diaphragm**: The diaphragm is a dome-shaped muscle. It contracts and expands the chest cavity, which aids in breathing.

**The digestive system** processes and absorbs food nutrients and eliminates waste products. Components include:

- **Mouth and teeth**: Mechanical and chemical digestion (by the teeth and saliva, respectively) starts in the mouth.

- **Stomach**: The stomach further breaks down food and initiates the digestion of proteins.
- **Small and large intestines**: These organs absorb nutrients from digested food.
- **Liver and pancreas**: The liver produces bile for fat digestion. The pancreas releases enzymes for carbohydrate, protein, and fat digestion.

**The endocrine system** regulates bodily functions through the secretion of hormones, which act as messengers to control growth, metabolism, and homeostasis. The main endocrine glands in the human body include:

- **Pituitary gland**: It is also called the *master gland*, and it controls the activities of other endocrine glands.
- **Thyroid gland**: Regulates metabolism and energy.
- **Adrenal glands**: They produce hormones involved in stress response and metabolism.
- **Pancreas**: This gland regulates blood sugar levels through insulin and glucagon.

**The immune system** defends the body against pathogens and foreign invaders, such as bacteria, viruses, and fungi. The components of the immune system include:

- **White blood cells**: White blood cells are vital to immunity and include lymphocytes and phagocytes.
- **Lymphatic System**: This system includes lymph nodes, the spleen, and tonsils, which filter and produce white blood cells.
- **Antibodies**: The immune system produces antibodies, which are small protein molecules that target and neutralize foreign substances.

**The urinary system** regulates fluid balance. It filters waste products from the blood and produces urine. Components include:

- **Kidneys** filter waste products and excess substances from the blood to form urine.
- **Ureters** serve as conduits for the urine to travel from the kidneys to the bladder.
- **The bladder** collects and stores urine until it is ready to be eliminated from the body through the urethra.
- **The urethra** is the passage through which urine is expelled from the bladder to exit the body.

**The reproductive system** facilitates the production of new offspring. The male reproductive system comprises the following:

- **The testes** are located in the scrotal sac. They are responsible for producing sperm and the male sex hormones.
- **The epididymis and vas deferens** store and transport sperm.
- **The penis** delivers sperm into the female reproductive tract.

The female reproductive system comprises the following:

- **Ovaries** produce eggs and the female sex hormones.
- **Fallopian Tubes** transport eggs from the ovaries to the uterus and are where fertilization occurs.
- **The uterus** is the organ where a fertilized egg implants and develops into a fetus.
- **The vagina** allows for copulation. It also serves as the birth canal during childbirth.

## Explanation of Anatomical Terms

Anatomical terms are specialized words and phrases used to describe the structures of the human body in terms of their relationship to the anatomical position, landmarks, and other organs. In anatomy, the anatomical position is a defined reference position used to identify and characterize different body parts and structures. It provides common reference points that identify and characterize the placements and relationships between various body parts and organs. A person in the anatomical position assumes an upright posture with their feet together or slightly apart and their arms by their sides. Their face and palms face front. The definitions of several common terminologies used in anatomy are provided here.

### Directional Terminology

Directional terms help locate and describe anatomical structures in relation to one another. They include the following:

- **Anterior and posterior**: These terms refer to the body's front (anterior) and back (posterior) sides. For example, the heart is anterior to the thoracic vertebrae.
- **Superior and inferior**: Superior denotes a structure situated above, and inferior indicates a position below. For example, the knee joints are inferior to the hip joints.
- **Proximal and distal**: These terms describe the relative position of structures and are usually used when discussing limbs and appendages. Proximal indicates a structure closer to the point of attachment. For example, the shoulder is

proximal to the hand. On the other hand, distal signifies a position farther from the attachment point.

- **Medial and lateral**: Medial refers to structures closer to the body's midline. Lateral indicates a structure farther away. For example, the big toe is medial to the little toe.
- **Dorsal and ventral**: In human anatomy, dorsal (posterior) refers to the back side of the body, while ventral (anterior) refers to the front side. However, in the context of four-legged animals, dorsal refers to the top, and ventral refers to the bottom.

### Planes of Reference

Anatomical planes are used to visualize and dissect the body. The planes include the following:

- **The sagittal plane** divides the body into right and left sides. The midsagittal plane precisely bisects the body into equal halves. The parasagittal planes create unequal divisions.
- **The coronal plane** is also known as the frontal plane. It segments the body into anterior and posterior sections.
- **The transverse plane** is also called the horizontal or axial plane. It slices the body into superior and inferior portions.

### Terms for Depth and Position

When discussing the depth and position of anatomical structures, the anatomical terms commonly used include:

- **Superficial and deep**: Superficial refers to structures closer to the body's surface, and deep describes structures situated farther beneath the surface. For example, the skin is a superficial structure. In contrast, muscles and bones are located deep under the skin.
- **Cranial and caudal**: These terms are particularly relevant when describing the position of structures in animals. Cranial denotes a structure closer to the head or upper part of the body. Caudal means it is closer to the tail or the lower part. For example, the eyes are cranial to the mouth, while the navel is caudal to the chest.

### Body Positions and Movements

Understanding how the body can be positioned and moved is essential for anatomical descriptions in clinical settings. Common terms include:

- **Prone and supine**: Prone describes a person lying face down, and supine means lying face up. These terms are used when positioning patients for procedures and examinations in healthcare settings. However, supination and pronation are terms related to the rotation of the forearm or foot. Supination of the forearm involves rotating it outward so the palm faces forward or upward, while pronation involves rotating it inward so the palm faces backward or downward. Supination of the foot involves lifting the outer edge of the foot, and pronation involves lowering the outer edge of the foot.
- **Flexion and extension**: Flexion is a movement that reduces the angle between two body parts. For example, bending the elbow or bringing the knee closer to the chest involves flexion. Extension is the opposite of flexion. It is a movement that generally increases the angle between two body parts (usually across the joint of a limb). Straightening the elbow or knee is an example of extension.
- **Abduction and adduction**: Abduction involves moving a body part (usually a limb) away from the body's midline along the frontal plane–for example, lifting the arm to the side. Adduction is the opposite of abduction. It involves moving a body part (usually a limb) toward the body's midline. Circumduction combines flexion, extension, abduction, and adduction. This results in a circular or cone-like movement. An example is the shoulder movement when making a windmill motion.
- **Internal and external rotation**: Internal and external rotation are anatomical movements that describe the rotation of a body part, usually a limb, around its longitudinal axis. Internal rotation involves the rotation of a bone or limb inward toward the midline of the body. In contrast, external rotation is the rotation of a bone or limb away from the body's midline.
- **Dorsiflexion and plantar flexion**: Dorsiflexion and plantar flexion are anatomical movements that describe the foot and ankle position along the sagittal plane. Dorsiflexion refers to the movement of the ankle joint, where the foot is flexed upward, which brings the toes closer to the shin. Plantar flexion is the opposite movement. It involves the extension of the ankle joint. The foot is pointed downward in plantar flexion, away from the shin.

## Evolving Medical Terminologies

Medical terminology continually evolves to keep pace with advances in healthcare, technology, and scientific discoveries. Healthcare professionals, researchers, and educators must continually update their knowledge and resources to keep up with changing language. This evolution is usually driven by factors such as:

- **Scientific advancements**: New diseases, treatments, and medical technologies necessitate the creation of new terms. For example, the development of gene-editing techniques like CRISPR has introduced new terminology into the field.
- **Globalization**: As medical knowledge is shared worldwide, there is a need for standardized terminology to ensure clear communication among healthcare professionals from different regions.
- **Cultural sensitivity**: Terminology is adjusted to respect cultural norms and values. For example, gender-neutral language may be adopted to promote inclusivity.
- **Regulatory changes**: Regulatory bodies may update terminology to align with new guidelines, such as the International Classification of Diseases (ICD) and Current Procedural Terminology (CPT) codes.

# Chapter 5: Introduction to ICD-10-CM

## Introduction

The translation of known medical conditions into codes began in the 1800s in England. Statistical data was collected into the London Bills of Mortality system, where information was used to determine causes of mortality in the seventeenth century. By 1937, the list morphed into the International List of Causes of Death. This valuable information has been used over the decades by the World Health Organization to discover international disease trends by tracking morbidity and mortality.

In 1977, there was global recognition of ICD-9-CM. This prompted the Federal National Center for Health Statistics to modify the available statistical study with reported clinical information in medical records. These modifications resulted in adopting ICD-9-CM as the national standard coding language for patient diagnosis, anomaly, and other injuries or reasons for requiring medical services and procedures. Although the ICD-9 CM was widely accepted, the version could not expand to cover a broader range of diseases because most categories were filled. There was also a lack of specificity and detail in the ICD-9-CM.

The tenth revision of the ICD (ICD-10) was endorsed by the Forty-third World Health Assembly in May 1990 and came into use in WHO Member States as from 1994. The ICD-10 is a detailed critical update that improved diagnosis and morbidity classification in the United States. Physicians, nurses, health information managers, coders, and all other healthcare providers rely on this standardized classification system to store and retrieve critical information related to selected diagnoses at different times. This includes a compilation of national morbidity and mortality statistics.

Generally, the ICD-10 code sets provide flexibility to accommodate public health care needs. It also includes future health needs and facilitates timely electronic claims processing by reducing requests for additional information to healthcare providers. Compared to ICD-9, the ICD-10 coding sets have unique improvements for basic healthcare exchanges, accidents caused by outside factors, mental illnesses, and preventive health.

## The ICD-10-CM

The ICD-10-CM, or International Classification of Diseases, Tenth Revision, Clinical Modification, is a globally recognized standard for classifying and coding diseases, health conditions, and related information. It provides a common language for health information used by healthcare professionals worldwide.

### Detailed Coding System

ICD-10-CM is known for its detailed and alphanumeric coding system. It consists of specific codes that provide a higher level of detail compared to its predecessor, ICD-9-CM. It captures added details on socioeconomics, ambulatory care conditions, problems related to lifestyle, and screening test results. This precision in coding allows for a more accurate representation of diagnoses and procedures.

### Up-To-Date

In the United States, the transition from ICD-9-CM to ICD-10-CM was mandated by the Health Insurance Portability and Accountability Act (HIPAA). The compliance deadline for this transition was October 1, 2015. The move to ICD-10-CM was driven by the need for a more comprehensive and up-to-date coding system. Medical terms and disease categories are constantly updated to reflect advancements in medical science and ensure clinical practices are aligned with current medical knowledge and standards.

### Expanded Code Set

ICD-10-CM features an expanded and updated code set that accommodates advancements in medical knowledge, technology, and terminology. This allows for a more accurate representation of a patient's health condition, which supports improved patient care and outcomes.

### Versatile Applications

Beyond its primary use in clinical settings for coding diagnoses and procedures, ICD-10-CM has versatile applications. It is employed in health statistics, epidemiology, reimbursement processes, healthcare research, and policy development. The standardized coding system facilitates communication, data analysis, and decision-making across various healthcare domains.

## Overview of ICD-10-CM Layout

The ICD-10-CM includes the official index, official conventions, and official guidelines designed to help track the correct diagnosis codes for each patient. The layout of ICD-10-CM includes several components to aid medical coders in accurately assigning diagnosis codes to each patient.

The first part of the code set comprises four sections.

- **Section I: Conventions, General Coding Guidelines, and Chapter-Specific Guidelines.** This section provides essential conventions and guidelines applicable to the entire code set. It includes chapter-specific guidelines for each section, which provide specific instructions for coding within different medical specialties.

- **Section II-IV** contains conventions, rules, and principles for selecting primary diagnoses, reports of additional diagnoses, and diagnostic coding and reporting of outpatient medical services.

The second part of the ICD-10-CM code set is the Alphabetic Index, which helps locate the necessary diagnosis codes and coding instructions. It consists of four parts:

- **Index of Diseases and Injury** lists diseases and injuries alphabetically. It also cross-references code numbers associated with specific conditions.
- **Index of External Causes of Injury** focuses on external causes of injuries, accidents, and other related events. It references codes related to external factors that result in injuries.
- **Table of Neoplasms** addresses neoplasms (tumors) and provides a structured table for coding these conditions. It helps to identify and code various types of tumors accurately.
- **Table of Drugs and Chemicals** contains information related to drugs and chemicals. It facilitates coding conditions and diseases caused by specific drugs or chemicals.

The Tabular List is the actual list of ICD-10-CM codes and descriptions, as well as instructions on how to apply the codes correctly. This list is organized into chapters based on body systems or conditions. Each chapter contains a range of codes listed in alphanumerical order.

- A00 – B99: Infectious and parasitic diseases.
- C00 – D49: Neoplasms.
- D50 – D89: Blood, blood-forming organs, and certain immune disorders.
- E00 – E89: Endocrine, nutritional, and metabolic diseases.
- F00 – F99: Mental, behavioral, and neurodevelopmental disorders.
- G00 – G99: Nervous system.
- H00 – H59: Eye and adnexa.
- H60 – H95: Ear and mastoid process.
- I00 – I99: Circulatory system.
- J00 – J99: Respiratory system.
- K00 – K95: Digestive system.
- L00 – L99: Skin and subcutaneous tissue.
- M00 – M99: Musculoskeletal system and connective tissue.

- N00 – N99: Genitourinary system (male and female).
- O00 – O9A: Pregnancy, childbirth, and the puerperium (six weeks post-childbirth).
- P00 – P96: Conditions originating in the perinatal period.
- Q00 – Q99: Congenital malformations, deformations, and chromosomal abnormalities.
- R00 – R99: Symptoms, signs, and abnormal findings not elsewhere classified.
- S00 – T88: Injury and poisoning.
- V00 – Y99: External causes of morbidity.
- Z00 – Z99: Factors influencing health status and contact with health services.

## Structure of ICD-10-CM Codes

The ICD-10-CM codes consist of a set of characters and a decimal point to indicate the position of the diagnosis in the ICD-10-CM. The first character of the code is a letter, which indicates the general category of the diagnosis. These include letters A- Z depending on the affected system of the body in the Tabular List.

The next set of characters are two numbers to narrow down the position of the code in the general listing. A decimal point immediately follows the two digits to separate the specific details of the condition from the general categories. The fourth character narrows the diagnosis to a specific detail, and the fifth and sixth characters provide even more specific information. A six-character code would appear as B02.123. The seventh character of the code includes additional information about a condition and when the encounter with the patient occurred.

The code range within a chapter is broken down into blocks. Each block consists of categories divided into subcategories of the ICD-10-CM Tabular List. For example, J45 is a category (Asthma), J45.2 is a subcategory (Mild Intermittent Asthma), and J45.22 is also a subcategory (Mild intermittent asthma with status asthmaticus). J45.901 is a six-character code for Unspecified asthma with (acute) exacerbation.

The seventh character is not always present in an ICD-10-CM code. However, it signifies laterality or whether the code represents an initial encounter, subsequent encounter, or sequelae arising from a condition. The seventh character is used to indicate the episode of care (such as initial encounter, subsequent encounter, or sequelae) and other specific information depending on the chapter. For injury codes, the seventh character can indicate the laterality or whether the code represents a right, left, bilateral, or unspecified side, but the specific values for these designations can vary depending on the code category.

Placeholder “X” is another character used in a diagnosis code. It allows the code set to expand in anticipation of the appropriate character code to give specific meaning. Therefore, medical coders must use the placeholder to preserve the code set’s structure until the specific diagnosis is made. If the code set is under six characters, the placeholder “X” is used for all the absent characters in the set—for example, T18.1XXS (foreign body in the esophagus, sequelae).

## Process of Diagnosis Code Selection

The ICD-10-CM coding book provides information required to code a patient’s condition based on notes provided in the medical record. The critical steps to make a code selection are as follows:

- **Check the diagnosis in the index**. All the diagnoses in ICD-10-CM are listed in the Alphabetical Index, with principal categories and subcategories. Carefully review the index to identify the condition of interest.
- **Trace the identified principal diagnosis to the proper code in the Tabular List**. Some codes have additional characters that cannot be determined if the search is limited solely to the principal category. Therefore, after identifying the condition in the index, follow the code to the Tabular List to complete it.
- **Report the identified code sequentially**. Unless otherwise stated, the code must be in the proper sequence in which the conditions are listed according to available medical information.

## Official Guidelines for ICD-10-CM Coding and Reporting

The Department of Health and Human Services created guidelines for coding and reporting using the ICD-10-CM. The American Hospital Association (AHA), the American Health Information Management Association (AHIMA), the Centers for Medicare and Medicaid Services (CMS), and the National Center for Health Statistics (NCHS) approved these guidelines.

### <u>Section I: Conventions, General Coding Guidelines, and Chapter-Specific Guidelines</u>

### Conventions for the ICD-10-CM

The ICD-10 CM is divided into an Alphabetical Index and a Tabular List. The Alphabetical Index consists of alphabetically ordered terms with the corresponding code. It comprises the Index of Diseases and Injury, the Index of External Causes of Injury, the Table of Neoplasms, and the Table of Drugs and Chemicals. The Tabular List is a structured compilation of medical codes split into chapters based on the body system or medical condition. The list enumerates categories, subcategories, and codes, which are characters that may be a number or a letter.

Categories are three-charactered and may be divided into subcategories of four or five characters. Further subdivision of a subcategory generates a code of three to seven characters. A category that is not further divided is equivalent to a code. A code that requires a seventh character is considered incomplete without the seventh character. The seventh character must always be the seventh position of a code. If a code that requires a seventh character is not 7 characters, a placeholder 'X' must be used to fill in the empty characters to meet the requirement.

In reporting, a placeholder "X" may fill in the empty characters to be considered valid. The ICD-10 CM uses an indented format for ease of referencing. A code may be titled *Other* or *Other specified* when the medical information does not match an existing code. These codes are designated in the Alphabetical Index under NEC (Not elsewhere classifiable) and represent diseases with no specific code. A code is classified as *Unspecified* when the information provided by the medical record is insufficient to assign to a more specific code in the Alphabetical Index.

A default code is listed next to a main item in the ICD10-CM Alphabetic Index. The default code of a condition is the most commonly associated term or the unspecified code of the disease condition. A condition documented in a medical record without further classification is assigned a default code. Code assignment should be based on the documentation in the medical record and the clinical criteria the healthcare provider uses to establish the diagnosis.

## General Coding Guidelines

The first step to locate a code in the ICD-10-CM is to identify the medical term in the Alphabetical Index based on available health information and then verify the identified code in the Tabular List.

It is essential not to be limited to the Alphabetical Index when locating a code in the ICD10-CM. The Tabular List is necessary for full code selection. This includes the applicable seventh character and laterality of the code.

Reporting of a diagnosis code is done to the maximum level of specificity as documented in the medical record provided, and this requires the highest number of available characters, which may be three to seven applicable characters.

The heading of the category consists of three characters. It may be divided further into a fourth or fifth character, subdivided to include a sixth character and a maximum of the seventh character where applicable.

A code is only valid if all the characters required for its complete coding are included, even though they are available on the ICD10-CM Tabular List. A combination code groups two diseases or just one diagnosis based on a concomitant complication or a secondary symptom. The inclusion and exclusion factors in the Tabular list are used to find combination codes.

When using a combination code, avoid ambiguity by using multiple codes when there is a code that identifies the elements that make up the diagnosis. A lack of specificity in a combination code to describe a disease should be identified promptly, and a secondary code should be assigned instead.

### Chapter-Specific Coding Guidelines

There are guidelines for specific conditions and diagnoses in addition to general coding guidelines. These chapter-specific guidelines apply to all healthcare settings. They are provided in the ICD-10-CM chapter-specific guidelines and should be applied accordingly.

## Section II: Selection of Principal Diagnosis

The Uniform Hospital Discharge Data Set defines the principal diagnosis of an inpatient as "that condition established after study to be chiefly responsible for occasioning the admission of the patient to the hospital for care." The definitions mentioned can be located in the Federal Register of July 31, 1980 (Volume 45, Number 147). Consistent and complete documentation of patient information in their medical record is essential to apply coding guidelines. For inpatients, a principal diagnosis is carefully made and reported in a standardized manner.

## Section III: Reporting Additional Diagnosis

For patients who require an additional diagnosis, reports are made under *Other diagnoses* and interpreted in terms of clinical evaluation, treatment, diagnostic procedures, extended hospital stay, or increased nursing care or monitoring requirement. Uniform Hospital Discharge Data Set defines all additional diagnoses as the conditions present at the time of admission, that occur later, or that affect the treatment or length of stay in the hospital. A diagnosis related to an earlier illness episode has no bearing on the current hospital stay and should be excluded.

These definitions help to report inpatient data elements in standardized forms. General coding guidelines should also be applied to outpatient services and hospital visits. Accurate reporting of diagnosis codes of ICD-10-CM includes specific diagnoses and broad descriptions of symptoms and reasons for an encounter. Some codes describe only symptoms and signs related to a particular entity before the healthcare provider confirms the diagnosis.

## Section IV: Diagnostic Coding and Reporting Guidelines for Outpatient Services

ICD-10-CM provides the Factors Influencing Health Status and Contact with Health Services codes in situations where the circumstances related to an injury are recorded as a diagnosis or problem. It is essential to code to the highest level of specificity. The use of the ICD-10-CM is supported by the medical records provided and all documented conditions that coexist at the time of the patient visit, mainly when these conditions directly affect patient care and treatment.

The first listed diagnosis is used instead of a principal diagnosis in an outpatient setting. A diagnosis may not be established in the first outpatient visit and sometimes takes two or more visits. General and specific disease guidelines take priority over outpatient guidelines.

# Chapter 6: Introduction to CPT, Surgery Guidelines, HCPCS Level II, and Modifiers

## Introduction to CPT

The Current Procedural Terminology is a definitive and all-inclusive compilation of medical codes. It is the go-to reference for reporting medical, surgical, and diagnostic procedures. It is also used to report services performed by healthcare providers to established entities such as health insurance companies, physicians, and accreditation organizations. The CPT code contains three categories of medical descriptors and nomenclature:

- **Category I** CPT codes are mandatory for reporting and reimbursements. They are a five-digit numerical code (for example, 12345). The codes are copyrighted, reviewed, and updated by the American Medical Association (AMA) yearly. For Medicare, there is support for CPT category I code and a separate code set, the Healthcare Common Procedure Coding System (HCPCS) Level II. The HCPCS II is owned by the Centers for Medicare and Medicaid Services (CMS) and is used for reporting and reimbursement.
- **Category II** CPT codes are optional performance tracking codes used for quality management purposes. While they were once associated with the CMS incentive-based program, Physician Quality Reporting System (PQRS), this program has been replaced by the Merit-based Incentive Payment System (MIPS) under the Quality Payment Program. The code is alphanumeric and consists of four digits followed by an "F" (for example, 1234F). These should be reported along with Evaluation and Management services or the Clinical service CPT Category I code.
- **Category III** CPT codes are temporary codes that the AMA assigns for emerging technologies, services, and procedures that may not yet have widespread usage or clinical efficacy data to warrant a Category I code. The code is alphanumeric, with "T" in the last position (for example, 1234T). These codes can be reported alone without a Category I CPT code.

### National Correct Coding Initiative

The CMS implemented the National Correct Coding Initiative (NCCI) to ensure accuracy and appropriateness. The NCCI identifies codes for procedures and services that are not to be separately reported because they are bundled (that is, one code is involved in the work of another code). Frequent unbundling of these may be characterized as fraudulent coding. The NCCI employs two types of edits to accomplish its objectives: procedural edits and edits designed to address medically unlikely scenarios.

**Procedure-to-procedure (PTP) edits** identify code pairs for specific procedures or services that should not be reported together under normal circumstances. These edits are designed to recognize instances where the work of one procedure is integral to or includes the work performed by another. Reporting both codes separately in such cases would be redundant and may result in incorrect reimbursement. For example, if a comprehensive surgical procedure includes the performance of a specific diagnostic test as an integral component, the NCCI PTP edits would discourage the separate reporting of both the surgical procedure and the diagnostic test. The NCCI contributes to accurate coding practices and ensures proper compensation by identifying and preventing such unbundling.

**Medically unlikely edits (MUE)** identify instances where the reported quantity of a service or procedure is deemed medically unlikely. MUEs are established based on clinical judgment and medical standards. They set thresholds for the maximum units or frequency of a specific code that can be billed on a single date of service. For example, suppose a particular medical procedure is considered unlikely to be performed multiple times on the same patient on the same day due to medical necessity or standard clinical practice. In that case, the MUEs will specify the maximum allowable units for that procedure on a given day.

## Sequencing CPT Codes

CPT code sequencing is vital for appropriate claim submission and reimbursement. When reporting different CPT codes, the sequencing will be done from the highest to lowest relative value, that is, based on relative value unit (RVU).

## CPT Category II Codes

CPT Category II codes and some HCPCS Level II codes are used to report performance measures and make up the Quality Data codes (QDC) for the Physician Quality Reporting System established by CMS. RVUs are not assigned to these codes. Rather, they are used to describe clinical components included in E/M Services, tests, and other procedures known as measurable data for quality patient care. The AMA also maintains these codes, but unlike Category I codes, CPT Category II codes are updated throughout the year.

## CPT Category III Codes

The CPT Category III codes are temporary codes used for data collection to assess credibility for more widespread usage. They are also used for documentation in the FDA approval process for new and emerging technologies, services, or procedures. RVU is not assigned for this code.

CPT Category III codes do not automatically become Category I codes upon FDA approval. Category III codes are used for emerging technologies, services, or procedures, and transition to Category I codes requires a separate review process by the CPT Editorial Panel, which considers factors such as widespread usage and clinical efficacy, not just FDA approval. If a Category III code is not accepted as a Category I code or renewed, it may be archived after five years.

## Surgery Guidelines

In reporting surgery procedures, some services are already billed into the code by default and, therefore, are not separately billable. These services include the following:

- Local infiltration, metatarsal/metacarpal/digital block, or topical anesthesia.
- One related evaluation and management visit on the day of or before the day of surgery, following the decision for surgery. This includes history and an exam.
- Immediate postoperative care, patient evaluation in the post-anesthesia recovery area, and usual postoperative follow-up care.
- Writing orders.

### Global Package for Surgical Procedures

A standard package of preoperative, intraoperative, and postoperative services is included when a patient pays for surgical procedures. The duration of the preoperative and postoperative services will depend on whether the service is classified as a major or minor surgery.

Also, these services may be provided in any service location. Visits by surgeons to patients in the intensive care or critical care unit are included in this package. If additional care services are needed, they should be reported separately. This includes complications, recurrence, or other diseases.

### Global Days for Surgery

The days for preoperative and postoperative services depend on whether the surgery is classified as a major or minor and is defined by Medicare. For minor surgeries, the preoperative period is the day of the procedure, and the postoperative period is either zero or ten days.

For major surgeries, the preoperative period is one day, and the postoperative period is ninety days. For endoscopic procedures, there is no associated postoperative period.

Although the CMS global package establishes postoperative periods of zero, ten, or ninety days, third-party payers can use different guidelines. The services included in the global package include:

- Preoperative visits covered by the respective classification of the surgery, i.e., minor or major procedure.
- Intraoperative services that are normal and essential parts customarily done for a surgical procedure.
- Complications care following surgery. This includes all medical and surgical services the surgeon provides postoperatively to treat complications without additional visits to the operating room.
- Follow-up visits related to postoperative recovery within the postoperative period.
- Postoperative pain management services provided by the surgeon.
- Other miscellaneous services required in the preoperative to postoperative period. These include wound care, wound site management, removal of wound dressing, and skin stitches. They also include urinary catheter insertion, irrigation, removal, and changing and removing tracheostomy tubes.

However, some services are not included in the global package and must be billed separately. These services include:

- The surgeon's initial consultation or evaluation of a patient to determine if surgery is needed.
- Any visit or surgical procedure performed that is unrelated to the diagnosis. The exception is if the visit was because of surgery complications.
- If there is treatment for the patient's underlying condition or any other treatment plan that is not a part of the normal postoperative recovery.
- Diagnostic tests and procedures and distinct surgical procedures performed during the postoperative period, which are not repeat operations or treatment of complications.
- Treatments for complications that require transport of a patient to the operating room are not included in the global package and must be billed separately. This includes treatment in the operating room, but does not exclude treatment in the patient's room, recovery area, minor treatment rooms, or intensive care unit if the procedure is performed there due to the critical nature of the patient's condition that precludes transport to the operating room.
- A second extensive procedure following an earlier, less extensive one, which failed.
- Organ transplantation immunotherapy management.

- Critical care services unrelated to the surgery, where the critically ill patient is constantly attended to by the physician or other qualified health practitioners.

## Healthcare Common Procedure Coding System (HCPCS) Level II

The Healthcare Common Procedure Coding System (HCPCS) Level II codebook is used as the procedure code set for healthcare practitioners, healthcare providers, and medical equipment suppliers. It is used when filing health plan claims for medical devices, drugs, transportation services, and other items or services rendered. Medical supplies may be covered by an HCPCS Level II code when they are not used in the physician's office. Manufacturers or brand names are not included when reporting HCPCS Level II.

### Understanding HCPCS Level II

The main body of the HCPCS Level II codebook has different classes of code divided by the types of services and products provided. The codes are discussed below.

**Permanent National Codes**: These are established codes that describe products and services. The codes are grouped in alphanumeric sections and are updated yearly.

**Miscellaneous National Codes**: These codes are used when no existing code describes the service or item being billed. They allow suppliers to bill for these items and services, but not all miscellaneous codes are specifically FDA-approved; the approval may pertain to the items or services being billed rather than the codes themselves.

**Temporary National Codes**: These codes are developed to meet specific operational requirements. These may include new health policy or legislative requirements. They are used at the discretion of the Centers for Medicare and Medicaid Services (CMS). Temporary codes give health plans the headwind to establish codes before the start of the calendar year (January 1) when the annual code update is done. When a temporary code becomes a permanent national code, the temporary code is deleted and cross-referenced to the new permanent code. The updating, addition, and deletion of temporary codes is done every quarter. There are different types of temporary codes, and they are used to report various types of services.

- **C code**: Required under Medicare Outpatient Prospective Payment System (OPPS) for hospital use.
- **G code**: Identifies professional healthcare procedures and services without existing CPT codes.
- **H code**: Mental health services for state Medicaid agencies, as it is mandatory for them by state law to have separate codes for these services.

- **K code**: Used by Durable Medical Equipment Medicare Administrative Contractors (DME MACs) when current national codes do not include codes for certain products and supplies needed for implementation of DME MAC medical review policy.
- **Q code**: For services not recognized by national Level II codes yet needed by CMS to facilitate claims processing. This includes drugs, biological, and other medical equipment.
- **S code**: Reports drugs, services, and supplies without existing national codes but are needed for policy implementation or to support claims processing not payable by Medicare.
- **T code**: For use by Medicaid agencies for items without permanent national codes but integral to Medicaid operating needs.

## HCPCS Level II Modifiers

Health planners may instruct service suppliers to include HCPCP Level II Modifiers alongside the HCPCS Level II code. This provides more information about the specified service or item. HCPCS Level II Modifiers are either two alphabetic characters or alphanumeric characters. They are needed to provide specificity in procedures done in paired organs such as fingers, eyelids, and arteries.

Modifiers help to prevent erroneous denial of filed claims and billings. These code components provide additional information to CPT and HCPCS Level II. This helps report specific service, procedure, or medical equipment alterations without changing the code's definition. Appropriate use of modifiers nullifies the need for a separate procedure list to describe the modifying circumstance.

Modifiers impact flexibility and clarity and can indicate any of the following:

- Both professional and technical components were required for a service or procedure.
- A service or procedure was performed by more than one physician or other qualified health care professional or in multiple locations.
- Only a part of a service was performed.
- A service was increased or reduced.
- A supporting service was performed.
- A bilateral procedure was performed.
- A service was performed more than once.
- Unusual events occurred.

Functional or pricing modifiers should be in the first position when reporting codes with multiple modifiers. This is to be followed by the informational modifiers. This sequence is necessary because payers consider functional modifiers to determine reimbursements. The informational modifiers help them clarify certain aspects of the services or procedures.

Examples of Modifier Codes and their functions are highlighted in the table below.

| Code | Function |
|---|---|
| 22 | • The provided service is greater than what is usually required for the listed procedure.<br>• The documentation must include the justification and need for the additional work. |
| 23 | • A procedure, normally done under local or no anesthesia, is done under general anesthesia because of unusual circumstances.<br>• Modifier is used only by anesthesiologists. |
| 24 | • A physician or other qualified healthcare professional performs evaluation and management services in the postoperative period unrelated to the original procedure. |
| 25 | • Significant and distinct evaluation and management service done on the same day of a procedure by the same physician or another qualified healthcare professional. |
| 26 | • The professional component of services that combines professional and technical components is reported separately. |
| 32 | • A mandated consultation and related services. |
| 47 | • Surgeon-provided anesthesia. This could be regional or local anesthesia done by the surgeon. |
| 50 | • Bilateral procedures performed during one operative visit. |
| 51 | • Multiple E/M services, physical medicine, rehabilitation services, or supplies are provided by a single provider in the same session. |
| 52 | • Indicates a partial reduction or exclusion of services/procedures at the discretion of physicians or healthcare professionals. |

| | |
|---|---|
| | • The code for the provided service is used with the modifier added to signify this. |
| **53** | • Signifies a discontinuation of a procedure by the physician or other qualified healthcare professional when there is reason to think there is a significant risk to the patient's well-being. |
| **54** | • A physician or other qualified healthcare professional only performs the surgical procedure. Here, the preoperative or postoperative management is provided by others. |
| **55** | • The service provider only performs the postoperative management for a patient.<br>• Useful when there is an existing Modifier 54. |
| **56** | • The provider only performs the preoperative management for a patient.<br>• Useful when there is an existing Modifier 54. |
| **57** | • An E/M service was provided on the day preceding or the day of surgery. This results in the decision to perform surgery. |
| **58** | • A procedure performed during the postoperative period by the same physician or other qualified healthcare professional was:<br>    • Planned or anticipated (not necessarily already planned) at the time of the initial surgery/procedure and performed more extensively than the original procedure.<br>    • A staged or related procedure performed during the postoperative period of the initial procedure.<br>    • Being done for therapeutic purposes following a diagnostic procedure that was part of the initial procedure.<br><br>• For each of these scenarios, Modifier 58 is reported. |
| **59** | • A service or procedure performed on a given day was separate from other E/M services provided on that day.<br>• It identifies services that are usually not reported together but are fitting to be reported together under the given circumstance. |
| **62** | • Two surgeons work together as primary surgeons, and each performs different parts of the procedure.<br>• The part of the surgery done by each surgeon is to be reported by each individual in the operative report. |

| | |
|---|---|
| | • Each must report the procedure with the same code with Modifier 62 added. |
| **63** | • A procedure is performed on an infant or neonate with a body weight less than four kg.<br>• Distinct due to increased complexity usually associated with this class of patients. |
| **66** | • Circumstances when highly complex procedures are performed by a surgical team. |
| **76** | • The same physician or other qualified health care professional does a repeat of a procedure or service. |
| **77** | • A repeated procedure or service initially done by another physician or other qualified health care professional.<br>• Modifier 77 is added to the code for the repeated procedure/service. |
| **78** | • An unexpected return of a patient to the operating room by the same physician or another qualified healthcare professional during the postoperative period.<br>• Describes a return due to complications during the global period of another procedure. |
| **79** | • A medical practitioner or any other qualified healthcare professional conducts a procedure unrelated to the primary procedure during the postoperative period. |
| **80** | • Assistant surgeon services. |
| **81** | • The minimum assistant surgeon services, i.e., another surgeon is called to assist for only a limited time. |
| **82** | • Modifier 82 is used when an assistant surgeon is necessary during a procedure where a qualified resident surgeon is not available. This modifier is specifically for cases where the primary surgeon requires the assistance of another surgeon for a procedure that is performed with a resident's help in a teaching setting. |
| **90** | • Laboratory procedures performed by: |

| | |
|---|---|
| | • Another person or entity other than where the patient is receiving treatment.<br>• The reporting physician.<br>• Other qualified healthcare professionals. |
| **91** | • A need to repeat a laboratory test on the same day to have subsequent test results.<br>• Not for use due to lost results, samples, or equipment. |
| **92** | • Laboratory testing is done with a portable, disposable, single-use analytic kit. |
| **99** | • Certain conditions where there is a need for two or more modifiers to delineate a service clearly. |

# Chapter 7: Integumentary System

## Introduction

The integumentary system is the outermost layer of the body. It is composed of the skin and its appendages to form a barrier between the environment and the internal organs of the body.

The objectives for this chapter include:

- Understand the anatomy of the skin and associated structures.
- Understand key terminologies used to describe conditions associated with the integumentary system.
- Learn common disorders of the integumentary system.
- Recognize common procedures carried out on the integumentary system.

## Examples of Words, Prefixes, and Suffixes

- Dermatitis (inflammation of the skin).
    - Prefix: derm- (skin).
    - Root: -at- (related to).
    - Suffix: -itis (inflammation).
- Epidermis (outer layer of skin).
    - Prefix: epi- (upon).
    - Root: derm- (skin).
    - Suffix: -is (pertaining to).
- Hidradenitis (inflammation of sweat glands).
    - Prefix: hidr- (sweat).
    - Root: aden- (gland).
    - Suffix: -itis (inflammation).
- Keratosis (abnormal thickening of the skin's outer layer).
    - Prefix: kerat- (horny tissue, keratin).
    - Root: none.
    - Suffix: -osis (abnormal condition).
- Lipoma (fatty tumor under the skin).
    - Prefix: none.
    - Root: lip- (fat).
    - Suffix: -oma (tumor, mass).
- Melanoma (skin cancer with pigment cells).
    - Prefix: none.

    - Root: melan- (black, dark).
    - Suffix: -oma (tumor, mass).
- Seborrhea (excessive secretion of sebum).
    - Prefix: none.
    - Root: seb- (sebum).
    - Suffix: -rrhea (flow, discharge).
- Subcutaneous (under the skin).
    - Prefix: sub- (under).
    - Root: cutane- (skin).
    - Suffix: -ous (pertaining to).
- Sudoriferous (sweat-producing).
    - Prefix: none.
    - Root: sudor- (sweat).
    - Suffix: -iferous (producing).
- Xeroderma (abnormally dry skin).
    - Prefix: xero- (dry).
    - Root: derm- (skin).
    - Suffix: -a is often used in the names of diseases or disorders.

## Anatomy of the Integumentary System

The integumentary system is the most extensive organ of the body. It is made up of the skin and divided into distinct parts. These include the epidermis, dermis, and hypodermis, hair, nails, and other associated glands. The epidermis is the outermost layer of the skin. It is in direct contact with the environment and contains a special type of cells that serves as a barrier. The epidermis layer differs in thickness based on the part of the body where it is present.

The dermis of the skin is the underlying tissue that serves as support to the epidermis. It contains blood vessels and provides nutrients to the epidermis through a vascular network. The hypodermis of the skin is commonly referred to as the subcutaneous layer. It is composed of fat cells and loose areolar tissue. This layer provides insulation for the other structures that lie beneath the skin.

Each hair on the body extends its root into the dermis. Hair is part of a unit composed of oil glands and arrector pili muscle. This is referred to as the pilosebaceous unit. The skin's exocrine glands produce different chemical substances that serve various functions. They include the sebaceous, sweat, ceruminous, and mammary glands. The nails at the tips of the fingers and toes are made of thick layers of keratin. Each nail growth begins proximally at the matrix and grows outward as it ages. The nails help improve the perception of sensation and movement.

The skin also serves as the first line of defense to prevent the entry of pathogens into the body. In the case of external trauma, the body relies on the healing process initiated by the integumentary system to restore damaged tissue and aid wound healing. The skin is also important for synthesis of vitamin D and regulation of body temperature to maintain homeostasis.

## ICD-10-CM Coding

The ICD-10-CM diagnosis codes for the skin are found mainly in the code category L00 - L99. This covers skin and subcutaneous tissue diseases. Other codes associated with the integumentary system are found in the chapters that cover neoplasms, injury, and poisoning. Infections of the skin and subcutaneous tissue can be found in categories L00 - L08.

L00 is the code for staphylococcal scalded skin syndrome. This is also known as Ritter disease. Impetigo is a common, highly contagious infection of the skin that usually presents in children. It is caused by a superficial bacterial infection and presents in affected patients with sores and yellow crusts on the face or other body parts. Impetigo is coded as category L01. Further subcategories include unspecified impetigo (L01.00), non-bullous impetigo (L01.01), Bockhart's impetigo (L01.02), and bullous impetigo (L01.03). Other classified cases of impetigo can be coded as L01.09.

Cutaneous abscesses of different body parts, either carbuncles or furuncles, can be found in category L02. This category excludes abscesses formed in the anal, genital, or rectal regions in both males and females. The organism that causes the carbuncles or furuncles reported can be coded by additional medical codes found in categories B95 - B96.

Cellulitis is a common acute bacterial infection of the affected area's deep dermis and surrounding subcutaneous tissue. The infection may be associated with the collection of pus or discharge. Lymphangitis is an infection of the lymphatic system that can spread proximally in a very short time. Cellulitis and acute lymphangitis are in the same category under ICD-10-CM diagnosis code L03.

L03 excludes cellulitis of the orbital region (H05.0-), which should be coded under category H05, not H00.0 as previously mentioned. H00.0 refers to Hordeolum and other deep inflammation of the eyelid.

Acute lymphadenitis is categorized separately as code L04. Inflammation of one or two lymph nodes in a specific body region is called lymphadenitis. This condition usually arises due to an infection that originates from another part of the body. Bullous skin disorders (L10 - L14) is a group of conditions that affect the skin. This results in blisters and bullae filled with fluid in the skin. The two main bullous disorders are pemphigoid (L12) and pemphigus (L10).

Other bullous disorders (L13) include dermatitis herpetiformis (L13.0), subcorneal pustular dermatitis (L13.1), and specified bullous disorders (L13.8). Further subcategories are based on additional provided details and found in the ICD-10-CM diagnosis code book.

Dermatitis is the term used to describe conditions that arise from skin irritation due to genetics, exposure to irritants or allergens, and infections that result from an overactive immune system. Eczema translates into 'itch that rashes.' It is the resulting rash that follows an itch that causes a patient to scratch or rub their skin.

There are numerous forms of dermatitis that affect the skin. They are listed in the following major categories:

- Atopic dermatitis (L20).
- Seborrheic dermatitis (L21).
- Diaper dermatitis (L22).
- Allergic contact dermatitis (L23).
- Irritant contact dermatitis (L24).
- Unspecified contact dermatitis (L25).
- Exfoliative dermatitis (L26).
- Dermatitis due to substances taken internally should include reactions to drugs or food, which can manifest as allergic contact dermatitis or other dermatological reactions. The correct classification would be L27, which covers dermatitis due to substances taken internally, including those caused by drugs and food, without excluding allergic or adverse reactions.
- Lichen simplex chronicus and prurigo (L28).
- Pruritus (L29).

Pruritus is an unpleasant feeling that evokes a desire to scratch the skin. It excludes neurotic excoriation (L98.1) and psychogenic pruritus (F45.8). The desire to scratch a lesion is commonly associated with many skin conditions. However, L29 includes those specific to the anus, pruritus ani (L29.0), pruritus scroti of the male scrotum (L29.1), pruritus vulvae of the female vulva (L29.2), unspecified anogenital pruritis (L29.3), other pruritus (L29.8), and unspecified pruritus (L29.9).

Urticaria is characterized by itchy pink papules and plaques that usually have central pallor. Urticaria and erythema are listed in code range L49 - L54. Some disorders of the skin and subcutaneous tissue are a result of radiation-related injuries (L55 - L59). Disorders of the skin appendages (L60 - L75) include those that affect the hair, nails, sweat glands, and sebaceous glands. Complications related to the skin and subcutaneous tissue during and after a medical procedure have codes from L76 to L76.82.

### Skin Grafting

To perform a skin graft, the surgeon must determine the area and size of the recipient site where the graft will be placed. Autografts are commonly used. For autografts, the skin placed over the defect is taken from the same patient at a different site on their body. Allografts are obtained from the body of another human donor. Xenografts are excised from an animal.

There have also been successful substitutes created for human skin types in laboratories as cultured tissues. A skin graft may be a full-thickness graft or a split-thickness graft. The extent of these grafts is reported in square centimeters ($cm^2$), not square meters, for both adults and children. The percentage of the body area affected in infants or children is assessed using the 'rule of nines' or the Lund and Browder chart, which is more detailed for pediatric patients. The site where the skin graft is to be placed requires preparation. The appropriate CPT codes are chosen based on the location and extent of the defect.

## Skin Flaps

A skin flap is the transfer of a section of skin with its blood supply to another defect. It is important to distinguish a skin flap from a pedicle flap.

### Pressure Ulcers

A pressure ulcer refers to a skin injury that breaks down toward the underlying tissue due to prolonged pressure on an area of skin. It results in ischemia which is disrupted nutrition and oxygen supply to the tissue. This subsequently causes tissue necrosis.

### Management of Burns

The choice of CPT code to report depends on the extent of the burn injury. The classification of burn injury is determined by the extent of body surface area affected as well as the depth of the injury. This percentage is usually calculated by the physician with use of a standard chart.

Major burns are managed in a high-dependency unit. It is important to prevent superimposed infections of burns. This is ensured through wound dressing or debridement (16020 - 16030). An escharotomy is a surgical incision created in necrotic tissue to relieve the pressure. The appropriate codes are found in the CPT codebook.

## Procedures on the Breasts

Patients with suspected breast cysts may require puncture aspiration for further investigation. Imaging guidance code should be included where applicable. A doctor may create an incision that extends deep into the breast tissue to drain an existing abscess or for other reasons. This procedure is referred to as a mastotomy.

Surgical removal of the breast due to an underlying malignancy or for cosmetic reasons is known as a mastectomy. Mastectomies are done for both men and women. In males, the surgical removal of enlarged breast tissue is a common cosmetic procedure. A mastectomy may be partial (19301) or radical (19306, 19307). It may be carried out alongside a lumpectomy. This should be reported with a single code of 19302.

A modified radical mastectomy (19307) involves the removal of the entire breast tissue and axillary lymph nodes, but unlike the radical mastectomy, it spares both the pectoralis major and minor muscles.

A mastopexy is the surgical lift of the breast. Reduction mammoplasty is the cosmetic reduction of breast tissue in a female. These procedures can be done to relieve complications associated with excessive breast tissue that causes pain in the shoulders, neck, or back.

Breast augmentation is the surgical reconstruction of smaller breasts to the desired size. Augmentation may involve the placement of an implant into the breast tissue. Some cases of ruptured implants have been reported. This requires the removal of existing implants. Not all cases permit the replacement of removed implants.

Reconstruction options are available to follow mastectomy or mastopexy. These options may be immediate or delayed depending on certain factors. Instead of an immediate reconstruction, a tissue expander may be placed and subsequently replaced with a permanent prosthetic material.

## Other Procedures

Cosmetic related procedures should also be considered. It is important to note that these procedures may be medical necessities that should be paid for by an insurance company. These procedures are found in the CPT codebook:

- Abdominoplasty.
- Ablation of superficial lesions.
- Blepharoplasty.
- Chemical peel.
- Cervicoplasty.

- Dermabrasion.
- Liposuction.

## Definitions of Important Terms

- Acne: A skin issue caused by infection of sebaceous glands.
- Albinism: Genetic disorder which causes the absence of melanin production.
- Arrector pili: The smooth muscle that pulls on hair follicles and makes hair stand up when it contracts.
- Basal cell carcinoma: Skin cancer that develops from the basal cells within the skin's epidermis.
- Bedsore: A decubitus ulcer, also known as a pressure sore or lesion, which develops on the skin when certain body areas begin to necrotize due to continuous pressure and insufficient blood flow.
- Callus: An area of skin thickening due to repeated abrasion.
- Corn: A type of callus that is painful and round, and forms on the toes due to pressure and friction.
- Cortex: The middle layer of keratinocytes in hair that can be seen in a hair bulb cross-section.
- Dermis: Skin layer just below the epidermis that consists mainly of connective tissue and contains various structures such as blood vessels, sweat glands, and hair follicles.
- Eczema: A skin condition that resembles a rash due to an allergic reaction.
- Epidermis: The outermost tissue layer of the skin.
- First-degree burn: A burn injury that affects only the epidermis.
- Fourth-degree burn: Burn injury that damages the full thickness of the skin, underlying muscle, and bone.
- Keloid: A type of scar that rises above the skin surface and has layers.
- Keratin: A structural protein that provides skin, hair, and nails with hard, water-resistant properties.
- Keratinocytes: The most predominant cell type in the epidermis that produces keratin.
- Meissner corpuscles: Also known as tactile corpuscles, these are receptors in the skin that respond to light touch.
- Medulla: The innermost keratinocyte layer that originates from the hair matrix.
- Melanin: The pigment responsible for determining hair and skin color.
- Melanocytes: Melanin-producing cells found in the stratum basale of the epidermis.
- Melanoma: A type of skin cancer that originates from the melanocytes of the skin.

- Melanosomes: Intercellular vesicles that transfer melanin from melanocytes into keratinocytes of the epidermis.
- Metastasis: The spread of cancerous cells from the initial location to other body parts.
- Nail bed: The layer of epidermis on which the nail body forms.
- Nail body: The main keratinous plate that forms the nail.
- Nail cuticle: Also known as the eponychium, this is a fold of epithelium that extends over the nail bed.
- Nail fold: The fold of epithelium that extends over the sides of the nail body and holds it in place.
- Nail root: The part of the nail from which the nail grows. It is situated in the epidermis.
- Rickets: Bone disease in children that is caused by deficiency of vitamin D and results in the weakening of bones.
- Sebum: An oily substance composed of lipids that lubricate the skin and hair.
- Second-degree burn: A partial thickness burn that affects the epidermis and a portion of the dermis.
- Squamous cell carcinoma: Skin cancer that originates from the epidermis.
- Sudoriferous glands: Another name for sweat glands.
- Third-degree burn: Burn that penetrates and destroys the full skin thickness.
- Vitiligo: Skin condition characterized by the inability of melanocytes in certain areas to produce melanin and is likely due to an autoimmune reaction. It causes patches of hypopigmentation on the skin.

# Chapter 8: Musculoskeletal System

## Introduction

This chapter examines the musculoskeletal system which comprises the bones and muscles of the body.

The objectives of this chapter are:

- Learn the parts of the musculoskeletal system.
- Learn the disorders associated with the musculoskeletal system.
- Recognize key terms related to the musculoskeletal system.
- Learn the appropriate use of HCPCS level II codes and modifiers.

## Examples of Words, Prefixes, and Suffixes

- Arthritis (inflammation of the joints).
    - Prefix: none.
    - Root: arthr- (joint).
    - Suffix: -itis (inflammation).
- Chondroma (benign cartilage tumor).
    - Prefix: none.
    - Root: chondr- (cartilage).
    - Suffix: -oma (tumor, mass).
- Myalgia (muscle pain).
    - Prefix: none.
    - Root: my- (muscle).
    - Suffix: -algia (pain).
- Myasthenia (muscle weakness).
    - Prefix: none.
    - Root: my- (muscle).
    - Suffix: -asthenia (weakness).
- Myositis (inflammation of muscle tissue).
    - Prefix: none.
    - Root: my- (muscle).
    - Suffix: -itis (inflammation).
- Orthopedics (branch of medicine related to the skeletal system and muscles).
    - Prefix: orth- (straight, correct).
    - Root: ped- (child, foot).
    - Suffix: -ics (pertaining to)

- Osteoporosis (condition of porous bones).
    - Prefix: none.
    - Root: oste- (bone).
    - Suffix: -porosis (condition).
- Scoliosis (abnormal curvature of the spine).
    - Prefix: none.
    - Root: scoli- (crooked).
    - Suffix: -osis (abnormal condition).
- Tendinitis (inflammation of a tendon).
    - Prefix: none.
    - Root: tendo- or tendin- (tendon).
    - Suffix: -itis (inflammation).
- Tenosynovitis (inflammation of tendon sheath).
    - Prefix: none.
    - Root: ten- (tendon).
    - Suffix: -synov- (synovial membrane) + -itis (inflammation).

## Anatomy of the Musculoskeletal System

The human body features 206 bones linked together by muscles, ligaments, tendons, and cartilage. This forms a framework to hold the body parts together. The human skeleton comprises an axial part and an appendicular part. The axial skeleton is the central part that begins from the skull and extends to the chest and spine with a limited range of movement. The appendicular skeleton includes bones of the arms, legs, and pelvis.

The bones are important storage vessels for calcium and other minerals. Within the long bones lies a strip of tissue referred to as the bone marrow. Hematopoietic cells are generated from bone marrow. Damage to these cells results in various forms of blood disorders. The long bones also have a wider area of attachment for muscles. The small bones in the hands and feet articulate with each other. They are lined with layers of cartilage which are lubricated by synovial fluid to prevent erosion and damage from overuse.

The muscles of the body help with movement and posture. There are various muscle types with different functions in specific body parts. The skeletal muscles are striated bands that are moved voluntarily to cause movement. The smooth muscles are visceral in the body's digestive system and blood vessels. The smooth muscles of the intestine help to propel food forward during digestion. The cardiac muscles are special muscle types specific to the heart. The synchronized action of cardiac muscles helps to pump blood.

## ICD-10-CM Coding

The codes for musculoskeletal system diseases are found in the chapter of the ICD-10-CM diagnosis code book that covers the Musculoskeletal System and Connective Tissue. You may also find other codes relevant to the musculoskeletal system in the chapters on symptoms, signs, and abnormal clinical and laboratory findings not elsewhere classified. M00 - M99 is the code range for diseases of the musculoskeletal system and connective tissue.

Arthropathies (M00 – M25) contain the ICD-10-CM diagnosis codes for infectious arthropathies, autoinflammatory syndromes, inflammatory polyarthropathies, osteoarthritis, and other joint disorders. M15 – M19 is the code set for osteoarthritis. It includes the diagnosis codes for polyosteoarthritis, osteoarthritis of the hip, knee, first carpometacarpal joint, and other unspecified osteoarthritis.

Systemic Lupus Erythematosus is an autoimmune condition coded under M32 in the ICD-10-CM, which falls within the range for systemic connective tissue disorders but specifically addresses Systemic Lupus Erythematosus. The choice of ICD-10-CM diagnosis code depends on the cause and the extent of organ involvement. Other categories found in this code set include polyarteritis nodosa and related conditions, other necrotizing vasculopathies (hypersensitivity angiitis, thrombotic microangiopathy, lethal midline granuloma, Wegener's granulomatosis, aortic arch syndrome, giant cell arteritis, microscopic polyangiitis, and other specified forms of necrotizing vasculopathies), dermatopolymyositis, scleroderma, and other systemic disorders of the connective tissue that are classified elsewhere.

Dorsopathies (M40 - M54) make up a group of diseases of the spine and paravertebral tissues. They are believed to result from increased load on the spine, impaired nutrition, and blood supply to the vertebrae and tissues. They can also result from shocks, falls from a height on the spine or legs, and other injuries. They include deforming dorsopathies, spondylopathies, and other forms of dorsopathies.

Soft tissue disorders (M60 - M79) make up the code range for disorders of the muscles, synovium, tendons, and other soft tissue disorders. Disorders of the muscles include inflammatory conditions, calcification or ossification of muscles, as well as other classified disorders of the muscles.

The ICD-10-CM diagnosis code category for other acquired deformities of the musculoskeletal system and connective tissue is M95.0 - M95.9. This includes deformities of the nose, ears, head and neck, chest and ribs, pelvis, and other specified acquired deformities of the musculoskeletal system.

Intraoperative and postprocedural complications and disorders of the musculoskeletal system not classified elsewhere (M96) include the following:

- Pseudarthrosis following arthrodesis or fusion, post-laminectomy syndrome, post-radiation kyphosis, post-laminectomy kyphosis, post-surgical lordosis, post-radiation scoliosis, bone fracture following implant.
- Fracture of the ribs, sternum, and thorax (M96.A) may be reported after cardiopulmonary resuscitation or chest compression.

Some of the codes related to the musculoskeletal system can be found in the category covering neoplasms (C00 - D49), congenital malformations, deformations, and chromosomal abnormality (Q00 - Q99). Code set S00 - T88 is for injuries due to external causes that affect the musculoskeletal system.

Fractures are pathological discontinuations of a bone. Further information related to fractures can be found in category S20 - S29 for thorax fractures, S30 - S39 for abdomen, lower back, lumbar spine, pelvis, and external genitals, S40 - S49 for shoulder and upper arm, and S50 - S59 for elbow and forearm. For accuracy, the medical coder should understand the use of a tabular list and ICD-10 CM diagnosis code index. Refer to the appropriate chapter for the proper allocation of codes.

## CPT Coding

The current procedural terminology code range for surgical procedures performed on the musculoskeletal system is 20100 – 29999. This code set is maintained by the American Medical Association and is available in the latest edition of the CPT codebook.

Code 20100 – 20999 applies to General Surgical Procedures on the Musculoskeletal System. The first code set for this category relates to wound exploration subsequent to trauma. This may be due to a penetrating gunshot or stab wound. The general excision procedures of the muscles include a biopsy of the muscles or bones. Other procedures include the introduction of diagnostic or therapeutic substances or the removal of foreign bodies in muscles or tendon sheaths.

Arthrocentesis, aspiration, or injection of major joints or bursa with diagnostic or therapeutic agents are found in the CPT code 20600 – 20615. Codes 20690 and 20692 describe the placement of external fixation devices. These may be uniplane or multiplane. The choice of stabilization method depends on the grade of fracture, type of fracture (comminuted, impacted, or spiral), and the location of the fracture.

Surgical procedures on the head are found in code sets 21010 – 21499. These procedures are performed on the skull, facial bones, and temporomandibular joint. Arthrotomy of the temporomandibular joint is reported as 21010. Excision procedures may be limited to the bones or tumors if present in the bones of the head. Codes 21076 – 21089 are used when describing professional services for rehabilitation of patients with oral, facial, and other anatomical deficiencies with use of prosthetic devices.

Surgical procedures on the soft tissues of the neck and thorax are within code set 21501 – 21899. Incision and drainage of abscess or hematoma in the soft tissues of the neck are described using code 21501. Biopsy or radical resection of tumors in the neck is reported under the code for excision. Surgeries performed on the back and flank are mostly excision procedures such as biopsy of superficial or deep tissues.

The surgical procedures on the vertebral column (spine) are within CPT code set 22010 – 22899. The vertebral column consists of the cervical, thoracic, and lumbar spine. When two primary surgeons are present for the excision of vertebra bodies, append the modifier 62 to the reported code.

Bone grafting procedures are reported separately and in addition to arthrodesis. Arthrodesis is the surgical immobilization of a joint intended to result in bone fusion at the site. Arthrodesis may be performed as a standalone procedure. It is essential to note the presence of possible combination procedures such as surgical sectioning of bone, treatment of fractures, and spinal corpectomy, or laminectomy. Refer to codes 22590 – 22632 to report arthrodesis.

Corpectomy is the removal of a vertebral body during a spinal surgery. Laminectomy is the excision of the vertebral lamina and commonly used to denote the removal of the posterior arch of the vertebrae.

Surgical procedures performed on the pelvis and hip joint are coded within the code range 26990 – 27299.

The code for prosthesis used should also be reported. Amputation procedures are reported based on the part of the body in which it is to take place. Amputation related to the foot can be found in code sets 28800 – 28825. This depends on the extent of the amputation. Application of casts and strapping (29000 – 29799) are reported along with the type of cast the physician or other healthcare provider applies. Refer to the CPT codebook for appropriate designation of codes for complex professional and technical surgical procedures performed on the musculoskeletal system.

## HCPCS Coding

Healthcare Common Procedure Coding System, Level II codes, are used for orthotic and prosthetic supplies. The common ones related to orthopedics and other musculoskeletal services are crutches, wheelchairs, canes, and traction devices. These supplies may be provided by the physician or an equipment provider that follows specific physician orders.

## Modifiers

The modifiers commonly used in orthopedic surgery include:

- Modifier RT, LT: To indicate the side of the body on which a procedure is being carried out.
- Modifier 50: To indicate that a procedure was done bilaterally.
- Modifier 58: To indicate a staged or related procedure or service by the same physician or qualified healthcare professional during the postoperative period of the first procedure
- Modifier 59: To indicate a distinct procedural service.
- Modifier 62: To indicate when two surgeons perform a surgery.
- Modifier 66: To indicate the surgical team that consists of three or more surgeons that may be required for more complex procedures.
- Modifier 80: To indicate an assistant surgeon.

Other modifiers can be found in the CPT codebook and should be applied properly for providers to pay for the correct procedure.

## Definitions of Important Terms

- Abduction: Movement of an extremity directed away from the body.
- Adduction: Movement of an extremity directed toward the body.
- Analgesia: To take away pain.
- Ankylosis: Abnormal stiffness of a skeletal structure.
- Appendicular skeleton: Pertains to bones of the arms and legs.
- Arthralgia: Pain in joints.
- Arthritis: Inflammation of the joints.
- Arthro: Associated with the joints of the body.
- Articulation: Point at which bones meet..
- Asthenia: Weakness or loss of strength.
- Atrophy: Shrinkage of muscle.
- Axial skeleton: Central axis of the body that includes the bones of the head, neck, chest, and back.
- Axial skeleton: Pertains to the bones of the skull, spine, ribs, and sternum.
- Belly: Bulky central body of a muscle.
- Bursa: Fluid-filled sacs that serve as a cushion in specific joints of the body.
- Burso: Associated with the bursa located between tendons and bones.

- Cartilage: Form of elastic connective tissue that is located at the edge of bones and the tip of the nose.
- Chondro: Related to the cartilages.
- Circular: Fascicles that are arranged in a concentric manner around an opening.
- Circumduction: Circular movement of the body that involves a combination of flexion, extension, adduction, and abduction motions.
- Deglutition: Process of swallowing.
- Diaphragm: Skeletal muscle that separates the thoracic and abdominal cavities. It is dome-shaped when at rest.
- Eversion: Outward turning of the foot away from the body.
- Extension: Backward bending movement of a part of the body.
- Extensor: Any muscle that increases the angle at the joint.
- Femoral triangle: Anatomical position at the intersection of the hip and the leg. It houses the femoral nerve, artery, and vein, as well as the pectineus and deep inguinal lymph nodes.
- Flexion: Forward bending of a body part.
- Flexor: Muscle that decreases the angle at the joint.
- Fracture: Bone break.
- Hamstring group: Three long muscles on the back of the leg.
- Hemarthrosis: Blood within joints.
- Hypertrophy: Increase in muscle size.
- Insertion: An end of a skeletal muscle attached to a bony structure as an anchor that moves when the muscle contracts.
- Inversion: Turning of the foot inward toward the midline of the body.
- Joint: Point of articulation of bones against each other.
- Ligaments: Tough elastic connective tissue that firmly adheres bones to other bones.
- Lumbrical: Muscles in the hand facilitate the flexion of each finger at the metacarpophalangeal joints and aid in the extension of each finger at the interphalangeal joints.
- Mastication: Action of chewing.
- Meniscus: C-shaped cartilage that serves as a shock absorber in joint spaces.
- Myalgia: Pain in the muscle.
- Myelo: Related to the bone marrow.
- Myo, Myoso: Pertains to muscles.
- Origin: End of a skeletal muscle attached to another structure as an anchor in a fixed position.
- Osteo: Related to the bones in the body.

- Osteoarthritis: A degenerative joint disease characterized by the breakdown of cartilage and underlying bone, which causes pain and stiffness, in the hips, knees, hands, and spine.
- Osteoporosis: Increased porosity of the bones that causes increased susceptibility to breakage.
- Pelvic girdle: The hips which serve as a foundation for the lower limbs.
- Perineum: Diamond-shaped region between the pubic symphysis, coccyx bones, and ischial tuberosities.
- Scoliosis: Abnormal lateral curvature of the spine accompanied by twisting.
- Synovial fluid: Lubricant found between joints that allows easy articulation.
- Synovial membrane: Lining of joints.
- Tendon: Fibrous connective tissue that keeps muscle attached to bone.

# Chapter 9: Respiratory, Hemic, and Lymphatic Systems

## Introduction

This chapter reviews the coding for the respiratory system, hemic system, lymphatic system, mediastinum, and diaphragm.

The objectives for this chapter include the following:

- Learn the basic anatomy and functions of the respiratory, hemic, and lymphatic systems.
- Understand how to apply CPT codes relevant to the respiratory, hemic, and lymphatic systems.
- Learn standard ICD-10-CM codes relevant to the respiratory, hemic, and lymphatic systems.
- Application of HCPCS level II codes to the respiratory, hemic, and lymphatic systems.
- Understand the use of CPT modifiers for services and procedures carried out on the respiratory, hemic, and lymphatic systems.
- Learn key terms associated with the respiratory, hemic, and lymphatic systems.

## Examples of Words, Prefixes, and Suffixes

- Dyspnea (difficulty breathing).
    - Prefix: dys- (difficult, painful).
    - Root: -pnea (breathing).
- Erythrocytosis (excessive red blood cells).
    - Prefix: erythro- (red).
    - Root: -cyt- (cell).
    - Suffix: -osis (abnormal condition).
- Hemoptysis (coughing up blood).
    - Prefix: hemo- (blood).
    - Root: -ptysis (spitting).
- Hemothorax (blood in the pleural cavity).
    - Prefix: hemo- (blood).
    - Root: thorac- (chest).
    - Suffix: -x (condition).
- Hemorrhage (excessive bleeding).
    - Prefix: hemo- (blood).
    - Root: -rrhage (bursting forth).

- Leukemia (cancer of the blood-forming tissues).
    - Prefix: leuk- (white).
    - Root: -emia (blood condition).
- Oxygenation (process of adding oxygen to the body).
    - Prefix: none.
    - Root: oxygen- (oxygen).
    - Suffix: -ation (process).
- Pneumonia (inflammation of the lungs).
    - Prefix: pneum- (lung).
    - Root: -onia (condition).
- Pulmonary embolism (blockage of a lung artery).
    - Prefix: pulmon- (lung).
    - Root: embol- (plug).
    - Suffix: -ism (condition).
- Thrombocytopenia (low platelet count).
    - Prefix: thrombo- (clot).
    - Root: -cyt- (cell).
    - Suffix: -penia (deficiency).

## Anatomy

### Respiratory System, Mediastinum, and Diaphragm

The respiratory system is the network of organs and structures that helps oxygenate tissues through blood circulation. The human respiratory system begins from the nose, through which air enters the respiratory system. The nostrils contain cilia that cover the surface of the nostrils and filter air.

The larynx is connected to the pharynx and trachea. It consists of cartilage secured by layers of muscle and ligaments. The epiglottis covers the larynx and prevents food or liquid entry into the trachea.

The vocal cords are also part of the larynx. These cords are separated by a small central opening called the glottis. Air enters the trachea from the nose and mouth through the glottis. The trachea is also called the windpipe of the respiratory system. It connects the mouth and nose to the lungs.

The trachea branches out into two main bronchi called the right and left main bronchus. The right main bronchus forms a more direct connection with the trachea. The right main bronchus divides into three secondary bronchi for the three lobes of the right lung, and the left main bronchus divides into two secondary bronchi for the two lobes of the left lung, which then further divide into segmental bronchioles. Each bronchiole terminates into alveolar sacs. The alveolus is the terminal unit of respiration. Gaseous exchange occurs at the alveolus through diffusion. Oxygen is exchanged for carbon dioxide across the alveoli and surrounding capillaries.

The human body has one lung on each side of the thoracic cavity. The right lung has three lobes and the left has two lobes. The lungs are protected by a serous membrane. This membrane includes two layers called the parietal pleura and visceral pleura. The space between each pleural membrane has minimal fluid for lubrication as the lungs expand when filled with air.

The mediastinum is a central space within the thorax that contains the heart, aorta, esophagus, trachea, and thymus gland. A thick muscle layer known as the diaphragm separates it from the abdomen. The mediastinum is divided into the superior, anterior, middle, and posterior mediastinum. The anterior mediastinum contains the thymus. The superior mediastinum contains the trachea, aorta, and esophagus. The heart is in the middle mediastinum. The posterior mediastinum contains the esophagus and descending aorta.

The diaphragm contracts during inspiration to allow air to fill the lungs. It relaxes to allow air to be pushed out of the thoracic cavity with exhalation. The diaphragm is the major muscle that controls respiration. It works alongside other accessory muscles of respiration, such as the intercostal muscles, scalene, trapezius, pectoralis, and sternocleidomastoid.

### Hemic and Lymphatic Systems

The hemic system performs the function of blood production. It consists mainly of the spleen and bone marrow. The spleen is located in the upper left quadrant of the abdomen and serves as a primary hematopoietic organ. The spleen produces antibodies, red blood cells, and other immune cells. It also destroys platelets and red blood cells in circulation that require breakdown. The spleen is a primary blood reserve in cases of hemorrhagic shock and can contain massive amounts of blood cells.

Bone marrow is found within many body bones, especially the ribs, vertebrae, sternum, and pelvic bones. Bone marrow produces red blood cells, white blood cells, and platelets. It also generates stem cells that develop into different blood cell types.

The lymphatic system is the network that collects lymph. Lymph is necessary to maintain the body's immune system. Lymph nodes are small structures found within the body where pathogens are removed during blood filtration. The lymphatic system connects through the spleen, thymus, tonsils, and Peyer's patches.

The spleen is the largest organ in the lymphatic system. The thymus is a structure in the anterior mediastinum that produces immune cells called T cells. T cells are essential to defend the body against invading pathogens and foreign materials. Peyer's patches are found in the intestine and especially in the wall of the terminal ileum of the small intestine. Their function is vital to maintain the immune system.

## ICD-10-CM Coding

When selecting the diagnosis code for conditions that affect the respiratory system, it is essential to refer to the index and verify the code with the tabular list in the ICD-10-CM diagnosis codebook. Code range J00- J99 contains diseases of the respiratory system. Other conditions that affect the respiratory system can be found in the first chapter. This includes A00 - B99 for infections and parasitic diseases and code range C00 - D49 for possible neoplasms that affect the respiratory system.

Acute upper respiratory tract infections are found in code range J00- J06. The common cold is J00 and includes acute rhinitis, coryza, infective nasopharyngitis, infective rhinitis, and acute nasal catarrh. The infective agent that causes the respiratory tract infection can be found in categories A00- B99.

Acute sinusitis (J01) is the inflammation of the sinuses. Croup (J05.0) is the inflammation of the larynx and trachea in children. Acute epiglottitis (J05.1) is a common condition reported in children that follows inflammation of the epiglottis. The causative infectious agent can be found in code range B95 - B97 and used as additional code for report.

Pneumonia is the inflammation of the alveoli of the lungs and surrounding tissue. It is often caused by infectious agents. The subcategories of pneumonia are based on the causative agents and are found in the code range J12- J18. Acute bronchitis and bronchiolitis are other acute lower respiratory infections (J20 - J22). Chronic lower respiratory diseases (J40 - J4A) include bronchitis, emphysema, bronchiectasis, asthma, and chronic lung allograft dysfunction.

Chronic obstructive pulmonary disease (COPD) is a treatable disease that is characterized by progressive airflow limitation and tissue destruction. It is further associated with structural lung changes due to the presence of chronic inflammation that follows prolonged exposure to noxious particles or gases, especially cigarette smoke.

Asthma (J45) is a form of chronic lung disease caused by inflammation and tightening around the airways that make it harder to breathe. The subcategories of asthma are based on the severity of presentation. Asthma can be mild intermittent (J45.2), mild persistent (J45.3), moderate persistent (J45.4), or severe persistent (J45.5).

Diseases of the blood, blood-forming organs, and certain disorders involving the immune mechanism are found in code range D50 - D89. Nutritional anemias cause a significant disease burden in the population. The forms of nutritional anemias include iron deficiency anemia (D50), vitamin B12 deficiency anemia (D51), folate deficiency anemia (D52), protein deficiency anemia (D53.0), scorbutic anemia (D53.2 - a form of megaloblastic anemia that responds to ascorbic acid alone), other specified nutritional anemias, and unspecified nutritional anemias.

Hemolytic anemias (D55 - D59) can arise due to enzyme disorders, thalassemia, sickle cell disorders, and other hereditary hemolytic anemias. This includes spherocytosis and elliptocytosis as well as acquired hemolytic anemias. Aplastic anemia (D60 - D64) is a syndrome of bone marrow failure. This is characterized by peripheral pancytopenia and marrow hypoplasia. It results in poor production of circulating blood cells and the inability of the body to perform its functions optimally.

Disseminated intravascular coagulation (DIC) is coded as D65, as it is a severe hematological condition that manifests as a widespread hypercoagulable state. It can cause both microvascular and macrovascular clotting and compromised blood flow. This results in multiple organ dysfunction syndrome. Other coagulation defects, purpura, and hemorrhagic conditions are found in category D65 - D69. Other disorders of blood and blood-forming organs can be found in the code range D70 - D77. Refer to the ICD-10-CM diagnosis codebook for the appropriate allocation of codes relevant to the hemic and lymphatic system.

## CPT Coding

### Respiratory System

The Current Procedural Terminology codes for the surgical procedures performed on the respiratory system are in the code range 30000 - 32999. The surgical procedures performed on the nose (30000- 30999) include incision procedures, excision procedures, introduction procedures, removal of foreign bodies on the nose, repair procedures of the nose, and destruction procedures on the nose. Endoscopic visualization of the accessory sinuses is in code range 31231 - 31298. The provider may insert an endoscope into the nasal cavity and use bipolar cautery to control bleeding in epistaxis, as reported in CPT code 31238.

Surgical procedures performed on the larynx are within the code range 31300 - 31599. The removal of the larynx with radical neck dissection and removal of lymph nodes and other adjacent tissues is an excision procedure of the larynx coded 31365. This procedure may be carried out for suspected neoplasm with accompanying biopsy. For CPT code range 31600 - 31614, incision procedures are carried out on the trachea and bronchi. An emergency tracheostomy done with a transtracheal approach should be reported as 31603.

For endoscopic procedures, the medical code is based on the anatomical site where the procedure takes place. A rigid or flexible bronchoscope inserted through the oropharynx and vocal cords and beyond the trachea into either the right or left main bronchi is termed a bronchoscopy. It is reported using CPT codes 31622 - 31661.

The code range for surgical procedures performed on the lungs and pleura is 32035 - 32999. Core needle biopsy on the pleura or lungs is performed with a specialized needle that easily obtains a core sample of tissue for histopathology. It is usually done with imaging guidance. Fine needle aspiration biopsy can also be carried out for cytological examination of cells obtained from aspirated material. Thoracoscopy (32601 - 32665) provides a view of the inside of the chest cavity using a fiberoptic endoscope. Video-assisted thoracic surgery (VATS) may include diagnostic thoracoscopy, but not all thoracoscopies are part of VATS procedures.

Surgical procedures on the mediastinum and diaphragm are found in the CPT code range 39000 - 39599. Mediastinotomy is performed via cervical or thoracic approach. When reporting the codes for repair of diaphragmatic hernias, the patient's age is considered. Repair may also follow acute trauma or chronic trauma.

### Hemic and Lymphatic System

The CPT codes relevant to the hemic and lymphatic system are found in the code range 38100 - 38999. Splenectomy is the removal of the spleen. This procedure may follow traumatic rupture of the spleen, hemolytic anemias, or cancer of the spleen. Complete excision of the spleen is coded using CPT code 38100.

Other procedures include general surgical procedures, transplantation, and post-transplantation cellular infusion procedures. Surgical procedures on the lymph nodes and lymphatic channels are also in this group.

## HCPCS Coding

Codes relevant to the respiratory system are found in the HCPCS level II, especially those for pulmonary rehabilitation (G0237 - G0239). The supplies used are reported separately and billed by individual providers.

## Modifiers

The CPT modifiers used to code the procedures performed on the respiratory system can be found in the CPT codebook. Most modifiers recur and can be reported depending on the information provided by the healthcare professional who writes the medical report for billing.

## Definitions of Important Terms

- Adaptive immune response: A relatively slow but precise and effective immune response controlled by lymphocytes.
- Alveoli: Small sacs that serve as the primary unit of exchange of oxygen and carbon dioxide in the lungs.
- Antibody: A form of antigen-specific protein secreted by plasma cells.
- Antigen: A protein molecule recognized by the receptors of B and T lymphocytes.
- B cells: Lymphocytes which eventually differentiate into antibody-secreting plasma cells.
- Bone marrow: Tissue in the center of bones that produces blood cells.
- Bronchi: Part of the respiratory tract that divides at the end of the trachea into a left and right portion.
- Bronchiole: Respiratory branches of main bronchi that are 1 mm or less in diameter. Each bronchiole terminates at an alveolar sac.
- Bronchoconstriction: Reduction in size of the bronchiole as a result of muscle contraction.
- Bronchodilation: Widening of the bronchioles that may follow administration of some drugs.
- Carina: Ridge-like cartilage that separates the left and right bronchi.
- Cilia: Tiny filaments that filter air entry through the nose and parts of the respiratory tract.
- Decortication: Process of separating the pleura from the lungs to help expansion of the lungs.
- Diaphragm: Muscle which separates the abdomen from the thorax. It is the primary muscle of respiration.
- Direct endoscopy: Use of endoscope to view the larynx directly.
- Empyema: Collection of pus in the pleura space.
- Epiglottis: A leaf-shaped lid made of elastic cartilage that protects the trachea from food and liquid.

- Glottis: The space between the vocal cords and the opening to the larynx. It is involved in phonation, the control of airflow during speech, and the regulation of sound volume.
- Hemic: Related to blood.
- Immune system: This consists of cells, barriers, organs, and soluble substances that combine to respond to infections of the body with pathogenic organisms.
- Indirect endoscopy: Use of mirrors along with a rigid laryngoscope to view the larynx.
- Innate immune response: This is the rapid but nonspecific immune response to an antigen.
- Larynx: Structure made of cartilage which connects the nasopharynx to the trachea. Also called the voice box.
- Lung: Primary organ of the respiratory system.
- Lymph: Fluid found within the lymphatic system.
- Lymphocytes: White blood cells characterized by a large nucleus and small rim of cytoplasm.
- Mucosa-associated lymphoid tissue (MALT): This is the lymphoid nodule associated with the mucosa of the digestive system.
- Nasopharynx: Portion of the pharynx that serves as an airway.
- Natural killer cell (NK): This is a form of cytotoxic lymphocyte for innate immune response.
- Pharyngeal tonsil: A structure of the immune system composed of lymphoid tissue and located in the nasopharynx.
- Pharynx: Region of the conducting zone which is lined with respiratory epithelium and located between the nose and the esophagus and trachea.
- Plasma cell: A well-differentiated B cell that is actively secreting antibody.
- Pleura: Serous membranous covering of the lungs.
- Pleural cavity: Space between the visceral and parietal pleura.
- Spleen: A secondary lymphoid organ located in the abdomen. It filters pathogens (white pulp) and removes damaged red blood cells and platelets from the blood (red pulp).
- Thoracic duct: A large lymphatic vessel that carries lymphatic fluid to the venous circulation from the lower limbs, left side of the head and thorax, and the left upper limb.
- Thymus: An organ of the lymphatic system where T lymphocytes mature. It is located in the upper anterior part of the chest cavity and plays a vital role in the development of the immune system, especially during early life. The thymus gradually decreases in size and function with age.
- Thyroid cartilage: Largest piece of cartilage that makes up the larynx and consists of two laminae.

# Chapter 10: Cardiovascular System

## Introduction

This section provides an overview of the cardiovascular system. Additional codes associated with the cardiovascular system are available in various chapters of the CPT codebook, with specific emphasis on the chapters that address radiology, medicine, and surgery.

The objectives of this chapter include:

- Understand the anatomy of the cardiovascular system.
- Learn key terms of the cardiovascular system.
- Learn how to select appropriate diagnosis code according to ICD-10-CM.
- Apply CPT modifiers and HCPCS level II codes.

## Examples of Words, Prefixes, and Suffixes

- Angioplasty (surgical repair of blood vessels).
    - Prefix: angio- (vessel).
    - Root: -plasty (surgical repair).
- Arrhythmia (irregular heartbeat).
    - Prefix: a- (without, lack of).
    - Root: rhythm- (rhythm).
    - Suffix: -ia (condition).
- Atherosclerosis (hardening of the arteries).
    - Prefix: athero- (fatty deposit).
    - Root: scler- (hardening).
    - Suffix: -osis (abnormal condition).
- Cardiogenic shock (shock due to heart failure).
    - Prefix: cardi- (heart).
    - Root: -genic (produced by).
    - Suffix: shock (condition of inadequate blood flow).
- Cardiomegaly (enlargement of the heart).
    - Prefix: cardi- (heart).
    - Root: -megaly (enlargement).
- Endocarditis (inflammation of the inner lining of the heart).
    - Prefix: endo- (within).
    - Root: card- (heart).
    - Suffix: -itis (inflammation).

- Hypertension (high blood pressure).
    - Prefix: hyper- (excessive).
    - Root: tens- (pressure).
    - Suffix: -ion (condition).
- Myocardial infarction (heart attack).
    - Prefix: myo- (muscle).
    - Root: cardi- (heart).
    - Suffix: -al (pertaining to), -ion (condition).
- Valvulopathy (disease of a heart valve).
    - Prefix: none.
    - Root: valvul- (heart valve).
    - Suffix: -opathy (disease).
- Thrombosis (formation of a blood clot).
    - Prefix: none.
    - Root: thromb- (blood clot).
    - Suffix: -osis (abnormal condition).

## Anatomy of the Cardiovascular System

The cardiovascular system is composed of the heart, arteries, and veins. The heart is a muscular organ in the thorax that pumps blood around the body. It is divided into four chambers that include the right atrium, right ventricle, left atrium, and left ventricle. The heart is surrounded by a protective layer of membrane called the pericardium.

The heart receives blood from the body through the superior and inferior vena cava. These great vessels empty deoxygenated blood into the right atrium. This blood is then pumped into the right ventricle for transport to the lungs through the pulmonary vessels.

After receipt of oxygen from the lungs, the blood is pumped back into the left atrium of the heart from the lungs. The oxygenated blood is then released into the left ventricle. The heart's contraction causes an outward flow of blood from the left ventricle into the aorta for distribution throughout the body. Each chamber is controlled by valves. Valves are leaflets at the opening of each chamber. There are four heart valves that include aortic, pulmonic, mitral, and tricuspid.

The heart is controlled by a highly specialized electrical conduction system that consists of nodes and fibers. The sinoatrial node is the heart's pacemaker. It located in the right atrium from where it generates electrical impulse. The impulses are passed to the atrioventricular node in the right atrium.

The AV node slows down the electrical impulse to allow the ventricles to fill with blood from the atria before they contract. The impulse then travels through the bundle of His that branch to the left and right. This terminates at Purkinje fibers at the surface of the ventricles. These fibers give the final signal for heart contraction.

Blood is supplied to the heart by two main coronary arteries that carry oxygenated blood from the aorta. The left and right coronary arteries further branch out to supply the myocardium of the heart. The occlusion of coronary arteries or conditions that cause spasms of these vessels can result in chest pain called angina.

Blood circulation in the body features a network of arteries and veins that supply tissues with adequate nutrients and oxygen. The arteries carry oxygenated blood away from the heart to the tissues. The veins carry deoxygenated blood from the tissues back to the heart.

The pressure within the veins is much lower. They contain less elastic tissue and smooth muscle. Valves help propel blood along the veins. The incompetence of these valves can result in stasis and pooling of fluid back into the tissues. This can form edema in severe cases. The capillaries are much smaller vessels with a single layer of epithelium where blood cells flow in a single file and gaseous exchange occurs.

## ICD-10-CM Coding

The diagnosis codes are found in the code range I00 - I99. Acute rheumatic fever (I00 - I02) is an abnormal immune response to infection caused by group A streptococcus. It may involve the heart (I01.0 - I01.9) or cause fever without the involvement of the heart.

Syndeham's chorea (I02.0, I02.9) is an abnormal movement reported in association with acute rheumatic fever. Chronic rheumatic heart disease results in damage to the valves of the heart and is reported with ICD-10-CM diagnosis code range I05 - I09.

Hypertensive heart disease refers to a myriad of symptoms and clinical signs caused by uncontrolled elevation of blood pressure. Damages to the atria, ventricles, valves, coronary vessels, and other blood vessels usually occur following a long-term elevation of blood pressure. The code range for hypertensive diseases is I10 - I1A. Essential hypertension (I10) is the single most common classification of hypertension reported due to structural changes of the heart in adults. Coding the underlying condition for secondary hypertension(I15) is also very important.

Hypertension may occur secondary to renovascular complications, endocrine disorders, or other specified causes. Hypertensive emergency (I16.1) is acute, marked elevation in blood pressure associated with signs of target-organ damage. Hypertensive urgency

(I16.0) is the presentation of markedly elevated blood pressure without any symptoms of end-organ damage.

Ischemic heart diseases (I20 - I25) are conditions affecting myocardial function due to the narrowing of the coronary arteries that supply the heart. They consist of angina pectoris, acute myocardial infarction, ST elevation, non-ST elevation myocardial infarction, complications following myocardial infarction, and chronic ischemic heart diseases. These diseases are also referred to as coronary artery diseases.

Pulmonary embolism (I26) is the sudden disruption of blood flow into the pulmonary artery or any branches by a thrombus that develops from a distant site to the cardiopulmonary circulation. In deep vein thrombosis (DVT), a thrombus develops within the deep veins. This is more common in the lower extremities. Other pulmonary heart diseases (I27) include primary and secondary pulmonary hypertension, kyphoscoliotic heart disease (I27.1), and other specified pulmonary heart diseases.

The other forms of heart disease are a broad range covered by ICD-10-CM diagnosis code range I30 - I5A. They include diseases of the pericardium, endocardium, myocardium, and valve disorders. They also include cardiomyopathies (I42), heart block, atrial fibrillation, heart failure, and other forms of arrhythmias that may not have specific descriptions.

Sudden cardiac arrest (SCA) - I46 is the sudden loss of all cardiac activity due to an irregular heart rhythm. It may be due to a known underlying heart condition or occur spontaneously due to a non-cardiac condition.

Heart failure (I50) is the inability of the heart to pump blood around the body due to complications of an underlying myocardial injury. Heart failure can be systolic or diastolic. It depends on a myriad of possible presentations of the patient.

Cerebrovascular diseases refer to a group of conditions that affect the blood vessels and blood supply to the brain. These conditions are classified in the ICD-10-CM under code range I60 - I69. Some of the billable codes are found in the categories of nontraumatic subarachnoid hemorrhage, intracerebral hemorrhage, cerebral infarction, occlusion and stenosis of cerebral arteries, and the sequelae of cerebrovascular diseases.

The I70 - I79 code range covers the diseases of arterioles, arteries, and capillaries. Atherosclerosis (I70) is a chronic inflammatory disease in which there is a buildup of plaques inside arteries that cause the vessels to harden. Aortic aneurysm and dissection, peripheral vascular diseases, arterial embolism and thrombosis, atheroembolism, and other disorders of the capillaries are coded based on information from the medical provider.

Diseases of the veins, lymphatic vessels, and lymph nodes not elsewhere classified in the ICD-10-CM diagnosis codebook are found in code range I80 - I89. Thrombophlebitis is the inflammation of the veins. Phlebitis and thrombophlebitis include diseases within the code range I80.0 - I80.9. This covers inflammation of superficial vessels of the lower extremities, femoral vein, other deep vessels of the lower extremities, as well as inflammation affecting veins in other sites which may or may not be specified. The appropriate code should be assigned based on the information provided by the medical provider.

Varicose veins are superficial tortuous veins. They arise due to impaired competence of the valves within the veins that normally serve for return of blood toward the heart. Varicose veins of the lower extremities (I83) may be asymptomatic or complicated by ulcer or inflammation. This code excludes varicose veins associated with pregnancy and puerperal period.

Esophageal varices (I85) are enlarged veins in the esophagus that may rupture and cause massive bleeding. While additional codes such as those from category F10 for alcohol abuse and dependence might be relevant in some cases, they are not universally applicable to all instances of esophageal varices and should be used based on the patient's specific clinical situation.

## CPT Coding

The Current Procedural Terminology code range for surgical procedures on the cardiovascular system is 33016 - 37799. Procedures performed on the pericardium are found in the CPT code range 33016 - 33050. Pericardiocentesis performed with imaging guidance is coded as 33016. Excision of cardiac tumors is in code range 33120 - 33130. Cardiac tumors may be intracardiac or extracardiac.

A pacemaker system with lead(s) includes a pulse generator that contains electronics, a battery, and one or two leads. An implantable defibrillator includes a pulse generator and electrodes. The CPT code range for pacemaker or implantable defibrillator procedures is 33202 - 33249.

Surgical procedures on cardiac valves (33361 - 33478) are performed on aortic valves, mitral valves, tricuspid, and pulmonary valves. The procedures may include repair, removal, or replacement. The code range for surgical procedures on the heart and great vessels of the cardiovascular system is 33300 - 33340. The codes used to report coronary artery bypass procedures with venous and arterial grafts during the same procedure should not be reported alone. These codes are add-on codes and range between 33517 - 33548.

Repair of complex cardiac anomalies are found between code range 33600 - 33697. The complete repair of tetralogy of fallot with pulmonary atresia, closure of ventricular septal defect, and reconstruction of conduit from right ventricle to pulmonary artery is a complex surgery for cyanotic heart disease. The appropriate CPT code assigned for this procedure is 33697.

Other complex surgical procedures include repair of transposition of great vessels (33770 - 33783), truncus arteriosus (33786 - 33788), and aortic anomalies (33800 - 33824). Other CPT codes can be found in the chapter that covers radiology procedures and services. Interventional procedures use minimally invasive methods to diagnose and treat diseases.

## HCPCS Coding

The codes for HCPCS level II are mostly for medications used in diagnosis. Pay close attention to the dosage for proper reporting.

G2066 is not a recognized HCPCS Level II code for Cardiac Device Evaluation for up to 30 days. HCPCS Level II codes for cardiac device evaluations start with 'C' or 'K' and should be verified in the most current HCPCS manual for accuracy. G9157 is the level II code for diagnostic cardiac Doppler ultrasound. This is the transesophageal Doppler measurement of cardiac output for monitoring purposes. This includes probe placement, image acquisition, and interpretation per treatment. G0422 - G0424 is the code range for cardiac and pulmonary rehabilitation services. These may involve ECG monitoring with or without exercise per session.

## Modifiers

The modifiers used in reporting CPT codes for the cardiovascular system are similar to those that recur in other chapters.

- Modifier 26 is the professional component appended when a qualified healthcare professional provides only the professional component of a service.
- Modifier TC is the technical component appended as appropriate. A qualified healthcare professional or physician may apply Modifier 26 and TC when both services are provided.
- Modifier 51 is used for multiple procedures performed during the same session.
- Modifier 58 is applied for procedures performed during the postoperative period. This is often planned prospectively at the end of the original procedure and is more extensive than the primary procedure.
- Modifier 59 is applied for distinct procedural services provided on the same day as the primary procedure.

- Modifiers 76 and 77 are used for repeat procedural services such as electrocardiography or echocardiography performed on the same day.

## Definitions of Important Terms

- Aneurysm: Abnormal bulging or swelling of a blood vessel.
- Angina: Chest pain due to reduced blood flow to the heart.
- Arrhythmia: Irregular heart rhythm.
- Arteriosclerosis: Progressive arterial thickening and hardening.
- Atherosclerosis: Accumulation of plaque in arteries.
- Aorta: Largest artery that conveys oxygenated blood from the heart.
- Bradycardia: Abnormally slow heart rate.
- Capillary: Microscopic vessel that facilitates nutrient and gas exchange.
- Cardiomyopathy: Disease of the heart muscle.
- Cardiovascular: Pertains to the heart and circulatory system.
- Coronary: Pertains to the heart's blood vessels.
- Diastole: Relaxation phase of the heart.
- Embolism: Blockage of a blood vessel by a clot or debris.
- Endocardium: Inner lining of the heart.
- Hemodynamics: Study of blood flow and pressure dynamics.
- Hypertension: Elevated blood pressure.
- Infarction: Tissue death due to lack of blood supply.
- Ischemia: Insufficient blood supply to tissues.
- Myocardium: Muscular tissue that forms the heart wall.
- Pericardium: Protective sac that envelopes the heart.
- Pulmonary: Related to the lungs.
- Regurgitation: Backflow of blood through a valve.
- Stenosis: Abnormal narrowing of a vessel.
- Systole: Contraction phase of the heart.
- Tachycardia: Abnormally fast heart rate.
- Thrombosis: Formation of a blood clot within a blood vessel.
- Vasoconstriction: Narrowing of blood vessels.
- Vasodilation: Widening of blood vessels.
- Vein: Blood vessel that carries blood toward the heart.
- Ventricle: Lower heart chamber that pumps blood.

# Chapter 11: Digestive System

## Introduction

The digestive system is made up of the alimentary tract and related organs.

The objectives of this chapter include:

- Learn key terms associated with the digestive tract.
- Learn the anatomy of the digestive system.
- Learn the CPT codes related to the digestive system.
- Understand the proper application of modifiers.

## Examples of Words, Prefixes, and Suffixes

- Gastroenteritis (inflammation of the stomach and intestines).
    - Prefix: gastro- (stomach).
    - Root: enter- (intestines).
    - Suffix: -itis (inflammation).
- Hepatitis (inflammation of the liver).
    - Prefix: hepat- (liver).
    - Root: -it- (related to).
    - Suffix: -is (inflammation).
- Cholecystectomy (surgical removal of the gallbladder).
    - Prefix: cholecyst- (gallbladder).
    - Root: -ectomy (surgical removal).
- Dyspepsia (indigestion or impaired digestion).
    - Prefix: dys- (abnormal, difficult).
    - Root: -pepsia (digestion).
- Colitis (inflammation of the colon).
    - Prefix: none.
    - Root: colon- (colon).
    - Suffix: -itis (inflammation).
- Gastrostomy (surgical creation of an opening into the stomach).
    - Prefix: gastro- (stomach).
    - Root: -nom- (related to a system or method).
    - Suffix: -y (process or procedure).
- Pancreatitis (inflammation of the pancreas).
    - Prefix: pan- (all).
    - Root: -creat- (related to the pancreas).
    - Suffix: -itis (inflammation).

- Proctology (study and treatment of disorders of the rectum and anus).
    - Prefix: proct- (rectum).
    - Root: -ology (study of).
    - Suffix: -y (process or procedure).
- Enterocolitis (inflammation of the small and large intestines).
    - Prefix: enter- (intestines).
    - Root: colon- (colon).
    - Suffix: -itis (inflammation).
- Gastrectomy (surgical removal of part or all of the stomach).
    - Prefix: gastro- (stomach).
    - Root: -ectomy (surgical removal).

## Anatomy of the Digestive System

The gastrointestinal tract that extends from the mouth to the anus makes up the digestive system. Food materials ingested through the mouth are processed along the digestive system and waste is generated out of the anus.

Within the mouth are the teeth, soft and hard palates, salivary glands, and other minor structures. The salivary glands produce saliva. Saliva contains enzymes that help break down some food particles. The mix of saliva with food particles makes swallowing easier.

The pharynx is located immediately after the mouth and keeps food out of the respiratory tract during swallowing. The esophagus is a long muscular tube that collects ingested particles into the stomach. The peristaltic movement of the esophagus helps in the easy swallowing of food.

The stomach processes ingested food from the esophagus into chyme. This is then passed into the duodenum. The stomach contains acid produced by special cells that line the stomach wall. This acidic environment is important to process food and prevent pathogenic colonization of the digestive tract.

The small intestine comprises the duodenum, jejunum, and ileum. The liver, gallbladder, and pancreas release secretions into the duodenum through ducts. This further aids food digestion. The ileum is the longest part of the small intestine and forms the end of the small intestine. Water reabsorption along the digestive tract mostly occurs in the large intestine. This is composed of the cecum, appendix, ascending colon, transverse colon, descending colon, sigmoid colon, rectum, and terminal anus.

The pancreas is a long, flat gland near the stomach and liver. It has both an exocrine and endocrine function. The exocrine part produces digestive enzymes important for metabolism. The endocrine pancreas produces insulin and glucagon which are important hormones to regulate blood glucose levels.

The liver is the largest organ of the digestive system. It is located in the right upper quadrant of the abdomen. The liver produces bile salt for the emulsification of fat. It also converts excess glucose into glycogen.

The gallbladder is a small sac-like structure found close to the liver. It receives bile and periodically empties it into the duodenum for proper fat metabolism.

## ICD-10 CM Coding

The codes for diagnosing diseases that affect the digestive system can be found in the chapter that covers the digestive system (K00 - K95). Other diseases not found here are coded in the chapters that cover neoplasms, congenital anomalies, signs, and symptoms.

Some other codes are found in the chapter Factors Influencing Health Status and Contact with Health Services. K00 - K14 is the category for diseases of the oral cavity and salivary glands. This category is mostly reported for dental disorders.

The category covers disorders of tooth development and eruption (K00), embedded (K01.0) and impacted teeth (K01.1), and dental caries (K02) which includes dental cavities, early childhood caries, pre-eruptive caries, recurrent caries, and tooth decay. Another disease of hard tissues of the teeth (K03) excludes bruxism (F45.8) and teeth grinding which is not otherwise specified (F45.8).

Diseases of the pulp (K04) cover the following code subcategories - pulpitis (K04.0), necrosis of the pulp (K04.1), pulp degeneration (K04.2), abnormal hard tissue formation in pulp (K04.3), acute and chronic apical periodontitis (K04.4, K04.5) periapical abscess (K04.6, K04.7), radicular cyst (K04.8), and other unspecified diseases of the pulp and other surrounding tissues (K04.9).

The other diseases of the oral cavity and salivary glands are gingivitis and periodontal diseases (K05), other disorders of gingiva and edentulous alveolar ridge (K06), other disorders of teeth and supporting structures (K08), cysts of the oral region NOS (K09), diseases of the salivary gland (K11), stomatitis and related lesions (K12), other diseases of the lips and oral mucosa (K13), and diseases of the tongue (K14).

K20 - K31 is the code range for diseases that affect the esophagus, stomach, and duodenum.

Gastroesophageal Reflux Disease (K21) is a common disorder of the gastroesophageal junction. This results in heartburn symptoms with complaints of burning chest pain and abdominal discomfort. It may be associated with esophagitis (K21.0).

An ulcer is a defect in the epithelial lining. It is most common in the stomach (K25) and duodenum(K26). Peptic ulcer diseases are responsible for a significant health burden in the population. Diseases of the appendix are found in code range K35 - K38. An acute inflammation of the appendix (K35) may be associated with generalized peritonitis (K35.2) or localized peritonitis (K35.3).

Hernia is the term used to describe an organ that protrudes abnormally through a defect or deficiency in the walls that surround it. Hernias can affect different body parts and are named based on the affected body part. Types of hernia include inguinal hernias (K40), femoral (K41), umbilical (K42), ventral (K43), diaphragmatic (K44), or other abdominal hernia (K45).

The other diseases that affect the digestive tract are:

- Non-infective enteritis and colitis (K50 - K52).
- Other diseases of the intestine (K55 - K64).
- Diseases of the peritoneum and retroperitoneum (K65- K68).
- Diseases of the liver (K70 - K77).
- Disorders of the gallbladder, biliary tract, and pancreas (K80 - K87).
- Other diseases of the digestive system (K90 - K95).

Liver cirrhosis is characterized by the fibrosis and formation of nodules in the liver due to a chronic injury that alters the liver's normal structure. The specific ICD-10-CM code for liver cirrhosis is K74.-, with further specification required based on the detailed diagnosis. Common causes of chronic liver injury include toxins, autoimmune conditions, and viral infections.

Chronic abuse of alcohol can also cause alcoholic liver disease (K70), with subcategories that include alcoholic fatty liver (K70.0), alcoholic hepatitis (K70.1), alcoholic fibrosis and sclerosis of the liver (K70.2), alcoholic cirrhosis (K70.3), and alcoholic hepatic failure (K70.4).

### Neoplasms of the Digestive Tract

Abnormal proliferation of cells of the digestive tract is classified based on whether it is malignant or benign. When coding for neoplasms that affect the digestive tract, it is important to note the affected part of the digestive tract reported by the attending physician. A family history of a neoplasm should be coded in addition to the reason for treatment.

### Congenital Disorders that Affect the Digestive System

Congenital disorders that affect the digestive tract can be categorized according to the affected part of the system. The appropriate code is based on the information provided by the medical professional.

## CPT Coding

The range of CPT codes for surgical procedures on the digestive system is 40490 - 49999. Coded as 40490, the biopsy of suspected lip lesions excludes procedures on the skin of the lips. To repair a lip through cheiloplasty, the CPT coding depends on the extent of repair which is 40650 – 40761. If the procedure is bilateral then it includes the modifier 50.

Tonsillectomy is removal of the tonsils and a procedure commonly performed in children. Adenoidectomy is the removal of the adenoids. The coding for these procedures depends on the patient's age, whether the procedure is primary or secondary, and the extent of the procedure.

For proper assignment of code, refer to the recent CPT codebook. Esophagoscopy is the direct visualization of the esophagus. This includes examination from the cricopharyngeus muscle to the gastroesophageal junction (43180 – 43232). This procedure may include a biopsy or resections within the esophagus.

Esophagogastroduodenoscopy is reported to examine the esophagus from the cricopharyngeus muscle. This forms the upper esophageal sphincter to the duodenum (43235 – 43259). Endoscopic retrograde cholangiopancreatography is a technique that combines the use of endoscopy and fluoroscopy to diagnose and treat certain problems of the biliary or pancreatic ductal systems. This is coded as 43260 - 43273.

A physician's skill and fluoroscopic guidance is required to place a nasogastric or orogastric tube. This includes image documentation and report and is coded as 43752. For expedient lavage and evacuation of stomach contents, a large bore gastric lavage tube is inserted orally through the esophagus into the stomach. This is called gastric intubation and is coded as 43753.

Laparoscopic fundoplasty (43280) always includes diagnostic laparoscopy. To close the hiatal hernia in laparoscopic fundoplasty, the esophagus and fundus are held aside. Sutures are placed in both crus diaphragmatic muscles below the esophagus, and the anterior and posterior walls of the fundus are wrapped and stitched around the esophagus.

Procedures carried out in the appendix are coded based on the indication for the surgery (44900 – 44960). Rectum examination which may include examination of a portion of the sigmoid colon is called proctosigmoidoscopy (45300- 45327). Sigmoidoscopy examines the entire rectum and a portion of the descending colon (45330 – 45350).

Colonoscopy examines the entire colon from the rectum to the cecum. This includes examination of the terminal ileum or small intestine that lies proximal to an anastomosis and can also be done through the stoma. The coding for an examination from the colostomy stoma to the cecum should be specified based on the details of the procedure. The codes 45378 - 45398 represent a range for colonoscopy procedures.

Procedures carried out on the liver are classified into incisions and excisions. These are 47000- 47015 and 47100 - 47130, respectively. A wedge biopsy of the liver is coded as 47100.

## HCPCS Coding

Codes G0104 - G0106 and G0120 - G0122 should be applied for sigmoidoscopy and colonoscopy of barium enemas.

## Modifiers

The common modifiers applied when coding for procedures carried out of the digestive system are:

- Modifier 51: This is used when the same provider performs multiple procedures on the same patient.
- Modifier 58: This is applied when the same physician carries out a staging procedure during the post-operative period.
- Modifier 78: This is used when there is an unplanned return to the operating room due to complications related to the procedure.
- Modifier 22: This is applied when additional work is required for a procedure that has already started.

## Definitions of Important Terms

- Absorption: Process of nutrients entering the bloodstream from the digestive tract.
- Anus: Outlet of the digestive tract through which waste is expelled.

- Appendix: Small pouch near the large intestine with an unclear function in digestion.
- Bile: Digestive fluid produced by the liver and stored in the gallbladder that aids in fat digestion.
- Cecum: Pouch-like structure that connects the small and large intestines.
- Chyme: Partially digested food mixed with digestive enzymes in the stomach.
- Colon: Part of the large intestine that is responsible for water absorption and formation of feces.
- Digestion: Process of breaking down food into smaller, absorbable components.
- Duodenum: First part of the small intestine where most digestion occurs.
- Enzyme: Biological molecule that speeds up chemical reactions in digestion.
- Esophagus: Tube that connects the mouth to the stomach and facilitates food passage.
- Feces: Solid waste material formed in the colon and expelled from the body.
- Gallbladder: Organ that stores bile and releases it to aid in fat digestion.
- Gastric: Pertains to the stomach.
- Gastritis: Inflammation of the stomach lining.
- Hepatic: Pertains to the liver.
- Ileum: Last part of the small intestine that connects to the large intestine.
- Insulin: Hormone that regulates blood sugar levels and is produced by the pancreas.
- Jejunum: Middle part of the small intestine that is involved in nutrient absorption.
- Lipase: Enzyme that breaks down fats into fatty acids and glycerol.
- Liver: Organ involved in the production of bile and various metabolic functions.
- Mucosa: Inner lining of the digestive tract that is involved in nutrient absorption.
- Pancreas: Gland that produces digestive enzymes and insulin.
- Pepsin: Enzyme in the stomach that breaks down proteins.
- Peristalsis: Wavelike contractions of the digestive tract muscles that aid in movement.
- Rectum: Last portion of the large intestine that stores feces before elimination.
- Saliva: Fluid in the mouth that contains enzymes that initiate digestion.
- Sphincter: Circular muscle that controls the passage of food between digestive organs.
- Ulcer: Open sore in the mucosa of the digestive tract.
- Villi: Small, finger-like projections in the small intestine that increase surface area for absorption.

# Chapter 12: Urinary System and Male Genital System

## Introduction

In this chapter, the structure of the urinary system and the male reproductive system is discussed. The urinary system comprises the kidneys, ureters, bladder, and urethra. These organs filter waste products away from the body.

The male reproductive system consists of all the body parts involved in production of semen and the process of fertilization. Medical coding is specific to each system and requires understanding of the basics to apply the rules of coding properly.

Objectives for this chapter include:

- Understand the basic anatomy related to the urinary and male genital system.
- Recognize key terms and essential terminologies.
- Define the common pathologies related to the urogenital system.
- Select relevant procedures and apply the CPT code that is associated.
- Application of ICD-10-CM and HCPCS Level II codes and guidelines for the urinary and male genital system.

## Examples of Words, Prefixes, and Suffixes

- Andropause (male menopause).
    - Prefix: andro- (man, male).
    - Root: paus- (cessation).
    - Suffix: none.
- Balanitis (inflammation of the glans penis).
    - Prefix: none.
    - Root: balan- (glans penis).
    - Suffix: -itis (inflammation).
- Cryptorchidism (undescended testicle).
    - Prefix: crypto- (hidden).
    - Root: orch- (testes).
    - Suffix: -idism (condition).
- Epididymitis (inflammation of the epididymis).
    - Prefix: epi- (upon).
    - Root: didym- (testis).
    - Suffix: -itis (inflammation).
- Hypospadias (abnormal opening of the urethra on the underside of the penis).

    - Prefix: hypo- (below).
    - Root: spad- (rent, tear).
    - Suffix: -iasis (presence of).
- Orchitis (inflammation of the testes).
    - Prefix: none.
    - Root: orch- (testes).
    - Suffix: -itis (inflammation).
- Penile prosthesis (artificial device implanted in the penis).
    - Prefix: none.
    - Root: pen- (penis).
    - Suffix: -thesis (placement).
- Prostatitis (inflammation of the prostate).
    - Prefix: none.
    - Root: prostat- (prostate).
    - Suffix: -itis (inflammation).
- Urethritis (inflammation of the urethra).
    - Prefix: none.
    - Root: urethr- (urethra).
    - Suffix: -itis (inflammation).
- Varicocele (dilation of veins within the spermatic cord).
    - Prefix: none.
    - Root: varic- (dilated vein).
    - Suffix: -cele (hernia, swelling).

## Anatomy and Medical Terminology

The urinary system filters waste products from the blood that pass through the kidneys from all over the body. This waste product is further filtered until urine is formed and released into the ureters. From there it is carried into the bladder for temporary storage until it is emptied through the urethra.

The term "nephrology" means the study of the kidney. A human body usually consists of two kidneys, two ureters, one bladder, and one urethra. The kidneys are located posteriorly within the abdominal cavity, behind a layer of the abdomen called the peritoneum. The peritoneum surrounds the intestines and other solid organs. The kidneys are solid, bean-shaped organs that average about 300 g in size in adults.

Each kidney is made up of units called nephrons. A nephron is a single unit that filters the blood through the glomerulus and tubule. The glomerulus is a roll of capillaries which are the smallest blood vessels in the body. The tubule directly collects the filtered urine from the glomerulus into the renal pelvis. Each renal pelvis empties into the ureters.

The ureters are paired, smooth muscular tubes that carry urine from the kidneys into the bladder. When urine flow is disturbed through the ureters due to a lower obstruction or an intrinsic structural problem, backflow may occur from the bladder towards the kidneys. This causes renal failure or the formation of stones.

The urinary bladder is a muscular organ that collects and stores urine produced by the kidneys through the ureters. It has a capacity of up to 300 -500 ml when expanded. An internal and external sphincter at the neck of the bladder controls the flow of urine outward through the urethra.

Through brain signals and voluntary control, the muscles of the bladder contract to release urine. The urethra is the outermost connection between the urinary bladder and the outside. It is about 20 cm long in an average adult male.

The male genital system refers to the reproductive organ in males which consists of the testes, epididymis and vas deferens, seminal vesicles, prostate, and bulbourethral glands. All except the prostate are paired.

Spermatozoa is produced by the cells in the testes. The testes are controlled by hormones produced within the brain. The other glands of the male reproductive system produce the remaining liquid component of the semen which is released into the urethra during ejaculation.

The penis is a fibromuscular part of the male reproductive system that comprises a shaft and a glans penis. It has an opening at the tip through which urine and semen exit the body.

## ICD-10-CM Coding

Diseases of the genitourinary system are generally listed under category N00 - N99.

### Glomerular Diseases

An inflammation of the glomerulus is called glomerulonephritis. It may be due to toxic insults from an external source or a primary abnormality of the kidney that predisposes it to damage. Glomerular diseases are specifically listed between N00 and N08.

Nephrotic syndrome (N04) is a common glomerulus disease characterized by facial puffiness and generalized fluid accumulation in the body. This includes the passage of frothy urine and worsening kidney function. Nephritic syndrome may be acute or chronic with passage of red blood cells in the blood due to failure of the glomerular filtration that follows damage.

### Renal Tubulointerstitial Diseases

Renal tubulointerstitial diseases (N10 – N16) are disorders that mainly affect the tubular system of the nephron. Primary infection of the kidneys is referred to as pyelonephritis and may result from a bacterial infection that ascends from the bladder towards the kidney. Acute pyelonephritis is a common disease with multiple complications and increased morbidity if left untreated.

Chronic tubule-interstitial nephritis is a condition due to injury of the tubules by toxic insults to the kidneys.

Hydronephrosis is the swelling of the kidney that follows the accumulation of urine due to an obstruction at the ureteropelvic junction (N13.0), ureteral stricture (N13.1), or renal and ureteral calculous obstruction.

Hydroureter is also a common diagnosis of abnormally enlarged ureters with fluid due to an obstruction of the outward flow of urine. Diseases of the kidneys may also be due to damage by contrast dye, heavy metals, or analgesics. This results in tubule-interstitial nephritis.

### Acute Kidney Failure and Chronic Kidney Disease

Acute kidney injury (N17.9) is a sudden deterioration of kidney function due to structural damage and loss of function with a fall in glomerular filtration rates and a rise in serum creatinine levels. This damage may be due to overwhelming infections, sudden blood loss, or persistent obstruction of urine flow from the urinary system.

By definition of the Acute Kidney Injury Working Group of KDIGO (Kidney Disease; Improving Global Outcome), acute kidney injury is diagnosed by an absolute rise in the serum creatinine levels by at least 0.3 mg/dl within 48 hours or a 50% increase in serum creatinine from baseline within seven days, or production of urine volume less than 0.5 mls/kg/hour for at least six hours.

Massive blood volume depletion is a common cause of acute kidney injury. This causes reduced blood supply and perfusion of the kidneys.

Chronic kidney disease is a persistent decline of renal function due to the death of nephrons and irreversible damage to the kidney structure. The Kidney Disease Outcome Quality Initiative (KDOQI) defines chronic kidney disease as renal damage or reduction in estimated glomerular filtration rates of less than 60 mls/minute/1.73 m2 for at least three months, regardless of the etiology. Chronic kidney disease is listed in the ICD-10-CM code description under N18.0 – N18.9.

Chronic kidney disease can be classified based on estimated glomerular filtration rate.

| Stage | Estimated Glomerular Filtration Rate (mL/min/m²) | Description |
|---|---|---|
| **Stage 1** | Greater than 90 | Renal damage with normal or increased eGFR |
| **Stage 2** | 60 - 89 | Mildly reduced eGFR |
| **Stage 3a** | 45 – 59 | Moderately reduced eGFR |
| **Stage 3b** | 30 -44 | Moderately reduced eGFR |
| **Stage 4** | 15 – 29 | Severely reduced eGFR |
| **Stage 5** | Less than 15 | End-stage renal disease |

### Urolithiasis

Urolithiasis is the formation of stones within the renal system. Stones may be found within the kidney or ureters. This causes severe pain as peristalsis occurs. This pain may be associated with blood in the urine and requires prompt intervention to reduce associated morbidity. Calculus of the kidneys and ureter are listed under N20. Calculus of the lower urinary tract (N21) includes those that affect the bladder, urethra, and other unspecified calculus of the lower urinary tract.

When a stone forms an obstruction at the level of the bladder, backflow of urine may accumulate towards the kidneys. This is a condition known as hydronephrosis. Another common cause of this obstruction is a neoplasm of the prostate known as benign prostatic hyperplasia.

Calculus of urinary tract in diseases classified elsewhere describes the manifestation of an underlying condition as a form of urolithiasis. Gout and schistosomiasis are diseases classified elsewhere with urinary system manifestation of stones.

### Other Diseases of the Kidney and Ureter

Malignant neoplasms of the kidneys are listed under category C64.0 - C65.9. Neoplasms that mainly affect the renal pelvis, ureters, and bladder are located between C65.0 - C67.9.

Disorders of the kidneys that result from impaired tubular function (N25) include nephrogenic diabetes insipidus and renal osteodystrophy. Secondary hyperparathyroidism may also arise from an impairment of renal tubular function (N25.81).

### Other Diseases of the Urinary System

Cystitis is the inflammation of the bladder (N30). This may be acute (N30.0) or chronic (N30.1). Cystitis is often associated with painful urination, an increase in the frequency of urination, urgency, pain in the suprapubic area, and sometimes hematuria.

Cystitis may also be due to irradiation as an intervention for neoplasm of the prostate (N30.4). Neuromuscular dysfunction of the bladder is also listed (N31) to include uninhibited neuropathic bladder (N31.0), reflex neuropathic bladder (N31.1), and flaccid neuropathic bladder (N31.2). Inflammation of the urethra is reported with code N34. Urethral strictures are reported within the N35 category.

### Disorder of the Male Genital System

The male genital system progresses from the testes to the urethra. The prostate is a commonly affected organ of the male genital system. Abnormal growth of cells that make up the prostate results in neoplasms. This is known as benign prostatic hyperplasia and is a common condition listed under ICD-10-CM code N40.

The disordered growth of the prostate may result in symptoms of the lower urinary tract (N40.1). This includes increased frequency, urgency and urge incontinence, hesitancy, dribble of urine, or pain during urination. These symptoms may occur due to obstruction of the neck of the bladder by an enlarged prostate which lies directly behind the bladder. This obstruction often results in stasis of urine within the bladder and an increased chance of development of a lower urinary tract infection.

Other inflammatory conditions associated with the prostate, such as prostatitis, abscess of the prostate, prostatocystitis, and granulomatous prostatitis, are characterized by an influx of inflammatory cells with various clinical presentations and treatments. Malignant neoplasms of the male genital system are listed under the category of neoplasms between C60.0 – C63.9.

Male infertility is the inability of a male to effectively fertilize an ovum after a specified period of unprotected sexual intercourse. Male infertility results from a range of underlying conditions such as azoospermia (N46.0) and oligospermia (N46.1). It may be due to extra-testicular causes, infection, obstruction of the efferent ducts, or radiation.

Male erectile dysfunction (N52) is the persistent failure to achieve or sustain an erection during sexual intercourse with one's partner. It may be due to a psychological condition or an underlying organ dysfunction. Other male sexual dysfunctions are classified as ejaculatory dysfunction (N53.1) which include retarded ejaculation (N53.11), painful ejaculation (N53.12), anejaculatory orgasm (N53.13), or retrograde ejaculation (N53.14).

Disorders of the scrotum include epididymitis (N45.1). This is the inflammation of the cordlike structure attached to the testis that results from the spread of infection of the urinary tract through the vas deferens. In some cases, infection reaches the epididymis through the lymphatics of the spermatic cord. Orchitis (N45.3) is an inflammation of one or both testes. This results in enlargement of the scrotum, lymph node swelling, blood within the semen, and painful urination or sexual intercourse.

## CPT Coding

The CPT coding of the urinary and male genital system covers medical procedures carried out on the kidneys, ureters, bladder, and urethra. Further, the CPT code describes whether the procedure is bilateral. If unilateral, it specifies which side is operated with the use of modifiers. The bladder and urethra are single structures. Therefore, no specificity is needed for billing.

## HCPCS Coding

Some supplies are specific for procedures carried out on the urogenital system. These supplies include catheters, medications, and trays for medical procedures.

The common HCPCS codes are those for catheterization supplies and chemotherapy medications used in managing prostatic neoplasm.

Injection Testosterone Cypionate is administered in conditions associated with decreased testosterone and is coded with HCPCS code J1071. Chemotherapy medications for prostatic cancer fall under codes J9217 – J9219. Supplies for urethral catheterization that include insertion trays, irrigation syringes, collection devices, and indwelling catheters with drainage bags are coded A4310 – A4360.

## Modifiers

In reporting some procedures, there may be a need to indicate more specific information with regard to the patient. Modifiers are the two-character codes added to a CPT code generated for a procedure or HCPCS code for further specificity.

These modifiers are essential to prevent wrong billing of a procedure when presented to the recipient of the report. A modifier is used to show any of the following:

- Increase (Modifier 22) or reduction in a procedure (Modifier 52).
- If a procedure is unilateral or bilateral (Modifier 50 is used for bilateral procedures and can be used as RT or LT for specific sides).
- Preventive services carried out (Modifier 33).
- Multiple procedures (Modifier 51).
- Repeat procedure by the same physician due to a recurring complaint that required the initial procedure (Modifier 76).
- Repeat of the same procedure by another physician or other qualified healthcare professional (Modifier 77).

## Definitions of Important Terms

- Bladder: Organ that stores urine.
- Bladder neck: Muscular area that connects the bladder and urethra.
- Cystectomy: Removal of the bladder.
- Cystitis: Inflammation of the bladder.
- Cystoscopy: Visual examination of the bladder.
- Dialysis: Artificial blood filtration for kidney failure.
- Glomerulus: Part of the kidney that filters blood.
- Hematuria: Blood in the urine.
- Hydronephrosis: Swelling of the kidney due to urine buildup.
- Incontinence: Inability to control urine flow.
- Interstitial cystitis: Chronic bladder inflammation.
- Ketones: Substances in urine during fat metabolism.
- Kidney: Organ that filters waste from the blood.
- Kidney stones (renal calculi): Hard deposits in the kidneys.
- Nephrectomy: Kidney removal.
- Nephritis: Kidney inflammation.
- Nocturia: Excessive urination at night.
- Pelvic floor: Muscles supporting pelvic organs that are involved in urinary control.
- Polyuria: Excessive urine production.
- Prostate: Gland that produces a component of semen.
- Prostatitis: Inflammation of the prostate gland.
- Pyelonephritis: Kidney infection.
- Renal artery: Blood vessel that supplies the kidney.
- Renal calculi: Kidney stones.
- Renal cortex: Outer region of the kidney that contains nephrons.
- Renal failure: Kidney dysfunction.

- Renal transplant: Replacement of a damaged kidney.
- Renin: Enzyme that regulates blood pressure and kidney function.
- Urea: Nitrogenous waste product in urine.
- Ureter: Tube that carries urine from kidney to bladder.
- Urethra: Tube that conveys urine out of the body.
- Urethral sphincter: Muscular valve that controls urine release.
- Urethral stricture: Narrowing of the urethra.
- Urethritis: Inflammation of the urethra.
- Urinary incontinence: Loss of bladder control.
- Urinary retention: Inability to empty the bladder completely.
- Urinary tract infection (UTI): Bacterial infection in the urinary system.
- Urodynamic testing: Assessment of bladder and urethra function.
- Urology: Medical specialty that focuses on the urinary system.
- Voiding dysfunction: Impaired ability to empty the bladder.

# Chapter 13: Female Reproductive System

## Introduction

This chapter examines the female reproductive system. The female reproductive system comprises all the organs and units involved in fertility and childbirth. The chapter also discusses the medical coding language for pregnancy, labor, and all the complications that arise from the female reproductive system.

Objectives for this chapter include:

- Learning the basic anatomy of the female reproductive system.
- Recognizing keywords and essential terminologies.
- Defining the common pathologies relating to the female reproductive system.
- Relevant procedures and CPT coding.
- Application of ICD-10-CM and HCPCS Level II codes and guidelines.

## Examples of Words, Prefixes and Suffixes

- Cervicitis (inflammation of the cervix):
    - Prefix: None.
    - Root: Cervic- (cervix).
    - Suffix: -itis (inflammation).
- Dysmenorrhea (painful menstruation):
    - Prefix: Dys- (difficult, painful).
    - Root: Men- (month, menstruation).
    - Suffix: -rrhea (flow, discharge).
- Endometriosis (abnormal growth of endometrial tissue outside the uterus):
    - Prefix: Endo- (within).
    - Root: Metri- (uterus).
    - Suffix: -osis (abnormal condition).
- Fallopian (relating to the fallopian tubes):
    - Prefix: None.
    - Root: Fallopi- (fallopian tubes).
    - Suffix: -an (pertaining to).
- Hysterectomy (surgical removal of the uterus):
    - Root: Hyster- (uterus).
    - Suffix: -ectomy (surgical removal).
- Mammogram (X-ray of the breast):
    - Prefix: None.

    - Root: Mamm- (breast).
    - Suffix: -ogram (record or image).
- Menopause (cessation of menstruation):
    - Prefix: None.
    - Root: Men- (month, menstruation).
    - Suffix: -opause (cessation).
- Oophorectomy (surgical removal of an ovary):
    - Prefix: Oophor- (ovary).
    - Root: -ectomy (surgical removal).
- Ovarian (relating to the ovaries):
    - Prefix: None.
    - Root: Ovari- (ovary).
    - Suffix: -an (pertaining to).
- Uterine (relating to the uterus):
    - Prefix: None.
    - Root: Uter- (uterus).
    - Suffix: -ine (pertaining to).

## Anatomy of the Female Reproductive System

The primary organ of the reproductive system in females is the uterus, otherwise referred to as the womb. The uterus is a muscular organ where an embryo is implanted after fertilization to support and provide all required nourishments. It measures about 5 cm by 7 cm on average before the development of pregnancy. The three parts of the uterus are the most superior fundus, mid corpus, and the lowermost cervix. The uterus connects to the vagina and the cervix.

The uterus has the widest portion extending into a fallopian tube on each end. The fallopian tubes are paired conduits for the eggs released by the ovary into the uterus. Fertilization also occurs in the widest part of the fallopian tube. The normal female body has two ovaries, the organs responsible for making eggs on either side of the uterus. The ovaries are suspended beside the fallopian tubes by suspensory ligaments connected to the internal layers of the pelvis and lower abdomen.

The ovaries are about 2-3 cm each in the pelvis cavity. Each ovary produces oocytes each month in a cycle regulated closely by hormones from the brain. The female reproductive system, therefore, requires proper functioning of the endocrine system for normal regulation.

The neck of the womb that forms the cervix leads into the vagina, which is a muscular canal about 10 cm long that terminates at the outside opening made up of the vulva.

This opening is termed the introitus. The vagina is the exit for menstrual blood from the uterus and the expulsion of a fetus during labor.

The structures that comprise the externally visible parts of the female reproductive system are called the vulva. The vulva comprises the labia majora, labia minora, mons pubis, clitoris, and vestibule. The paired glands found at the vaginal opening include the Bartholin gland and the Skene's gland. The Bartholin gland is located on either side of the lower part of the introitus of the vagina. The Skene's glands are also known as the lesser vestibular glands, and they are located near the lower end of the urethra. These glands secrete fluid for lubrication of the vestibular area.

The female perineum is the area between the bone of the pubic symphysis anteriorly and the tailbone or coccyx posteriorly. The perineum forms the birth canal during labor, and there may be complications resulting from disparities in the size of the perineum to the size of the fetus.

## ICD-10-CM Coding

Diagnosis codes for the female reproductive system are found in categories for the urogenital system (N70 – N77, N80 – N98. Disorders of the breast N60-N65). Disorders associated with pregnancy, childbirth, and the puerperium are listed in chapter O (O00 – O9A).

## Inflammatory Disease of Female Pelvic Organs

Inflammation of the fallopian tubes is known as salpingitis and is often caused by an ascending infection from the outermost part of the female genital system. Acute salpingitis (N70.01) is often caused by bacterial infections originating from the vagina and ascending to the fallopian tubes.

This may also cause lower abdominal cramps, painful sexual intercourse, fever, or nausea. If left untreated, acute salpingitis can become chronic and cause infertility or scarring of the fallopian tube, which is a risk factor for the formation of ectopic pregnancy. Oophoritis (N70.02, N70.12, N70.92) is also a pelvic inflammatory disorder specific to the ovary and may be present alongside salpingitis, with general diagnosis code N70 and further categorization depending on specificity.

Endometritis is the inflammation of the uterine body (N71), excluding the cervix. Myometritis is the inflammation of the muscular layer of the uterus. Depending on the patient's presentation, it can be either purulent, suppurative, or non-specific.

Cervicitis (N72) is the inflammation of the cervix, which may be associated with an eversion of the margins forming an ectropion or associated with inflammation of the body of the uterus, erosion of the cervix, hyperplasia, or an ulcer in longstanding cervicitis.

The Bartholin gland may develop a cyst or abscess. This results in an inflammation of the gland, which can be suppurative, hypertrophic, or exudative (N75.8).

All other inflammation of the vagina and vulva are listed under ICD-10-CM beginning with diagnosis code N76. Acute inflammation of the vagina is termed vaginitis (N76.0). Acute inflammation confined to the vulva is listed as acute vulvitis with ICD-10-CM diagnosis code N76.2.

Fournier gangrene is a serious bacterial infection that affects the genital region, perineum, and perianal region. It can result in the death of tissue due to restricted blood flow and is more common in men than in women. The correct ICD-10-CM code for Fournier gangrene is N49.3. This condition is identified by the ICD-10-CM code N76.82 in the diagnosis codebook. Ulceration of the vulva due to the manifestation of an underlying disease in a female patient is listed with N77.0.

Endometriosis (N80) is a condition characterized by the growth of endometrial tissue outside the normal uterine cavity. This causes severe pain, heavy menstrual periods, and in some cases, infertility. Endometriosis commonly affects other organs in the pelvis, such as the ovaries (N80.1), and some cases involve deposition of the endometrial tissue in the pelvic peritoneum (N80.3), pelvic brim (N80.38), intestines (N80.5), ureters (N80.A5), bladder (N80.A), or cardiothoracic space (N80.B).

Genital prolapse may manifest in females (N81) as a downward displacement of the normally suspended organs through the vagina and, in some cases, through the rectum. This downward displacement can occur due to trauma sustained during childbirth or instrumentation. Another possible complication of the genital tract is an abnormal connection of the epithelial linings of different parts of the female genital tract.

Most commonly, this abnormal connection forms between the vagina and the urinary system (N82.0, N82.1). However, a fistula may also form between the vagina and intestine (N82.2, N82.3) or directly with the skin (N82.5). A commonly reported cause of fistula formation is prolonged obstructed labor with poor obstetric interventions.

Common non-inflammatory disorders of the ovary are follicular cysts (N83.0), corpus luteum cysts (N83.1), and ovarian torsion (N83.51). Torsion may be reported to involve the fallopian tube (N83.52) or may involve the ovary, the fallopian tube, and the ovarian pedicle (N83.53).

The disorders specific to the cervix are usually discussed separately. An important condition associated with the cervix is dysplasia (N87). Dysplasia of the cervix is the abnormal growth of squamous epithelial cells of the cervix in the pre-malignant phase, which means the cells are yet to penetrate the basement membrane that lines the cervix.

Malignant conditions associated with the female genital tract are listed in the second chapter of the ICD-10-CM diagnosis codebook in categories C51 – C58. Neoplasms affecting the uterine cervix are listed under category C53.

Fibroids are benign neoplasms of the uterine smooth muscle, which may be asymptomatic or characterized by symptoms such as abnormal uterine bleeding, painful menstrual flow, or lower abdominal swelling, with possible infertility by direct or indirect causality.

Amenorrhea is an abnormal cessation of menstruation during the reproductive cycle of a female, which may be primary amenorrhea in females who have never had a menstrual flow in their lives (N91.0) or secondary when a female does not have a menstrual flow for an extended period during her reproductive years (N91.1). Oligomenorrhea (N91.3, N91.4, N91.5) is irregular and infrequent menstrual blood flow in a female.

Abnormally heavy menstrual bleeding is a disorder of the female reproductive system termed menorrhagia (N92) and may be associated with a regular menstrual cycle (N92.0) or an irregular menstrual cycle (N92.1).

Vaginismus (N94.2) is a disorder of the female genital tract characterized by an involuntary spasm of the muscles of the pelvic floor that results in the tightening of the walls of the vagina, which can be associated with painful penetrative sexual intercourse. Other causes of pain associated with the female genital tract include Mittelschmerz (pain experienced during ovulation period- N94.0), dyspareunia (pain associated with penetrative sexual intercourse- N94.1), dysmenorrhea (pain associated with menstrual blood flow – N94.4, N94.5, N94.6), vulvodynia (complex pain syndrome characterized by generalized pain in the vulva region following application of pressure, with a normal appearing vulva - N94.81).

However, in middle-aged females, the permanent cessation of menstrual blood flow for twelve months or more due to hormonal changes is termed menopause, and it is associated with psychological, urogenital, and variable systemic changes due to a reduced circulating estrogen level in the female body. Menopause and other perimenopausal disorders are listed under the ICD-10-CM category N95.

According to the ICD-10-CM code index, recurrent pregnancy loss is the spontaneous ejection of a dead or non-viable fetus, at roughly the same developmental stage, in three or more successive pregnancies. Recurrent pregnancy loss is coded as N96.

Infertility is the inability to conceive, and in a third of reported cases, it is mainly due to the female partner as a result of hormonal, post-infectious, environmental, or lifestyle factors. ICD-10-CM has classified female infertility under category N97. It is further categorized based on the location of its origin within the female genital tract. The categorization is done from the fallopian tubes down to the body of the uterus.

Artificial methods of fertilization are fraught with many complications. Infections (N98.0), ovarian hyperstimulation (N98.1), problems while attempting to introduce a fertilized ovum into the uterus after in-vitro fertilization (N98.2), complications during fertilization (while attempting to introduce the embryo in embryo transfer) (N98.3), and other complications related to artificial fertilization (N98.8) have been reported.

Pregnancy is a physiological condition following conception up to termination. On average, a complete pregnancy lasts for forty weeks and is classified into three trimesters. Each trimester lasts thirteen to fourteen weeks, and various disorders are associated with the different trimesters of pregnancy—the ICD-10-CM categories O00 – O9A contain codes for all disorders associated with pregnancy, childbirth, and the puerperium.

The puerperium is the post-delivery period and includes all the events that occur during the following six weeks (O85 – O92). Puerperal sepsis (O85) is a febrile illness that occurs in the immediate period after childbirth due to inflammation affecting the female genital tract with pathogenic colonization that may be life-threatening. Other puerperal infections (O86) include infection of an obstetric surgical wound (O86.0), genital tract (O86.1), urinary tract (O86.2), or of an unknown origin (O86.4). Infection may arise from the breasts during pregnancy or lactation, with or without purulent collection (O91).

Complications of labor and delivery listed in the ICD-10-CM code (O60 – O77) include preterm labor, failed induction of labor, prolonged labor, abnormalities with the forces of labor, obstructed labor, and labor complicated by complications of the umbilical cord or bleeding.

Blood loss after a vaginal delivery that is more than 500 mL or more than 1000 mL after a cesarean delivery is referred to as postpartum hemorrhage (O72). Any blood loss that results in hemodynamic instability in a mother following childbirth is also classified as postpartum hemorrhage (PPH). PPH may occur in two phases - primary or secondary. Primary postpartum hemorrhage is the initial stage that happens during the first twenty-four hours after giving birth. After twenty-four hours, any bleeding that occurs is regarded as a secondary postpartum hemorrhage.

Some complications are reported due to the administration of general, regional, or local anesthesia or other forms of sedation during labor and delivery (O74).

Close fetal heart rate monitoring is important during labor and delivery, and any abnormalities detected need to be evaluated (O76) to prevent fatal complications.

## CPT Coding

Current Procedural Terminology coding for the female genital system can be found labelled between codes 56405 – 58999 in the CPT code book 2023. This includes surgeries, diagnostic investigations, anesthesia administered, and all medical services offered to patients with conditions affecting the female reproductive system.

Procedures are generally classified as any of the following: incision, destruction, excision, repair, endoscopy, introduction, manipulation, laparoscopy, and other procedures that cover those associated with in-vitro fertilization.

The CPT codes for the procedures related to maternity care and delivery are listed between codes 59000 – 59899 and cover fetal invasive services, vaginal delivery, antepartum care, cesarean deliveries, abortions, and other procedures relating to maternity care and delivery.

## HCPCS Coding

The Healthcare Common Procedure Coding System for the female reproductive system is a collection of codes representing procedures, services, products, and supplies used by healthcare professionals.

G0101 is the HCPCS code for cervical and vaginal screening with specific coverage for pelvic and clinical breast examination. G0141 – G0148 are specific screening cytopathology listings for the cervix and vagina that may require collecting samples from smears by a supervising physician.

Other non-specific services such as patient transportation, trays required for procedures during pregnancy and childbirth, administration of medications for managing cancers related to the female reproductive system, and all other possible services are found in the appropriate code category of the HCPCS database.

## Modifiers

Modifiers are recurrent across most body systems and are used to provide accurate information regarding the procedure being reported. Modifiers are the two-character codes added to a CPT code generated for a procedure or HCPCS code for further specificity. These modifiers are essential to prevent wrong procedure billing when presented to the report recipient. A modifier is used to show any of the following:

- Modifier 50 is used for bilateral procedures.
- Preventive services are reported under Modifier 33.
- Modifier 51 is used for multiple procedures performed on one patient.
- Modifier 76 is used for a repeat procedure by the same physician due to a recurring complaint that required the procedure the first time, such as a repeat myomectomy by the same gynecologist.
- Modifier 77 is used when another gynecologist repeats the same procedure.

## Definition of Important Terms

- Antepartum: The period of pregnancy before labor begins.
- Amenorrhea: Absence of normal menstrual blood flow.
- Bartholin gland: Paired glands located in the vulva which produce lubrication for the vagina.
- Colposcopy: Use of a magnifying instrument termed a colposcope to view the cervix and the tissues of the vagina and vulva.
- Dysmenorrhea: Painful menstruation.
- Dyspareunia: Pain during sexual intercourse.
- Endometriosis: Abnormal implantation of tissue of the endometrium outside the uterus.
- Fertilization: The process of fusion of a sperm cell with an oocyte.
- Gynecology: The study of disorders of the female reproductive system.
- Hysterectomy: The surgical removal of the uterus due to a pathology.
- Laparoscopy: Insertion of a flexible instrument through the abdominal wall without opening the abdomen to facilitate viewing of the abdominal and pelvic organs.
- Menarche: The attainment of first menstruation in a female at puberty.
- Menopause: The permanent cessation of menstrual blood flow in a woman after an absence of one full year, especially in middle-aged women.
- Menorrhagia: Excessive menstrual blood flow.
- Oocyte: An immature egg produced by the ovary.
- Pap smear: Papanicolaou smear is a procedure for screening cervical cancer by collecting cervix cells with a special brush for microscopy.

- Postpartum: The period immediately following childbirth and lasting six weeks.
- Salpingo-oophorectomy: The process of surgically extracting both the ovary and the fallopian tube.
- Tubal ligation: A method of permanent contraception done by surgically closing the fallopian tubes in a female.

# Chapter 14: Endocrine and Nervous System

## Introduction

In this chapter, we discuss the endocrine system as well as the nervous system. The endocrine system is a network of organs and important glands that produce chemical substances that control the human body's metabolism, growth, and reproductive development.

Objectives for this chapter include:

- Understanding the anatomy of the endocrine and nervous systems.
- Recognizing relevant terminologies related to the endocrine and nervous systems.
- Application of ICD-10-CM codes for these systems.
- Discussing the use of CPT codes relevant to the endocrine and nervous systems.
- Application of modifiers and use of HCPCS Level II codes and guidelines.

## Examples of Words, Prefixes and Suffixes

- Adrenaline (hormone produced by the adrenal glands):
    - Prefix: None.
    - Root: Adren- (adrenal gland).
    - Suffix: -ine (a suffix denoting a substance).
- Endocrinology (study of the endocrine system):
    - Prefix: Endo- (within).
    - Root: Crin- (separate, secrete).
    - Suffix: -ology (study of).
- Hypothalamus (brain region controlling the endocrine system):
    - Prefix: None.
    - Root: Hypothalam- (below the thalamus).
    - Suffix: -us (pertaining to).
- Insulinoma (tumor of the pancreas producing insulin):
    - Prefix: None.
    - Root: Insulin- (insulin).
    - Suffix: -oma (tumor, mass).
- Myelin (fatty substance covering nerve fibers):
    - Prefix: None.
    - Root: Myel- (marrow, spinal cord).
    - Suffix: -in (a suffix denoting a substance).
- Neuropathy (disease affecting the nerves):

    - Prefix: Neuro- (nerve).
    - Root: -pathy (disease).
- Neurotransmitter (chemical messenger in the nervous system):
    - Prefix: Neuro- (nerve).
    - Root: Transmit- (send across).
    - Suffix: -er (one who does).
- Parathyroid (glands next to the thyroid, regulating calcium):
    - Prefix: Para- (beside).
    - Root: Thyroid- (thyroid gland).
    - Suffix: None.
- Pituitary (pea-sized gland at the base of the brain):
    - Prefix: None.
    - Root: Pituit- (pituitary gland).
    - Suffix: -ary (pertaining to).
- Thyroidectomy (surgical removal of the thyroid gland):
    - Prefix: None.
    - Root: Thyroid- (thyroid gland).
    - Suffix: -ectomy (surgical removal).

## Anatomy and Medical Terminology

The endocrine system comprises important glands that produce and secrete hormones into the blood toward target organs. Secreted hormones help regulate the body's growth and development and other metabolic functions important for a balanced system.

The thyroid gland is located in the anterior part of the neck of a normal human body. It secretes the thyroid hormones, which are important in regulating the body's basal metabolism. Disorders that cause abnormal decreases or increases in thyroid hormones cause serious metabolic consequences.

The parathyroid glands are a part of the endocrine system comprising four similarly shaped small organs just behind the thyroid gland. These glands produce the parathyroid hormone, which controls the level of calcium and phosphate circulating in the body.

The pancreas is located in the abdomen and performs both endocrine and exocrine functions. The pancreatic islets of Langerhans are composed of cells that produce insulin and glucagon, which are important in regulating blood glucose levels.

The adrenal glands are paired organs located at the apex of each kidney. The adrenals comprise an inner medulla part that secretes epinephrine and norepinephrine. The outer cortex of the adrenals secrete glucocorticoids, mineralocorticoids, and the precursors for reproductive hormones.

The thymus is an immune function organ that produces thymosin to stimulate immune cells, which help protect the body against diseases. The organ is mainly active in young children and becomes smaller after puberty, to be gradually replaced by fat in adulthood.

The brain contains the pineal gland, which secretes the melatonin that regulates the circadian rhythm, and the pituitary gland. The pituitary gland is divided into anterior and posterior pituitary. Together, they produce several hormones that serve as precursors for other hormones generated by some body organs.

The nervous system comprises the central nervous system and the peripheral nervous system. The central nervous system includes the brain and the spinal cord. The cerebrum is the largest part of the brain, occupying most of the skull. It is further divided into lobes – frontal, parietal, temporal, and occipital lobes. The cerebellum occupies the lower part of the brain below the occipital lobe.

The brainstem consists of the pons, medulla oblongata, and midbrain and connects the brain to the spinal cord. The spinal cord is the structure that conveys information from the brain to the peripheral parts of the body. It also serves as a conduit for information received from the peripheral parts of the body back to the brain.

The neuron is the smallest unit of the nervous system. Each neuron is composed of a cell body, axon, and dendrites. Signals are sent from one nerve to another, separated by a terminal space called a synapse. Chemicals secreted at these ends are referred to as neurotransmitters and serve as messengers for regulating function within the nervous system.

## ICD-10-CM Coding

The disorders associated with the endocrine system are found in the ICD-10-CM chapters E00 -E89.

### Thyroid Gland

Disorders of the thyroid gland are categorized between ICD-10-CM E00 – E07.

Goiter is the pathological enlargement of the thyroid gland due to a disorder of the production of thyroid hormones. Goiter may be toxic or non-toxic based on the clinical presentation. Thyrotoxicosis (E05) is the clinical manifestation of an abnormal increase in circulating thyroid hormone levels.

Thyroiditis (E06) is an inflammatory thyroid disease that can be acute, subacute, or chronic. Thyroiditis may be due to an underlying autoimmune condition or drug-induced.

## Diabetes and Glucose Regulation

Diabetes mellitus is a group of chronic metabolic disorders caused by defects in the production or action of insulin. This results in a persistent hyperglycemic state with a varying range of complications affecting the body's organs. Diabetes mellitus is listed between categories E08 –E13.

Type 1 diabetes mellitus (E10) is a subtype of diabetes mellitus due to insulin deficiency, which manifests as early onset hyperglycemia with life-threatening metabolic complications. Some of the major complications categorized under Type 1 diabetes mellitus in the ICD-10-CM diagnosis codebook include diabetic ketoacidosis, kidney complications, ophthalmic complications, neurological complications, circulatory complications, and other specified complications related to the skin or joints.

Hypoglycemia is a complication of diabetes mellitus management due to insulin therapy or other factors affecting glucose levels. Hypoglycemia without coma in type 1 diabetes mellitus is coded as E10.649. Type 2 diabetes mellitus (E11) is the subtype of diabetes mellitus that is not insulin dependent as there is a characteristic insulin resistance in peripheral tissues.

Diabetes mellitus may also be drug or chemical-induced (E09) or due to an underlying condition (E08). Other disorders affecting secretion by the pancreas (E16) include hypoglycemia, abnormal glucagon secretion, gastrin, and other drug-induced hypoglycemic manifestations. Disorders of the parathyroid glands can either be due to elevated levels of circulating parathyroid hormone causing hyperparathyroidism (E21) or reduced levels of parathyroid hormones resulting in hypoparathyroidism (E20).

## Pituitary Gland

Increased function of the pituitary gland (E22) causes elevated levels of circulating hormones released by the pituitary gland. It can result in acromegaly (E22.0), hyperprolactinemia (E22.1), syndrome of inappropriate secretion of antidiuretic hormone (E22.2), and other forms of hyperfunction of the pituitary gland.

Reduced function of the pituitary gland (E23) may manifest as hypopituitarism (E23.0), diabetes insipidus (E23.2), or other hypothalamic dysfunction (E23.3). Diabetes insipidus is a disease caused by reduced production of antidiuretic hormones or poor kidney response to the antidiuretic hormone. This causes excessive passage of urine and thirst.

Cushing's syndrome (E24) is characterized by excess levels of circulating cortisol in the body from endogenous or exogenous sources. It results in facial puffiness, elevated blood pressure, high blood sugar, stretch marks, weight gain, and severe fatigue.

## Adrenal Gland

Adrenogenital disorders (E25) are syndromes causing virilization that result from defects in the synthesis of hormones produced by the adrenal glands. These disorders may be congenital or acquired. Hyperaldosteronism (E26) is the overproduction of aldosterone by the cortex of the adrenal glands. It causes sodium retention and excretion of potassium. This causes elevated blood pressure and hypokalemia. Conn's syndrome (E26.01) is a form of primary hyperaldosteronism with persistent hypertension, headaches, and muscle weakness. Other adrenal gland disorders (E27) are found between subcategories E27.0 – E27.9. This includes adrenocortical insufficiency, Addisonian crisis, and adrenomedullary hyperfunction.

## Sex Hormones

Dysfunction of the ovaries caused by hormonal imbalances are listed in ICD-10-CM category E28. These disorders include estrogen excess (E28.0), androgen excess (E28.1), polycystic ovarian syndrome (E28.2), primary ovarian failure (E28.3) and premature menopause (E28.31).

Some endocrine disorders directly affect the testicles in males. This causes hyperfunction (E29.0) or hypofunction (E29.1). Puberty is a period experienced by adolescents. It includes multiple endocrine changes. Changes in the normal hormonal balances may cause delayed puberty (E30.0) or precocious puberty (E30.1). Multiple endocrine neoplasia are syndromes of polyglandular dysfunction listed in the ICD-10-CM subcategory E31.2.

## The Thymus

The body's immune system includes the thymus gland as an essential lymphoid organ. This gland is an indispensable component of the immune system. Diseases of the thymus gland are found in category E32.

## The Nervous System

Diseases of the nervous system are categorized in ICD-10-CM chapter G00 – G99. Meningitis is the inflammation of the meninges. It may occur due to bacterial infiltration, viral, parasitic, or other specified causes between categories G00 –G03.

Other inflammatory processes affecting the brain and its surrounding structures are encephalitis, myelitis, and encephalomyelitis (G04). They are often caused by pathogenic invasion of the central nervous system, toxins, autoimmune diseases, or many other conditions.

Localized purulent material that results from an ongoing infection is known as an abscess. Abscesses may be found in intracranial (G06.0), intraspinal (G06.1), extradural, or subdural (G06.2) spaces of the nervous system.

Some systemic atrophies mainly affecting the central nervous system (G10-G14) include Huntington's disease, hereditary ataxia, spinal muscle dystrophy, post-polio syndrome, and other atrophic disorders classified elsewhere.

Huntington's disease (G10) is a familial disease of autosomal dominant inheritance with progressive onset of neurological symptoms of chorea and dementia and worsening decline with poor prognosis. Extrapyramidal and movement disorders (G20 - G26) include Parkinson's disease, secondary Parkinsonism, and other degenerative diseases of the basal ganglia. Parkinson's disease (G20) is a progressive degenerative disorder resulting from the loss of dopamine-producing neurons in the substantia nigra, and manifesting with neurological symptoms such as tremors, rigidity, and abnormal posture. The disease may or may not be associated with abnormalities with movement, referred to as dyskinesia. Dystonia (G24) is a movement disorder causing involuntary muscle contraction across various muscle groups.

Alzheimer's disease is a degenerative disease of the nervous system. It is characterized by senile plaques, neurofibrillary tangles, and severe cortical atrophy. These degenerative changes in the brain cause a decline in cognitive functioning in older adults and progressive dementia with memory loss, confusion, and changes in language, behavior, and personality. It is a common neurodegenerative disorder seen in older adults. Alzheimer's disease may be early onset (G30.0) or late onset (G30.1).

Demyelinating central nervous system diseases are found in ICD-10-CM categories G35-G37. Multiple sclerosis (G35) is an autoimmune disorder characterized by the destruction of the myelin sheath layer with pathological findings of multiple areas of demyelination throughout the central nervous system. Myelin is the lipid-containing sheath of nerves, serving as an insulator and important for the fast transmission of nerve signals. The description should emphasize that demyelination can occur in both the white and gray matter of the central nervous system. Multiple sclerosis is a chronic disease with clinical manifestations of visual disturbances, muscle weakness, paresthesia, dysarthria, and a long line of neurological symptoms.

Epilepsy (G40) is a disorder of the central nervous system caused by excessive abnormal neuronal discharge in the brain, which causes sensory or motor neurological dysfunction manifesting as seizures, abnormal body movements, or impaired consciousness.

Migraines are mainly associated with recurrent pulsatile headaches (G43) and may be associated with aura. Other headache syndromes are found in category G44.

Disorders associated with nerves, nerve roots, and plexuses are found between G50 -59. This includes mononeuropathies of both upper and lower limbs.

Myasthenia gravis (G70.0) is a chronic autoimmune disorder of the neuromuscular system due to the blockage of acetylcholine receptors by autoantibodies at neuromuscular junctions.

Cerebral palsy (G80) is a group of heterogeneous non-progressive motor disorders due to irreversible brain injury that occurs during the period of birth of an individual and up to the first few years of life.

Cerebral palsy ranges from minor difficulties in fine movement to severe muscle spasticity across all limbs. The disease has no cure. However, there are options for management to improve the quality of life of an affected individual. Forms of cerebral palsy are spastic quadriplegic, spastic diplegic, spastic hemiplegic, athetoid, and ataxic cerebral palsy, with different clinical manifestations specific to each subtype. Other paralytic syndromes of the nervous system are hemiplegia, hemiparesis, paraplegia, or quadriplegia.

Hydrocephalus (G91) is an abnormal accumulation of cerebrospinal fluid produced within the brain's ventricles. Hydrocephalus may be present at birth. This causes an unusually large head. It may also be acquired later in life. Acquired hydrocephalus may cause headaches, vomiting, blurred vision, or permanent brain damage if no intervention is made.

Cerebrovascular diseases are a group of disorders that occur due to problems affecting the brain's circulatory system. They are found in ICD-10-CM category I60 - I69. Long-standing elevated blood pressure is a well-recognized cause of damage to the blood supply network of the brain. Stroke may occur due to bleeding within the brain cavity or sometimes a sudden flow disruption to a brain region. This results in cerebral infarction (I63).

Cerebral infarction is defined as ischemia of the brain due to an insufficiency in arterial or venous flow of blood. This causes focal neurological deficit.

Other cerebrovascular diseases (I67) are cerebral aneurysm (I67.1), cerebral atherosclerosis (I67.2), progressive vascular leukoencephalopathy (I67.3), hypertensive encephalopathy (I67.4), thrombosis within the intracranial venous system (I67.6), cerebral arteritis (I67.7), and other specified cerebrovascular diseases (I67.8).

## CPT Coding

### Procedures for the Endocrine System

Procedures related to the endocrine system are those limited to organ incision and excision or laparoscopic interventions for disorders of some endocrine glands.

Procedures relating to the thyroid gland are within CPT codes 60000 – 60300. Incision and drainage of thyroglossal cysts are found under code 60000. For a thyroid lobectomy, the thyroid gland is exposed by a transverse cervical incision, and the superior and inferior thyroid vessels are ligated. Following ligation, the surgeon severs the isthmus of the thyroid gland, which allows the entire resection of each thyroid lobe (60220).

Adrenal gland excision may follow a diagnosis of an adrenal gland tumor. Partial or complete adrenalectomy done as open surgery is found as CPT code 60540. The dissection and removal of the adrenal gland under laparoscopic guidance is listed as code 60650. Other unlisted endocrine glands or organ procedures are in a general category listed as code 60699.

### Procedures for the Nervous System

Procedures related to the skull, meninges, and brain are grouped between 61000 and 61315. A burr hole is a surgical procedure to relieve intracranial pressure due to accumulation of hematoma, brain abscess, or cysts. The different burr hole procedures can be found between 61105 – 61253.

The surgical creation of an opening in the skull to access the cranial lobe is known as craniotomy or craniectomy (61304 – 61576). Some lesions are found in the skull base and require surgical management (61580 – 61619), which may be categorized according to approach procedure, definitive procedure, or repair/reconstruction of defects following definitive procedures. Surgeries done for aneurysms, arteriovenous malformation, or vascular diseases, as well as craniotomy appropriate for the procedure, are found in CPT codes 61680 – 61702.

A cerebrospinal fluid shunt is a surgical intervention for hydrocephalus, and the various approaches for a CSF shunt are described by CPT codes 62180 – 62258. A ventriculostomy (62223) is the surgical creation of an opening in the ventricle of the brain to allow CSF release through a shunt into the peritoneal cavity.

Every surgery associated with the spinal cord and peripheral nerves is also found under codes for the nervous system procedure, with extensive descriptions associated with every listed surgical intervention of the nervous system in the CPT code book.

## HCPCS Coding

Healthcare Common Procedure Coding System covers codes directly and indirectly related to the endocrine and nervous systems. The HCPCS codes mainly report medications used for specific conditions of both systems. Some supplies for neurological surgery procedures are found between codes. Recent technological advancements for these procedures can also be found in the HCPCS level II codebook. Refer to the HCPCS index for the location of specific codes assigned.

## Modifiers

Being familiar with the modifiers needed for reporting endocrine and nervous system-related procedures and services is important.

- Modifier 22 is designated for reporting more procedural services offered to a patient than previously listed.
- Modifier 50 is applied when a procedure is carried out bilaterally. However, this modifier is limited to paired structures in the body.
- Modifier 52 is used to reduce the services a physician provides or cancel the procedure before completion.
- Modifier 53 describes the discontinuation of services due to unexpected circumstances.
- Modifier 59 is applied when the same physician or other qualified healthcare professional carries out an unrelated procedure during the postoperative period.
- Modifier LT or RT differentiates procedures on the left from those on the right side.
- Modifier 62 is appended when two surgeons mainly work together to complete a procedure.

- Modifier 77 is used to report a repeat of the same procedure by another physician or other qualified healthcare professional due to a similar complaint.

## Definition of Important Terms

- Acromegaly: Condition marked by increased production of growth hormones.
- Adenoma: Benign growth of glandular tissue.
- Adrenaline: Hormone responsible for the body's fight or flight response.
- Alzheimer's disease: Progressive neurodegenerative disorder.
- Amyotrophic lateral sclerosis (ALS): Progressive nervous system disease.
- Aphasia: Difficulty with the use of language caused by a lesion in the brain.
- Axon: The part of a neuron that sends signals to other nerves.
- Bradykinesia: Slowed movement.
- Brainstem: Lower part of the brain connecting cerebrum and spinal cord.
- Cerebrospinal fluid (CSF): Liquid protecting the brain and spinal cord.
- Cushing's syndrome: Disorder caused by prolonged exposure to high levels of cortisol.
- Dementia: General term for the loss of cognitive function.
- Diabetes mellitus: Chronic condition characterized by elevated blood sugar levels.
- Endocrine system: Collection of glands producing hormones.
- Epilepsy: Disorder of abnormal electrical discharge from the brain.
- Glasgow Coma Scale: Classifies the extent of head injury.
- Goiter: Enlargement of the thyroid gland.
- Hemiplegia: Paralysis affecting one half of the body.
- Hypothyroidism: Underactivity of the thyroid gland.
- Hyperthyroidism: Overactivity of the thyroid gland.
- Insulin: Hormone regulating blood sugar levels.
- Islets of Langerhans: Cell clusters in the pancreas producing hormones.
- Meningitis: Inflammation of the meninges.
- Migraine: Intense, throbbing headache.
- Multiple Sclerosis (MS): Immune system attacks the protective covering of nerve fibers.
- Myasthenia Gravis: Autoimmune neuromuscular disorder.
- Neuralgia: Pain along the course of a nerve.
- Neuropathy: Pathological disturbance of the peripheral nervous system.
- Pancreas: Produces insulin and digestive enzymes.
- Parathyroid gland: Regulates calcium and phosphorus balance.
- Parkinson's disease: Neurodegenerative disorder affecting movement.
- Pineal gland: Produces melatonin, influencing sleep-wake cycles.

- Pituitary gland: Controls other endocrine glands.
- Permanent national codes: Describe the products and services.
- Pineal gland: Produces melatonin, influencing sleep-wake cycles.
- Pituitary gland: Controls other endocrine glands.
- Seizure: Sudden, uncontrolled electrical activity in the brain.
- Stroke: Sudden interruption of blood supply to the brain.
- Synapse: Junction between two nerve cells transmitting nerve impulses.
- Thymus gland: Important for immune system development.
- Ventriculostomy: Opening into the brain ventricles to relieve pressure.

# Chapter 15: Eyes and The Auditory System

## Introduction

This chapter examines the disorders affecting the eyes and ears, as listed in the ICD-10-CM codebook. It also discusses how to report important CPT codes and peculiarities associated with the modifiers.

## Examples of Words, Prefixes and Suffixes

- Audiogram (record of hearing):
    - Prefix: None.
    - Root: Audi- (hear).
    - Suffix: -gram (record).
- Auricle (external part of the ear):
    - Prefix: None.
    - Root: Auric- (ear).
    - Suffix: -le (small).
- Cochlear (relating to the cochlea of the ear):
    - Prefix: None.
    - Root: Cochle- (cochlea).
    - Suffix: -ar (pertaining to).
- Lacrimal Gland (gland producing tears):
    - Prefix: None.
    - Root: Lacrim- (tear).
- Ophthalmoscope (instrument for examining the eye):
    - Prefix: Ophthalm- (eye).
    - Root: -scope (instrument for viewing).
- Optometrist (healthcare professional specializing in eye care):
    - Prefix: Opto- (vision).
    - Root: Metr- (measure).
    - Suffix: -ist (one who specializes).
    - Suffix: -al (pertaining to).
- Otitis Media (inflammation of the middle ear):
    - Prefix: Otitis- (ear).
    - Root: Medi- (middle).
    - Suffix: -a (condition).
- Retinopathy (disease of the retina):
    - Prefix: Retin- (retina).

        - Suffix: -opathy (disease).
- Tympanoplasty (surgical repair of the eardrum):
    - Prefix: Tympan- (eardrum).
    - Suffix: -plasty (surgical repair).
- Visualize (to form a mental image):
    - Prefix: Visu- (sight).
    - Suffix: -ize (to make or do).

## Anatomy of the Eyes

The eyeball is the organ of sight. The tough white membrane of the eye is the sclera, which is covered by a thin protective layer that also lines the eyelids inside. The eye's transparent central part is the cornea, which directly overlies the colored iris. The pupil is the aperture through which light enters into the eye.

The average vertical diameter of the eyeball is 24 mm, weighing about 7.5 g each. The ciliary muscle helps control the light that enters the eye through the pupils. The retina is the innermost eye layer directly behind which the choroid lies. The choroid is the posterior part of the uvea, a layer of blood vessels. The ciliary body is an anterior continuation of the choroid, which secretes aqueous humor. The retina contains rods and cones, photosensitive cells that convert light into chemical energy.

## Anatomy of the Ears

The human ear is the organ of hearing and maintaining equilibrium. It is divided into an outer, middle, and inner ear. The outer ear comprises the external pinna and a short auditory canal, which terminates at the tympanic membrane.

The middle ear is a narrow cavity with three tiny bones (ossicles) - malleus, incus, and stapes. These bones conduct sound waves from the tympanic membrane to the inner ear.

The inner labyrinthine ear is a system of fluid-filled passages within the temporal bone. The vestibule and semicircular canals help to maintain postural equilibrium, and the cochlea is a highly specialized organ of hearing. The inner ear directly interacts with the vestibulocochlear nerve.

## ICD-10-CM Coding

The ICD-10-CM code for eye and ocular adnexa diseases is found in chapters H00 – H59.

The disorders of the eyelid, lacrimal system, and orbit are found in H00 – H05. Hordeolum is an acute infection of the eyelid. This causes pain and swelling. The infection may result in the purulent collection of the sebaceous gland of Zeis along the eyelid margin (Hordeolum externum – H00.01) or the Meibomian gland on the conjunctival aspect of the eyelid (Hordeolum internum – H00.02).

Chalazion (H00.1) is the most common inflammatory lesion found on the eyelid. This causes painless cysts due to blockage of the Meibomian gland.

Other eyelid inflammation (H01) includes blepharitis, allergic dermatitis, xeroderma, and other non-infectious eyelid disorders.

The lacrimal gland is a small tear-producing gland situated at the upper outer region of the orbit. Pathological conditions associated with the lacrimal apparatus are found in category H04. These conditions include dacryoadenitis, dacryops, dry eye syndrome, lacrimal cysts, and lacrimal gland atrophy.

Epiphora (H04.2) is the excessive production of tears due to increased production or poor drainage and remains a common cause of presentation at ophthalmology clinics.

Visual disturbances include disorders resulting in amblyopia, also called lazy eye, a sight disorder due to interruption of the normal visual pathway during development, transient visual loss, or diplopia (double vision caused by misalignment of both eyes), amongst others found in category H53.

Blindness refers to impaired light perception and can be partial or total, as seen in patients without light perception. Blindness and low vision are categorized under ICD-10-CM code H54.

Glaucoma is also a commonly reported eye disorder. It arises due to a persistent increase in the pressure within the intraocular space, predisposing to optic nerve and retina damage. It can occur mainly with angle closure caused by obstruction of the flow of aqueous humor. Glaucoma may also occur secondary to trauma affecting the eye or inflammation of the eye. All forms of glaucoma are found coded under categories H40 and H42.

Cataract is a disorder of the eye characterized by opacification of the lens. Increasing age (H25) is one of the most common causes of cataracts. Cataracts may also be found in young people, as seen in infantile and juvenile cataracts. They may also occur secondary to trauma to the eye. Cataracts due to an underlying condition would be found in the main condition category. An example is diabetes mellitus with cataracts, found in subcategory E08.36.

Conjunctivitis (H10) is an inflammation of the mucous membrane that lines the inside of the eyelid and the anterior surface of the sclera. Acute atopic conjunctivitis is a commonly reported disorder of the conjunctiva that occurs due to an allergic reaction.

Strabismus is a condition in which one eye is turned in a different direction from the other. It may be paralytic (H49) due to oculomotor nerve palsy (H49.0), trochlear nerve palsy (H49.1), or abducens nerve palsy (H49.2). Another form of strabismus is ocular misalignment with excessive convergence of the visual axes, which results in a cross-eye presentation (H50.0).

Refraction and accommodation disorders are the most common causes of the use of prescription eyeglasses. Hypermetropia (H52.0) is also called long-sightedness. Myopia (H52.1) is a disorder of refraction resulting in shortsightedness. Astigmatism (H52.2) is an unequal curvature of the lens causing lack of focus of the light entering the eyes on to the retina.

Presbyopia (H52.4) is the loss of accommodation due to loss of elasticity of the eye lens, as seen in older people.

## Diseases Affecting the Ear and Auditory System

Diseases affecting the ear can be found between H60 - H95. Otitis externa (H60) is an inflammation of the external ear extending to the ear canal. It may be associated with the formation of abscesses or cellulitis.

Wax impaction (H61.2) is a common complaint in otolaryngology. It may affect both ears and cause ear ringing or hearing loss if left unattended.

Otitis media is an inflammatory process of the middle ear which may be associated with the formation of pus or due to allergic reactions. Non-suppurative otitis media and other associated classifications are coded under category H65. Suppurative otitis media and unspecified otitis media are coded in category H66.

Mastoiditis (H70) is an inflammation of the mastoid bone, which is one of the bones of the head in close relation to the ear, lying just below it. It can occur acutely or sometimes result in chronic hearing problems.

A perforation of the tympanic membrane (H72) is also a commonly reported cause of impaired hearing. Further classification is based on the location or extent of the opening. Otosclerosis is the formation of spongy bone in the labyrinth capsule of the inner ear (H80). This results in hearing loss.

Disorders affecting the vestibule of the ear (H81) cause dizziness and imbalance. Other disorders affecting the ear and mastoid process can be found listed accordingly in the ICD-10-CM codebook.

## CPT Coding

Specialists usually report codes for procedures performed on the ears and eyes found in the CPT codebook. Surgeries performed on the eye may range from laser procedures to open eye removal in the setting of a tumor or other disorders causing irreversible disfiguring. The procedures performed on the eye and ocular adnexa are between 65091 and 68899. Those related to the auditory system are between 69000 and 69979.

### Procedures of the Eye

Evisceration (65091, 65093) is the removal of the contents of the eyeball that spares the outer part of the sclera. This allows for the implantation of a prosthetic eyeball with proper fitting and easy movement in the eye socket with the muscles of the eye.

Enucleation of the eye (65101 – 65105) removes the eyeball and the muscles, nerves, and blood vessels surrounding the eye. Exenteration of the eye (65110 – 65114) is the removal of the eyeball and its contents, the surrounding fat and muscle layers, and the orbital bone.

An implant may be placed following the removal of the eyeball to protect the void created. Laser surgeries are preferred to open procedures. An ocular implant is placed within the muscular cone, while an orbital implant is placed outside the muscular cone. Secondary implant procedures range from modification of an ocular implant (65125), insertion of an ocular implant after evisceration or enucleation (65130), or removal of an ocular implant (65175).

Foreign body removal from the eye is classified based on the anatomical position: external eye, intraocular – anterior chamber, posterior chamber.

Lacerations directly affecting the inner eye structures are found in the chapter covering the eye and ocular adnexa, unlike lacerations affecting the eyelid, which are found in the integumentary system.

Procedures of the anterior segment include those involving the cornea (excision, removal, or transplant). Keratoplasty is a corneal transplant using fresh or preserved grafts obtained from donors (65710 – 65757).

Cataract surgeries include incision of the lens or removal through iridectomy, lateral canthotomy, iridotomy, anterior capsulotomy, enzymatic analysis, posterior capsulotomy, or pharmacological agents. Intraocular lens procedures for cataracts are lens removal procedures that may include prosthesis insertion.

Goniotomy (65820) is the creation of a surgical opening to relieve intraocular pressure from glaucoma within the anterior chamber. It is another minimally invasive procedure with an external approach, which uses an aqueous shunt. It involves the application a drainage device through the trabecular meshwork.

Retinal detachment can be repaired (67107) by procedures such as scleral buckling or vitrectomy. Scleral buckling involves indenting the sclera to close breaks and flatten the retina, while vitrectomy involves removing the vitreous gel and repairing the retina with lasers or cryotherapy, and replacing the gel with a gas or silicone oil.

The ocular adnexa consist of the extraocular muscles of the eye, and strabismus surgeries are carried out for the horizontal and vertical extraocular muscles. The orbit is made of the bony structures surrounding the eyeball, and orbitotomy can be performed for exploration, excision, or decompression.

Incision procedures of the eyelids include those for abscess drainage (67700) or incisional biopsy (67810). Other CPT codes for the eye are for procedures on the conjunctiva and lacrimal system.

Blepharoplasty is the surgical removal of the skin of the eyelid, and the procedure is found in the integumentary chapter. However, when blepharoplasty is accompanied by the removal of structures within the eye, the CPT codes are listed in this section.

## Procedures for the Ear

The procedures carried out on the ear are listed according to their anatomical position. The outer ear is mostly affected by conditions requiring simple interventions such as incision and drainage of abscesses (69000 – 69020), ear piercing (69090), excision procedures for the tissue of the external ear, and removal of a foreign body or impacted ear wax from the auditory canal.

Myringotomy is the creation of an incision on the ear drum and may include aspiration and inflation of the Eustachian tube. The insertion of a ventilating tube into the opening of the tympanum is a tympanostomy (69433 – 69436), and the repair of a perforated eardrum using a graft is tympanoplasty (69635 – 69646).

A cochlear implant is introduced into the inner ear (69930) by attaching an internal coil to the temporal bone and the temporalis muscle. Vestibular and auditory testing are found in the medicine chapter of the CPT codebook. This includes all diagnostic and screening procedures performed by physicians or audiologists.

## HCPCS Coding

The HCPCS codes for the eye and auditory system report drug supplies for managing associated disorders. The codes include visual aids, glasses, contact lenses, hearing aids, and other prosthetic devices. Screening codes for glaucoma are G00117 (for screening high-risk patients by an ophthalmologist or optometrist) or G0118 (for screening high-risk patients under the supervision of an optometrist or ophthalmologist).

The medical devices used for procedures relating to the eyes and ears are prescribed and coded independently based on the particular disorder and the specific device or supply used. The drug injection supplies for procedures are important to note and are located within the Table of Drugs, which can be confirmed in the HCPCS codebook.

## Modifiers

The eyes and ears are bilateral organs, and therefore require proper identification of the side that a procedure is being carried out on for reporting. The common modifiers used include modifier 50 for bilateral procedures, LT for procedures on the left eye and RT for procedures on the right eye. E1 and E2 represent the upper and lower left eyelids respectively. E3 and E4 represent the upper and lower right eyelids. If a patient has aphakia (that is, absence of the crystalline lens in their eyeball), they are represented with VP.

## Definition of Important Terms

- Accommodation: Adjustment of the ciliary bodies to allow or filter light entering the eyes.
- Acuity: Sharp vision.
- Acoustic Neuroma: A tumor of the cells of the auditory nerves. They are also referred to as a vestibular schwannoma.
- Aqueous humor: The clear fluid behind the cornea of the eye, lying just before the iris.
- Astigmatism: Impaired vision.
- Audiogram: Graphical measurement of the sensitivity to sound.
- Blepharitis: Inflammation of the eyelids.
- Cataract: Complete or partial opacity of the lens in the eye.
- Cerumen: Soft wax produced by the glands in the ear.

- Choroid: Vascular membrane in the eye between the retina and sclera. It minimizes the diffusion of light in the eyes.
- Cochlea: A coiled tube in the ear where sound is converted into nervous impulses.
- Convex: Bulging outward.
- Deafness: Loss of hearing.
- Dilation: To become wider.
- Diplopia: Double vision.
- Eardrum: The sensitive membrane protecting the middle ear, also called the tympanic membrane.
- Esotropia: Abnormal turning of the eyes inward toward the nose.
- Eustachian tube –A tubular link between the middle ear and nasopharynx. It helps to balance the atmospheric pressure to the middle ear pressure.
- Exotropia: An outward deviation of the eye.
- Hemianopsia: Blindness affecting half of the visual field of one or both eyes.
- Incus: One of the small bones of the middle ear, lying between the malleus and stapes.
- Iris: A muscular diaphragm that regulates the pupillary diameter and forms the colored part of the eye.
- Malleus: One of the tiny bones of the middle ear attached to the eardrum.
- Myringotomy: Surgical opening of the eardrum.
- Nystagmus: Involuntary movement of the eyeball.
- Ossicles: Refers to the malleus, incus, and stapes, the three small bones in the middle ear.
- Otitis: Inflammation of the ear.
- Otoscope: Instrument used to examine the ear.
- Papilledema: Swelling of the optic disc.
- Photophobia: Pain in the eye that results from exposure to light. It might also mean a morbid fear of light.
- Presbyopia: Loss of elasticity of the eye lens.
- Ptosis: Drooping of the eyelid.
- Pupil: The opening within the eye that allows light in.
- Refraction: The bending of light as it passes from one medium to another, which enables the focusing of images onto the retina in the eye.
- Retina: The light-sensitive area of the eye responsible for vision.
- Sclera: The white outer fibrous membrane of the eye. It is overlaid by the conjunctiva to protect the eyeball.
- Stapes: The third small bone in the middle ear that transmits sound from the incus to the cochlea.
- Strabismus: Abnormal alignment of the eye.
- Tinnitus: A ringing sensation in the ear.

- Tonometry: Measurement of the intraocular pressure.
- Vertigo: Dizzy sensation causing loss of balance.
- Vestibule: The part of the ear connecting the semicircular canals to the cochlea, which helps with balance.
- Vitreous humor: Fluid within the posterior chamber of the eyes.
- Xerophthalmia: Excessive dryness of the conjunctiva and cornea of the eyes.

# Chapter 16: Anesthesia

## Introduction

Anesthesia is the medical practice used to keep patients from experiencing pain or discomfort during invasive procedures like dental treatments, biopsies, screening and diagnostic testing, and surgery. Anesthesia is central to medical practice because it guarantees improved health outcomes and helps patients live longer, healthier lives.

The codes pertaining to anesthesia are arranged by anatomical location, starting with the head. The phrase "not otherwise specified" is also seen in several anesthetic codes. In the event that a specific code is not available, this phrase permits the codes to be supplied for the concerned anatomic region. For instance, anesthetic operations performed on the male genitalia are coded as 00920. However, this code specifically pertains to anesthesia for procedures on the male genitalia excluding penile prosthesis, circumcision, and destruction of lesion of penis, which have their own specific codes. Open urethral procedures, if not specifically listed, should be coded using the most accurate and specific code available.

As for medical coding, the CPT codes list covers anesthesia services in conjunction with procedures on specific body areas such as the head, neck, spine, and spinal cord. This also includes the upper leg or the elbow. Sometimes, a code listed under a body part grouping may be specific to a procedure, such as the endoscopic retrograde cholangiopancreatography (ERCP).

However, for unlisted anesthesia procedures, those that do not have a specific and appropriate CPT code available, the code set includes 01999. The old coding pattern is determined by looking under the former CPT codes 00100 - 00210 section's anesthesia section and then looking under the appropriate anatomic heading. This is pending till the new anesthesia codes become familiar.

Codes are only sometimes found under the surgical description, and the coder may need to default and move backward to find the most accurate description. For example, the code ranges for anesthesia for a mastectomy are not listed as 'Mastectomy' but rather under 'Breast.'

Coders are also aided by anesthetic "crosswalk" books. Crosswalk books "crosswalk" (transpose) known surgical codes to a suitable anesthesia code. The coder must choose the code with the highest base unit and the most appropriate code to report when the crosswalk provides more than one code.

## Types of Anesthesia

There are three primary types of anesthesia: general, regional, and monitored anesthesia care (MAC).

**General anesthesia** induces a total loss of consciousness in the patient. It renders them completely unconscious and unaware during the surgical procedure. This type of anesthesia is usually administered through inhalation or intravenous (IV) medications. General anesthesia ensures that the patient feels no pain and is in a state of deep sleep throughout the surgery. It is commonly used for complex or invasive surgical procedures.

**Regional anesthesia** blocks sensation in a specific body region during procedures like limb or obstetric surgeries. It allows the patient to remain conscious while preventing pain in the targeted area. Various techniques fall under regional anesthesia, including:

- **Spinal anesthesia:** Injection of anesthetic medication into the spinal fluid to numb the lower half of the body.
- **Epidural anesthesia:** Injection of anesthetic into the epidural space surrounding the spinal cord, commonly used for pain relief during childbirth or certain surgeries.
- **Nerve block or local nerve block:** Injection of anesthetic near a specific nerve or group of nerves to block sensation in a localized area.

**Monitored anesthesia care (MAC)** is a form of anesthetic service where the patient is lightly sedated, or in some cases, not sedated at all. Patients often commence surgery with only the local anesthesia provided by the surgeon and can respond to verbal commands. This form of anesthesia also requires that the patient's airways are maintained spontaneously. An anesthesia provider monitors this service and should always be prepared to convert MAC to general anesthesia if necessary.

Generally, monitored anesthesia care (MAC) differs distinctly from moderate sedation. It may also involve the administration of sedatives, analgesics, hypnotics, anesthetic agents, or other medications necessary for patient safety, all of which are based on each patient's health status. In this case, the patient does not lose consciousness, is still readily arousable, and can maintain an open airway.

The patient's anesthesia plan is determined on a case-by-case basis. When using monitored anesthesia care, the provider must be qualified and always prepared to convert to general anesthesia if necessary. If the patient loses consciousness and the ability to respond purposely, the anesthesia care, in this instance, is a general anesthetic.

Monitored anesthesia services should also be paid for in the same way as general or regional anesthesia services. However, many insurance companies request special modifiers to identify the service as monitored anesthesia care. Monitored anesthesia care and other modifiers are subsequently discussed in other parts of this book, specifically in the healthcare common procedure coding system (HCPS).

## Direction, Supervision, and Monitoring

In anesthesia, medical direction occurs when the anesthesiologist is involved in two, three, or four anesthesia procedures simultaneously, a single anesthesia procedure simultaneously, or a single anesthesia procedure with a qualified anesthesia resident, CRNA, or anesthesiologist assistant.

According to the Centers for Medicare and Medicaid Services, some vital steps must be followed when an anesthesiologist is medically directing. Also, it is the rule that while medically directing, anesthesiologists should not provide other services to other patients. However, there are some exceptions to the services they can provide in a way that does not affect their ongoing primary ability at that particular time.

## Post-Operative Pain Management

Anesthesia is about preventing pain, so it is not out of order. It is a specialty that is an essential part of postoperative pain management. In this instance, the surgeon may request postoperative pain management and then be billed separately by the anesthesiologist if the anesthesia for the surgical procedure is not dependent on the efficacy of the regional anesthetic technique.

Nerve block codes are used as an adjunct to general anesthesia, especially if the placement is for postoperative pain management. Nerve block codes are not reported separately if the block is the mode of anesthesia for a procedure being performed. For instance, an axillary block is used during a carpal tunnel surgery, and a code from the anesthesia section is reported. Thus the axillary block is not additionally reported with a separate code.

Coding as a whole, or in this particular instance, depends largely on the medication injected, the site of the injection, and the placement of either a single injection block or a continuous block by catheter. The CPT codes reported are unique and are appended to signify that the service is separate and distinct from the anesthesia care provided for the surgery.

When ultrasound or fluoroscopic guidance is utilized for pain management procedures and appropriately documented, the codes are reported separately with the professional component unless the code selected includes image guidance (fluoroscopy, ultrasound, or CT). There are distinct diagnostic codes for acute pain. There are also codes for the continuous infusion of anesthetic agents by catheter (including catheter placement) in the management of post-operative pain.

## Anesthesia Coding Terminology

**One-lung ventilation (OLV)**: This is when one lung is ventilated, and the other is collapsed temporarily to improve surgical access to the lung. For this, several anesthesia codes separately identify the utilization of one-lung ventilation.

**Pump oxygenator**: This refers to instances where a cardiopulmonary bypass (CPB) machine is used to function as the heart and lungs during heart or great vessel surgery.

**Intraperitoneal**: This is action within the peritoneal cavity, where organs in the upper abdomen include the stomach, liver, gall bladder, jejunum, spleen, and transverse colon. Examples of lower abdominal organs within the peritoneal cavity include the appendix, cecum, ileum, and sigmoid colon.

**Extraperitoneal (or retroperitoneal)**: This means "outside or behind" the peritoneum or the peritoneal cavity. Extraperitoneal organs are in the lower abdomen and include the ureter and urinary bladder. The adrenal glands, kidneys, and lower esophagus form the extraperitoneal organs of the upper abdomen. Also located in the retroperitoneum are the aorta and the inferior vena cava.

**Radical**: This is when an extensive and demanding surgery is needed to correct a severe condition. Conditions such as cancer are an example of this.

**Diagnostic or surgical arthroscopic interventions**: These are procedures performed on the temporomandibular, shoulder, elbow, hip, knee, wrist, and ankle joints. Coders, in this instance, can only assign a diagnostic code.

## ICD-10-CM Coding

In line with the general norms of anesthetic services provided to patients during surgery, the preoperative diagnosis is used for coding purposes, as it reflects the condition that led to the surgery. However, if the diagnosis changes based on intra-operative findings, the postoperative diagnosis should be coded. For example, if a patient is admitted with pain in the lower quadrant and subsequently has an appendectomy, the postoperative diagnosis may be acute appendicitis.

## CPT Coding

This code range includes anesthesia CPT codes. The American Medical Association (AMA) maintains the current procedural terminology (CPT) code set. This code list covers a range of anesthesia services provided in conjunction with procedures on specific body areas. Additionally, billing codes for anesthesia are available for services pertaining to radiological procedures, obstetric operations, and burn excisions or debridements.

At the end of the anesthesia procedure code list, a group of other codes, as mentioned earlier, cover services for nerve blocks and the daily hospital management of epidural continuous drug administration. Arterial catheters, central venous lines, and pulmonary arterial catheters such as the Swan Ganz catheter are not included in the base unit value of the anesthesia code. Services included with the base unit value of anesthesia codes reported are:

- Every customary visit both before and after surgery.
- Anesthetic management throughout the operation.
- Fluids and blood products administered during the procedure.
- Non-invasive observations such as temperature checks, pulse oximetry, electrocardiography, blood pressure monitoring, capnography, and mass spectrometry.

Base values are not stated individually in the CPT code. Rather, the complexity of the technique conducted is used by the American Society of Anesthesiologists (ASA) to define the base unit values for anesthetic codes. Determining the base value for anesthesia codes is the first step in calculating anesthesia charges and expected payments. Time reporting is the second step.

Anesthesia time begins when the anesthesiologist starts to prepare the patient for the induction of anesthesia in the operating room or equivalent area. Pre-anesthesia assessment time is not part of the reportable anesthesia time. The anesthesia time ends when the anesthesiologist is no longer in personal attendance and generally is reported when the patient is safely placed under postoperative supervision. Time, in this instance, does not need to be continuous.

For example, an axillary block may be performed in a holding room before surgery. If the axillary block is considered the mode of anesthesia, then the time for the placement of that block is counted. The anesthesiologist may then leave, and when the patient is brought to the operating room, the anesthesiologist counts the anesthesia again. In all, the time for the block is then added to the total anesthesia time for the case.

Time reporting might also vary, and there is no national guideline to introduce some processes to the whole action. Time units are added to the base unit value as is the 'norm in the local area.' For example, insurance companies like Medicare may report the exact time without rounding it up to the nearest five minutes, while some other insurance companies might process the anesthesia time reported in increments. That is, from the exact time to ten, twelve, and fifteen minutes or some other format of time increment.

Before rounding up this section, it is best to state that multiple surgical procedures may be performed on a single patient during anesthesia administration. Whenever this occurs, the surgery represents the most complex procedure because this service carries a higher base unit value. Anesthesia time should always be reported as usual, from when the anesthesiologist begins to prepare the patient until the patient is safely placed under postoperative supervision.

## Qualifying Circumstances

In anesthesia, qualifying circumstances are codes simply assigned to report anesthesia services performed under extremely difficult circumstances that massively affect the character of an anesthesia service. These circumstances include patients less than one year old, patients more than seventy years old, and patients with unique risk factors. Qualifying circumstances are reported as add-on codes (that is, as qualifiers for other anesthetic procedures).

The ASA assigns base unit values for the qualifying circumstances, even though they are not listed in the CPT. Medicare and some insurance companies may not provide additional payment for codes related to qualifying circumstances. There are different codes for reporting in these kinds of circumstances. However, all reported codes must be backed up by sufficient evidence in the documentation.

Qualifying circumstances are important to the calculation for anesthesia services. For Medicare payers, the formula is given as BASE + TIME multiplied by the Medicare conversion factor for the region. For non-Medicare payers, the formula is given as BASE + TIME + PHYSICAL STATUS MODIFIERS + QUALIFYING CIRCUMSTANCES multiplied by the CONVERSION FACTOR.

## Definition of Important Terms

- Analgesia: The relief of pain without causing unconsciousness.
- Anesthesia: Loss of feeling or sensation in a part or whole body. Usually drug-induced.

- Apnea: Cessation of respiration.
- Arrhythmia: Variation from the normal rhythm of the heart.
- Asystole: Absence of contractions of the heart.
- Ataractic: A tranquilizer.
- Basal narcosis: A state of unconsciousness produced before surgical anesthesia.
- Blood-brain barrier: The membrane that divides the brain from the blood. Water, respiratory gases, glucose, alcohol, certain medications, and general anesthetics can all pass through it.
- Bradycardia: Abnormally low heart rate.
- Bradypnea: Abnormally low respiratory rate.
- Bronchospasm: Constriction of the air passages in the lungs.
- Cyanosis: Bluish discoloration of the skin and mucous membranes due to insufficient oxygen.
- Defibrillation: Restoring normal heart rhythm in ventricular or atrial fibrillation.
- Defibrillator: An instrument that restores normal heart rhythm by applying a high-voltage electric current.
- Dyspnea: Difficult or labored breathing.
- Dysrhythmia: Disturbance of a regularly occurring pattern.
- Emesis: The act of vomiting.
- Epidural: Outside the dura mater. An epidural analgesia is a form of pain relief obtained by injecting a local analgesic into the epidural space to block the spinal nerves.
- Hyperpnea: Excessive but not necessarily rapid breathing, which can occur in various physiological states.
- Hypertension: Persistently high blood pressure.
- Hypotension: Persistently low blood pressure.
- Hypoxia: Inadequate oxygen in the tissues.
- Intravenous: Administered into a vein.
- Laryngitis: Inflammation of the voice box.
- Laryngospasm: A reflex prolonged contraction of the laryngeal muscles. This may be associated with the clumsy passing of endotracheal tubes.
- Narcosis: A state of stupor or unconsciousness produced by drugs.
- Neuroleptic: A drug that acts upon the nervous system.
- Premedication: Drug(s) given preoperatively to reduce fear and anxiety and to facilitate the induction, maintenance, and recovery of anesthesia.
- Pulse oximetry: Measurement of oxygen concentration in the blood.
- Sedative: A sleep-inducing drug used to lessen excitement and reduce tension.
- Soporific: Sleep-inducing.
- Tachycardia: Abnormally fast heart rate.
- Tranquillizer: A drug that eases fear and anxiety without inducing sleep.

# Chapter 17: Radiology

## Introduction

Radiology is a diagnostic aspect of medicine. It is a branch of medicine that utilizes radiation to treat and diagnose diseases. Through radiology, physicians are able to visualize and identify the internal bodily structures correctly. This imaging technology involves the use of a wide variety of advanced applications. Some of these include computerized axial tomography (CAT or CT scan), magnetic resonance imaging (MRI), positron emission tomography, ultrasound technology, and the relatively new fields of radiation oncology and nuclear medicine. Radiology is a cardinal part of improving healthcare outcomes in that the visualization of the body's internal structures is made possible, and the concerned healthcare practitioners can make a more informed diagnostic decision.

## Anatomy and Medical Terminology

The body is separated into different planes. The frontal and sagittal planes are the two most well-known planes. The anterior and posterior portions of the body are separated by the frontal plane. The right and left halves of the body are separated by the sagittal plane.

The last is the transverse, also known as the axial or horizontal plane, which divides the body into the upper (superior) and lower (inferior) halves. There is also the mid-sagittal plane, which divides the body into equal portions of right and left. The main positional terms that are of significance to the field of radiography are highlighted below.

- **Anatomic position**: The subject being erect, facing forward, having the arms rotated outward with the palms forward, the hands open with the thumbs pointed out, and the feet together.
- **Supine**: The supine position involves the patient lying on their back with face up. This position is also known as the dorsal recumbent.
- **Lateral position**: Here, the subject's side is placed next to the film. This can also be performed with the position of staying erect lateral or lateral decubitus (lying down by the side).
- **Prone position:** This refers to lying face down on the front of the body. This position is also known as the ventral recumbent.
- **Oblique position:** This position requires a bit of explaining. Here, the subject lies at an angle that cannot be described as prone or supine. For example, the right anterior oblique (RAO), left anterior oblique (LAO), right posterior oblique (RPO), or left posterior oblique (LPO). In oblique positions such as right anterior

oblique (RAO) and left anterior oblique (LAO), the terms 'anterior' and 'posterior' refer to the part of the body that is angled towards or away from the X-ray film.

The different forms of projections indicating the path of the X-ray beam are explained below.

- **Anteroposterior (AP)**: In this position, the X-ray beam enters the front of the body (anterior) and exits the back of the body (posterior).
- **Posteroanterior (PA):** In this projection, the X-ray beam enters the back of the body (posterior) and exits through the front of the body (anterior).
- **Lateral**: Here, the beam enters just one side of the body and exits through the other. Lateral projections are named after the side of the body next to the film.
- **Oblique**: In this projection, the X-ray beam enters at an angle that cannot be seen as frontal or lateral.

## Supervision and Interpretation, Imaging Guidance

In X-ray services, it is ideal for imaging to be required, especially during the performance of specific procedures. Some imaging procedures may even require mild surgical techniques to access the imaged area. It is not necessary to report image guidance services separately if they are already included in the base service.

There are also CPT codes that usually define descriptors and also serve as guidelines when imaging guidance is required. If a surgical procedure does not include imaging, the imaging guidance is labeled as 'radiological supervision and interpretation' and may be reported for the portion of the service that requires imaging.

Codes for radiologic supervision and interpretation (S&I) are utilized to denote the direct monitoring of the radiologic component of a procedure by one or more physicians and the analysis of the results. Billing for the supervision aspect of the system may be performed simultaneously or by another physician. This is mostly done to prevent mix-ups or clinical errors in the discharge of medical duties.

In some instances, the cardiologist may, for example, bill for supervision (remember the 'S') of the S&I code we mentioned earlier, and a radiologist then accounts for the interpretation (the 'I') of the code. Both physicians should also use a -52 modifier indicating a reduced service of only one supervision or performance (USC, Office of Culture and Ethics, 2014).

## The Administration of Contrast Material(s)

Contrast materials in radiology refer to using material administered intra-articularly, intrathecally, and intravascularly for imaging enhancement. For intra-articular injection, it is essential to use the appropriate joint injection code. If a radiographic arthrography is performed, make sure the arthrography supervision and interpretation code for the relevant joint are applied.

If the computed tomography or magnetic resonance arthrography is performed without radiographic arthrography, ensure to use the appropriate joint injection code, the appropriate CT or MR code ('with contrast' or 'without followed by contrast'), and the correct guidance code for needle placement for contrast injection.

Intravascular contrast material is administered during 'with contrast' CT, computed tomographic angiography (CTA), magnetic resonance imaging (MRI), and magnetic resonance angiography (MRA) examinations. Only oral and rectal administration do not qualify as a study 'with contrast.' One common use of the oral means of administering contrast in radiology is using the barium meal to provide more details when images of the digestive system are to be taken.

## Written Reports

In some circumstances, it is ideal to have written reports (handwritten or electronic) duly signed by the interpreting individual. This report should be considered an important part of a radiologic procedure or interpretation. Regarding CPT descriptors for imaging services, 'images' in the context of radiology must contain anatomical information that is considered unique to the patient for which the imaging service is provided. 'Images' in this context refers to shots or images acquired in either an analog (film) or digital (electronic) manner.

## Foreign Body/Implant Definition

In radiology, any object intentionally placed by a physician or the attending or supervisory healthcare professional for diagnostic, therapeutic, or other purposes is considered an implant. An object that is unintentionally placed, either by trauma or accidental ingestion, is regarded as a foreign body. If an implant has shifted from its original position due to trauma or structural damage, and it is no longer functional or poses a threat to the patient, it may require attention. Unless the instructions in the CPT indicate otherwise or there is a specific CPT code available to describe the removal of the broken/moved implant, this would also meet the criteria of a foreign body for coding purposes.

## Types of Radiological Services

In the CPT codebook, the radiology section is divided into the following subsections.

- Bone/Joint Studies.
- Breast, Mammography.
- Diagnostic Radiology (Diagnostic Imaging).
- Diagnostic Ultrasound.
- Nuclear Medicine.

- Radiation Oncology.
- Radiologic Guidance.

## The Components of a Radiology Service

Many codes within diagnostic radiology reports stipulate the supervision and interpretation of a service. These (S&I) codes contain both the technical and professional components. Hence, a surgeon performs a procedure, and a radiologist provides the radiological supervision and interpretation.

The surgeon reports the surgery code whenever this occurs, and the radiologist says the supervision and interpretation code. In some instances, if a physician gives the injection and another provides the imaging supervision and report, each physician should report the service that has been performed. If one physician conducts the entire procedure, the physician should register both sides.

Parenthetical instructions guide the supervision and interpretation code when looking at the surgical procedure. Always remember that the radiologist billing the supervision and interpretation must be present during the process, and there must also be a written report.

## Diagnostic Ultrasound

Diagnostic ultrasound involves using sound waves to grasp or better visualize internal structures. Different ultrasound scans exist. This includes A-mode (A-scan), B-mode (B-scan), M-mode, and real-time scans. The A-mode (amplitude mode) is a one-dimensional scan usually only seen in ophthalmic ultrasounds.

A professional medical coder must understand the different types of radiology scans to choose the appropriate codes.

Doppler ultrasound studies blood flow using sound waves that penetrate solids or liquids. Ultrasound codes can be reported as complete or limited, depending on the extent of the procedure performed.

Abdominal ultrasound scan includes the visualization of solid abdominal organs like the liver, spleen, pancreas, and kidneys. These structures are divided into intraperitoneal and retroperitoneal aspects, depending on their relationship to the peritoneum, a layer of soft tissue protecting the abdominal content. For the pelvis, ultrasound imaging is divided into obstetrics and non-obstetrical. The non-obstetrical pelvic ultrasounds are transvaginal ultrasound and ultrasound of the uterus. A transvaginal ultrasound is done early in pregnancy to visualize the early stages of pregnancy, including the embryo or fetus, and the uterus.

## CPT Coding

The CPT code range for all radiology procedures is from 70010 to 79999. Diagnostic imaging procedures are classified based on the anatomical location in which the process is carried out.

CPT codes 70010 - 70559 are for diagnostic imaging of the head and neck. These diagnostic images may be used to determine the presence of a fracture using plain X-rays of the bones of the face or jaw. These images are also applied for dental diagnosis and procedures.

Some diagnostic images are also generated to diagnose disorders associated with structures in the neck. This includes the pharynx, larynx, and other associated systems. Radiological images of the head and neck also include computed tomography (CT) scans and magnetic resonance imaging (MRI).

Codes 71045 - 71555 represent diagnostic radiology procedures of the chest. Plain chest radiographs can be obtained in different views, and the appropriate codes depend on the number of views. Other chest radiology images are computed tomography with or without contrast and magnetic resonance imaging in tumor settings.

Diagnostic imaging of the spine and pelvis is represented by 72020 - 72295, and this code range extensively covers imaging of the entire spine and pelvis as well as different modalities of diagnostic radiology applied. Other categories of diagnostic radiology procedures are those for the upper and lower extremities (73000 - 73725), abdomen (74018 - 74190), gastrointestinal tract (74210 - 74363), urinary tract (74400 - 74485), heart (75557 -75574), vascular system (75600 - 75989), and others not specified (76000 - 76499).

Gynecological and obstetrical diagnostic radiology procedures (74710 - 74775) are used intrapartum and antepartum to diagnose complications with the fetus or mother. Diagnostic ultrasound procedures are separate under code sets 76506 - 76999. The codes for ultrasound procedures are also grouped based on the anatomical locations.

Radiological guidance for delicate procedures, including fluoroscopy, computed tomography, and magnetic resonance guidance, is included within specific codes in the range 70010 - 79999, but not all codes within this range are for guidance equipment. Fluoroscopy guidance, computed tomography guidance, and magnetic resonance guidance are specifically coded in separate categories. Fluoroscopic guidance is used for inserting catheters into vessels, placing needles, and localizing previously inserted needles or catheters. A fluoroscope generates continuous X-ray images on the screen for monitoring. Computer tomography guidance is used to localize radiation beams to ensure direct targeting of tumors, placement of radiation therapy fields, and monitoring of ablation of parenchymal tissues.

Mammography and other breast-related radiological procedures are coded 77046 - 77067. Screening mammograms are always bilateral. Diagnostic mammograms can be unilateral based on the focus of symptoms. A radiologist can apply computer-aided detection to interpret diagnostic mammograms using software that analyzes prior algorithms.

Radiology can be applied to studying bones or joints (77071 - 77092) to detect abnormalities related to the growth or spread of chronic diseases such as cancer. Bone age studies are performed on children to estimate their skeletal system's maturity based on their bones' growth plate appearances. Discrepancies in bone length can also be identified using bone length studies. A dual energy X-ray absorptiometry (DEXA) scan is commonly carried out to determine bone density and screen for osteoporosis or osteopenia.

Radiology has been used to manage cancers in order to reduce the spread, and in some cases, cure the underlying cancer. Radiation oncology treatment has multiple subcategories, and these include the following:

- Clinical treatment planning for radiation treatment (77261 - 77299).
- Medical radiation physics, dosimetry, treatment devices, and special services for radiation treatment (77295 - 77370).
- Stereotactic radiation treatment delivery (77371 - 77387).
- Radiation treatment delivery (77399- 77417).
- Neutron beam treatment delivery (77423- 77425).
- Radiation treatment management (77427 - 77499).
- Proton beam radiation treatment delivery (77520- 77525).
- Radiation hyperthermia treatment (77600- 77615).
- Clinical intracavitary radiation hyperthermia treatment (77620).
- Clinical brachytherapy radiation treatment (77750 - 77799).

Nuclear medicine is the aspect of radiology that examines the use of radioactive materials and the radiation emitted from the body by these tracers to diagnose and treat diseases. Procedures associated with nuclear medicine are found in CPT code 78012 - 79999 and further classified into diagnostic and therapeutic procedures.

A radiologist billing for supervision and interpretation of a radiological procedure must be present at the time of the process and should provide a written report. Contrast materials will be coded separately from the radiological procedure using HCPCS level II. This is to be reported by the facility, except when the physician owns the equipment and the procedure is performed in the physician's office. Do not code for the difference when it is given orally or rectally.

## Modifiers

The modifiers most commonly applied when coding for radiology procedures are:

- Modifier 26 is used to indicate the professional component of a service when only the interpretation and report are provided by the physician.
- Modifier TC is the technical component of a procedure, and it includes the equipment cost and related supplies, as well as the cost of keeping a technician.

A qualified healthcare professional is expected to interpret the images generated and write a report for the patient following a procedure. A facility can bill for professional and technical components if both services are offered. Other relevant modifiers are for repeat procedures by the same physician (modifier 76) or another physician (modifier 77) and functions specific to different sides of the body (RT or LT).

## Definition of Important Terms

- Angiography: The injection of contrast material into the body to view the blood vessels.
- Brachytherapy: Using catheters, needles, and other materials to put radiation into the body.
- Cholangiography: The imaging of the bile duct system.
- Colonoscopy: The direct visualization of the colon using an endoscope passed through the rectum.
- Computed tomography: The use of special equipment to take images along an axis of the body. The photos are cross-sectional and used to study possible pathologies in the body's organs.
- Cystography: Radiographic imaging of the bladder
- Dacryocystography: Radiographic imaging of the lacrimal ducts.

- Discography: Radiographic imaging of the spinal vertebra disc.
- Dosimetry: Calculation of doses of radiation
- Doppler: An ultrasound used to examine the blood flow across specific body tissues.
- Echocardiography: The use of sound waves to generate images of the heart and all the structures within it.
- Fluoroscopy: An X-ray image generated continuously to view the movement of an injected substance through the body.
- Hysterosalpingography: A fluoroscopic procedure to view images of the uterus and fallopian tubes of a woman following the administration of contrast dye to determine the patency of the reproductive tract.
- Intravascular: Into a blood vessel, which may be an artery or a vein.
- Intrathecally: Into the subarachnoid space or cerebrospinal fluid through the vertebra.
- Intra-articular: Into a joint.
- Lymphangiography: The diagnostic imaging of the lymphatic system is generated using a special dye and imaging equipment such as X-ray or CT after the injection of a contrast dye into the lymph vessels.
- Magnetic resonance imaging: Using specified equipment to convert protons into images of the body in slices. The images are viewed in three-dimensional slides from different angles. An MRI may be performed with or without contrast.
- Myelography: Radiographic imaging of the spinal cord.
- Pyelography: Radiographic imaging of the renal pelvis following injection of radio-opaque substance through the ureters or directly into a vein.
- Sialography: Radiographic imaging of the salivary gland and ducts.
- Urography: Radiographic imaging of the kidney and ureters.
- Venography: Radiographic imaging of the veins following administration of contrast dye.

# Chapter 18: Pathology and Laboratory

## Introduction

This chapter discusses pathology and laboratory services as applied to the human body. The process or analyzed substances define these services.

The objectives of this chapter include:

- Learning key terms related to pathology and laboratory studies.
- Understanding the appropriate application of ICD-10-CM diagnosis code guidelines.
- Understanding how to report CPT codes.
- Identifying the relevant HCPCS level II codes and use of modifiers.

## Examples of Words, Prefixes, and Suffixes

- Chemopathology (Study of chemical changes in diseases):
    - Prefix: Chemo- (chemical).
    - Root: -path- (disease).
    - Suffix: -ology (study of).
- Cytogenetics (Study of chromosomes and their abnormalities):
    - Prefix: Cyto- (cell).
    - Root: Genet- (origin, development).
    - Suffix: -ics (study of).
- Cytopathology (Study of diseases at the cellular level):
    - Prefix: Cyto- (cell).
    - Root: -path- (disease).
    - Suffix: -ology (study of).
- Hematology (Study of blood and blood disorders):
    - Prefix: Hemat- (blood).
    - Root: -ology (study of).
- Histopathology (Study of tissues at the microscopic level):
    - Prefix: Histo- (tissue).
    - Root: -path- (disease).
    - Suffix: -ology (study of).
- Immunohistochemistry (Detection of antigens in tissues using antibodies):
    - Prefix: Immuno- (immune system).
    - Root: Histo- (tissue).
    - Suffix: -chemistry (study of chemical processes).

- Microbiology (Study of microorganisms):
    - Prefix: Micro- (small).
    - Root: Bio- (life).
    - Suffix: -ology (study of).
- Pathophysiology (Study of the functional changes associated with diseases):
    - Prefix: Patho- (disease).
    - Root: Physi- (nature, function).
    - Suffix: -ology (study of).
- Serology (Study of blood serum and immune responses):
  - Prefix: Sero- (serum).
  - Root: -logy (study of).
  - Suffix: None."
- Virology (Study of viruses):
    - Prefix: None.
    - Root: Vir- (virus).
    - Suffix: -ology (study of).

## Anatomy

Pathology is the study of disease conditions, specifically the causes of diseases, manifestation, progression, and effect on normal function. Laboratory refers to the tests performed in a medical laboratory. These tests are carried out on clinical specimens and provide more information on disease conditions. Laboratory tests are either quantitative or qualitative. The tests may be gross or microscopic. Gross examination of a specimen is the inspection of a specimen before slide sectioning. Microscopic examination is the examination of a specimen under a microscope.

## ICD-10-CM Coding

The ICD-10-CM diagnosis code range relevant to pathology and laboratory can be found in code range R00–R99 for symptoms, signs, and abnormal clinical and laboratory findings. R70–R79 examines abnormal findings on examination of the blood without diagnosis. These abnormal findings include:

- Elevated erythrocyte sedimentation rates and abnormality of plasma viscosity.
- Abnormal red blood cell count.
- Elevated blood glucose level.
- Abnormal serum enzyme levels (for example, transaminase and lactic acid dehydrogenase).
- Inconclusive laboratory evidence of HIV.

- Other abnormal immunological findings in serum (for example, raised antibody titer).
- Other abnormalities of plasma proteins (for example, albumin, globulin, alpha-fetoprotein).
- Findings of drugs and other substances not usually found in the blood.
- Other abnormal findings of blood chemistry.

R80–R82 covers abnormal findings on examination of urine without diagnosis. Proteinuria is the presence of protein in urine. Glycosuria is the presence of glucose in the urine.

R83–R89 is the code range for abnormal findings on examination of body fluids, substances, and tissues without diagnosis. These findings may be from analysis of cerebrospinal fluid, respiratory secretions, digestive and other abdominal secretions, fluids from male or female genital organs, and those in other body fluids and substances.

Abnormal levels of tumor markers such as cancer antigen 125, carcinoembryonic antigen, prostate-specific markers, or other tumor markers are found in the ICD-10-CM code range R97.0–R97.8 codebook. Some other important ICD-10-CM diagnosis codes relevant to this chapter can be found under the last category in the ICD-10-CM diagnosis index: Factors Influencing Health Status and Contact with Health Services (Z00–Z99).

Z00–Z13 covers codes for persons who encounter health services solely for examination. Various health conditions can be screened in categories Z11, Z12, and Z13. Blood type is reported under ICD-10-CM category Z67. Blood type can be Type A, B, O, or AB.

## CPT Coding

The Current Procedural Terminology code for Pathology and Laboratory services extends from 80047 to 89398. The services in Pathology and Laboratory are to be provided by a physician or technologists under the supervision of a primary physician. Separate entries should designate multiple procedures performed on the same day.

A service rarely provided or has unusual results may require a special report. The information provided should include a proper definition or description of events that led to the need for the procedure. Also, note the time, effort, and equipment necessary to provide the service. If a service offered is not listed in the current codebooks, the appropriate "Unlisted Code" and an accompanying special report should be indicated.

## Organ or Disease-Oriented Panels (80047–80081)

These panels have been designed solely for coding and should not be interpreted as clinical parameters. Each panel identifies the defined components of that panel, and the components are not intended to limit the performance of other tests. If there is an overlap of tests belonging to each panel, assign the code that incorporates a greater number of tests to fulfill the video definition. The remaining tests can be reported using an individual test code for each of them.

An obstetric panel (80055) is a standard group of tests carried out during antenatal booking. It includes a complete blood count, hepatitis B surface antigen, rubella antibodies, qualitative syphilis tests, antibody screening, ABO blood typing, and Rhesus D blood typing.

## Therapeutic Drug Assays (80143–80377)

A therapeutic drug assay is performed to monitor the clinical response to a known prescribed medication. The two major categories for drug testing are:

- Presumptive drug class (procedures for identifying possible use or non-use of a drug class).
- Definitive drug class (qualitative or quantitative tests for identifying possible use or non-use of a specific drug).

Therapeutic drug assays require whole blood, serum, plasma, or cerebrospinal fluid. The examination is quantitative, and coding is by the parent drug. The metabolites of the drug are included in the code.

80143 is the code assigned for the therapeutic drug assay of acetaminophen. Some codes are now out of numerical sequence. 80204–80285 are out of numerical sequence, and Drug Assay Procedures 80305–80377. Zonisamide (80203) is the last drug on the therapeutic drug assay list.

## Evocative/Suppression Testing Procedures (80400–80439)

The test panels in this sequence follow the administration of evocative or suppressive agents and the baseline and subsequent measurements of their effects on chemical constituents of interest. An example is the ACTH stimulation panel for adrenal insufficiency, which must include Cortisol (82533 x 2). The " x 2" refers to the number of times the test for a particular analyst is performed.

## Clinical Pathology Consultations (80503–80506)

A pathology clinical consultation is a service that is inclusive of a written report. A pathologist renders this in response to a request from a physician or other qualified healthcare professional related to clinical assessment, evaluation of pathology and laboratory findings, or other relevant clinical or diagnostic information that requires additional medical interpretative judgment.

When pathology and laboratory findings are reported without medical interpretative judgment, it is not considered a pathology clinical consultation. The following criteria must be met before reporting a pathology clinical consultation service:

- The pathologist renders a pathology clinical consultation at the request of a physician or other qualified healthcare professional at the same or another institution.
- The pathology clinical consultation request is related to pathology and laboratory findings or other relevant clinical or diagnostic information that requires medical interpretative judgment.

The selection of the appropriate level of pathology clinical consultation services may be based on the total time spent on the consultation date or the level of medical decision-making defined for each service rendered.

### Elements of Medical Decision-Making

The elements of medical decision-making include:

- The number and complexity of problems addressed.
- The amount and/or complexity of data to be reviewed and analyzed.
- The risk of complications and/or morbidity or mortality of patient management.

The level of medical decision-making is based on two of the three elements above. It is classified into straightforward, low, moderate, or high levels. Refer to Chapter 19 for further details.

## Urinalysis Procedures (81000–81099)

This includes laboratory services that require urine collection for dipstick analysis, microscopy, or volume measurement.

## Molecular Pathology Procedures (81105–81479)

These procedures involve nucleic acid analysis to detect genetic variants that may indicate germline conditions. It is also applied for procedures to test for histocompatibility antigens (HLA). The choice of code to be assigned depends on the specific gene that is being analyzed. There are specific guidelines that should be noted for these code sequences.

Codes 81105–81168 are followed by 81170–81189 in numerical sequence, where 81173 and 81174 fit within this range according to the CPT codebook organization. Refer to the CPT codebook for updated versions and note the other codes that are now out of numerical sequence. Compared to tier 1 treatments, tier 2 molecular pathology procedures are carried out in smaller numbers but are nonetheless therapeutically beneficial.

## Genomic Sequencing Procedures and Other Molecular Multianalyte Assays (81410–81471)

The methods for genetic analysis are described in this code set. These DNA/RNA analytic techniques simultaneously assess numerous genes or genetic areas relevant to a clinical condition. These processes might be directed toward a particular set of genes or genetic components.

## Multianalyte Assays with Algorithmic Analyses (81490–81599)

These procedures utilize multiple results from analysis panels of different types. This includes molecular pathology, fluorescent in-situ hybridization, and non-nucleic-based assays.

The format for code description of Multianalyte Assays with Algorithmic Analyses should include the following in the correct order:

- Disease type.
- Materials analyzed.
- Number of markers.
- Methodology.
- Number of functional domains.
- Specimen type.
- Algorithm result type.
- Report.

## Chemistry Procedures (82009–84999)

Examination materials can be from any source unless otherwise specified in the description provided for the code. The test is usually quantitative unless otherwise specified.

## Hematology and Coagulation Procedures (85002–85999)

Bleeding time is reported using the appropriate code based on the specific procedure performed. For example, the Duke method and the Ivy method for measuring bleeding time might have different codes. Refer to the segment covering transfusion medicine for blood banking procedures.

## Immunology Procedures (86000–86849)

This code range covers all procedures relevant to immunology and autoimmune conditions and includes some specific antibody and antigen testing as well as tissue typing services.

## Transfusion Medicine Procedures (86850–86999)

This code range covers all screening tests on collected blood and blood products prepared for transfusion procedures.

## Microbiology Procedures (87003–87999)

This code range includes bacteriology, mycology, parasitology and virology. There are two forms of identification of microorganisms: Presumptive and Definitive identification.

- Presumptive identification of microorganisms is defined as the identification of colony morphology and growth on selective media or gram stain.
- Definitive identification is the identification of an organism up to the genus or species level, which would require additional testing.

## Anatomic Pathology Procedures (88000–88099)

Include more than just postmortem exam services; they also encompass various surgical pathology procedures performed on surgical specimens and biopsies. Modifier 90 is used for lab tests performed by a party other than the treating or reporting physician.

## Cytopathology Procedures (88104–88199)

These procedures involve examining cells from bodily tissues or fluids to determine a diagnosis. More specific details are found in each code listed in this category.

## Cytogenetic Studies (88230–88299)

Cytogenetic studies are the branch of biology that focuses on the study of chromosomes and their inheritance. It explains the roles of chromosomes in disease and heredity.

## Surgical Pathology Procedures (88300–88399)

A specimen is a submitted tissue that requires examination and pathologic diagnosis. If two or more specimens are collected from the same patient, each should be assigned an individual code to indicate the proper level of service rendered. The services are divided into Levels I–VI. The codes are specific to collected specimens.

## In Vivo Laboratory Procedures (88720–88749)

The code stands for laboratory services carried within a living person. It includes transcutaneous testing procedures.

## Other Pathology and Laboratory Procedures (89049–89240)

Refer to this code range for other procedures not found in different sequences.

## Reproductive Medicine Procedures (89250–89398)

All procedures relevant to reproductive medicine are found among these coding sequences.

## Proprietary Laboratory Analysis (PLA) CPT codes

Proprietary Laboratory Analysis (PLA) CPT codes are an addition to the standard CPT code set for laboratories and manufacturers that wish to identify their tests more specifically. The American Medical Association CPT editorial panel has approved this alphanumeric code set, which can be found between code range 0001U–0419U. An example is PLA code 0061U, which describes BCR–ABL1 major and minor breakpoints fusion transcripts by the University of Iowa Department of Pathology on whole blood or bone marrow aspiration specimens.

## HCPCS Coding

The Healthcare Common Procedure Coding System codes set specifically for Pathology and Laboratory services are P2028–P9615.

- P2028–P2038: Laboratory tests of blood and hair.
- P3000–P3001: Pap Smears.
- P7001: Urine Bacterial Culture and Sensitivity Study.
- P9010–P9100: Blood and Blood Products, with Associated Procedures.
- P9603–P9604: Specimen Collection, Travel Allowance.
- P9612–P9615: Specimen Collection, Catheterisation.

## Modifiers

The majority of modifiers used specifically for pathology and laboratory CPT codes include the following:

- Modifier 9: Reference (outside) laboratory. This Modifier is used when any party other than the primary physician or qualified healthcare personnel performs a laboratory test.
- Modifier 91: Repeat Clinical Laboratory test. This Modifier is applied when the same laboratory test is repeated on the same day on the same patient to obtain multiple results. It is important to note that this Modifier does not apply for a rerun of tests to confirm initial tests due to technical problems or for other reasons when a normal single result is required. This Modifier is also approved for hospital outpatient use.
- Modifier 92: Alternative Laboratory Platform testing. This Modifier applies when a transportable kit or instrument performs the exact laboratory testing to be reported. The instrument consists of a whole or partial single-use disposable analytical chamber.

## Definition of Important Terms

- Abscess: A collection of pus in a small cavity following bacterial infiltration of damaged tissue.
- Agglutination: Abnormal clumping together of cells, especially within blood or blood products.
- Anaplasia: The loss of differentiation of cells within a tissue.
- Antigen: A protein that causes an immunological response when introduced into the body.
- Apoptosis: The programmed death of cells.

- Bacteremia: The presence of bacteria within the blood.
- Benign: Favorable, not malignant.
- Biopsy: The removal of tissue from a living body for examination to establish a diagnosis.
- Blood Urea Nitrogen: The serum concentration of urea, an indicator of renal function.
- Caseous: Cheese-like.
- Coagulate: Causing clot by converting a liquid into a gel or solid.
- Congestion: Abnormal accumulation of fluid in a tissue.
- Creatinine: An amino acid serving as an energy source for muscles. Blood levels indicate renal function.
- Cytology: The study of cell structure, function, and pathology related to cells.
- Edema: Excess fluid accumulation.
- Exudate: Fluid in the body with a high concentration of cellular debris following inflammation.
- Fibrin: An insoluble protein essential for blood clot formation.
- Granuloma: Small aggregation of inflammatory cells.
- Hematology: The study of blood and its components.
- Hematoxylin: A histological stain derived from the logwood tree that is used to stain cell nuclei blue in tissue sections.
- Hematoxylin and Eosin: A staining method used for examining tissues.
- Immunology: The study of the immune system and its functions.
- Metabolism: The chemical processes within a living organism to maintain life.
- Microbiology: The study of microorganisms.
- Molecular Diagnostics: The measurement of DNA, RNA, or other metabolites to detect abnormal changes.
- Mycology: The study of fungal organisms.
- Necrosis: The death of cells or tissues due to injury, disease, or lack of blood supply.
- Neoplasm: An abnormal mass or tumor resulting from uncontrolled cell growth.
- Oncology: The study and treatment of tumors or cancer.
- Panel: A group of tests performed together.
- Parasitology: The study of parasites.
- Pathogen: A microorganism or agent causing disease.
- Pathology: The study of the nature and causes of diseases.
- Plasma: The liquid blood component that carries cells and other substances throughout the body.
- Prognosis: The likely course and outcome of a disease.
- Qualitative: Tests to determine the presence of a substance in a given sample.
- Quantitative: Tests to detect the amount of a substance in a sample.

- Semi-quantitative: Tests that identify the amount of a substance within a specified range but do not recognize the specific quantity of the substance in the given sample.
- Serology: The study of blood serum, especially immune responses and antibodies.
- Thrombus: A blood clot that has developed inside a blood vessel and is still attached to its original location.
- Virology: The study of viruses.

# Chapter 19: Evaluation and Management

## Introduction

Evaluation and management (E/M) codes are essential in determining the provider's services a patient will assess. It includes an assessment of the patient's condition and the management plan for the patient.

## Categorization of E/M Services

E/M services are categorized regardless of whether they are outpatient or inpatient care. First, the patients are classified as either *new* or *established*. This is based on CPT Guidelines, which asserts that:

- **New patient**: This patient has not received any professional services from a physician, other qualified healthcare provider, or another physician or other healthcare provider of the same specialty or subspecialty who is a member of the same group practice during the previous three (3) years.
- **Established patient**: This patient has received professional services from a physician, another qualified healthcare professional, or another physician or other qualified healthcare professional of the same specialty and subspecialty who belongs to the same group practice within the past three years.

It is important to note that *where* the patient is seen does not impact categorization as new or established. When working with physicians, advanced practice nurses and physician assistants are considered to be working in the same specialty and subspecialty as the physician.

## Key Components for Determining Overall E/M Service Level

- Patient's history.
- Examination.
- Level of medical decision-making.

### <u>Patient History</u>

This is the section that tells us the patient's details. A patient's history can be divided into three sections:

- History of presenting illness.
- Review of systems.
- Past, family, and social history.

## History of Presenting Complaint (HPI)

This evaluates/elaborates the complaint of the patient and may include references to the location of the symptom, when symptoms started, severity (usually graded on a scale of 1–10), associated complaints, what worsens or makes it better (modifying factors), and any pattern to symptom or relation to any time of the day.

## Review of System

This is the section where the physician addresses other body parts or systems that have been/might be affected by the presenting complaint.

## Past Family and Social History

This assesses the patient's past medical history and presence of any pre-existing health conditions, family history of health conditions, and the use of alcohol or tobacco.

## Examination

This is the physical or clinical assessment of the patient's bodily parts or affected areas. The organs and systems are systematically organized. Hence, the approach to examination is usually either as body areas (head (including face), neck, chest (including breast, axilla, and extremities), abdomen, genitalia, groin, back (including spine)), or organ system (cardiovascular, respiratory, genitourinary, musculoskeletal, ear, nose, and throat (ENT)). All these respective systems will be addressed later in appropriate sections of this study guide.

In the selection of an Evaluation and Management code, you must ascertain that the physician or health care professional has conducted a medically appropriate examination for the patient based on their complaint.

## Levels of Medical Decision-Making

This is the process by which a physician or qualified healthcare practitioner can establish a diagnosis, evaluate the patient's clinical status, and select the appropriate management plan. The four different levels of Medical Decision-Making are:

- Straightforward.
- Low.
- Moderate.
- High.

Three elements must be considered in determining the MDM Level for a patient.

- The number and complexity of problems addressed during the visit.
- The amount and/or complexity of data to be reviewed/analyzed. This considers test results, medical records, and discussion of care plans with a physician or other qualified healthcare professional.
- The risk of complications, morbidity, or mortality associated with patient management. This includes all considered care options, irrespective of whether this was ultimately selected for the patient.
- In deciding to place a case into an MDM level, it must meet or exceed at least two elements for that level.

| Element | The Problem Addressed During the Visit | Amount and Complexity of Data to Be Reviewed | Risk of Complications, and/or Morbidity or Mortality |
|---|---|---|---|
| **Straight** | • Minimal.<br>• **1** (one) self-limited or minor problem. | Minimal or none. | Minimal risk of morbidity from additional diagnostic testing or treatment. |
| **Low** | Low.<br><br>• **2** or more self-limited or minor problems.<br>• **1** stable chronic illness.<br>• **1** acute uncomplicated illness or injury.<br>• **1** stable acute illness.<br>• **1** acute uncomplicated illness or injury requiring hospital inpatient or observation level of care. | Limited.<br><br>Must meet the requirement for at least 1 out of 2 categories:<br><br>**Category 1:** Tests and documents.<br><br>Any combination of 2 of the following:<br><br>• Review of prior external notes from each unique source.<br>• Review of the result(s) of each unique test.<br>• Ordering of each unique test.<br><br>**Category 2:** Assessment requiring an independent historian. | Low risk of morbidity from additional diagnostic testing or treatment. |
| **Moderate** | Moderate. | Moderate. | Moderate risk of morbidity from |

| | | | |
|---|---|---|---|
| | • **1** (one) or more chronic illnesses with exacerbation, progression, or side effects from treatment.<br>• **2** or more stable, chronic illnesses.<br>• **1** undiagnosed new problem with unknown prognosis.<br>• **1** acute illness with systemic symptoms.<br>• **1** acute complicated injury. | Must meet the requirement for at least 1 out of 3 categories:<br><br>**Category 1:** Tests, documents, and independent historian(s).<br><br>Any combination of 3 of the following:<br><br>• Review of prior external notes from each unique source.<br>• Review of the results of each unique test.<br>• Ordering of unique test.<br>• Assessment requiring independent historian.<br><br>**Category 2:** Independent interpretation of test.<br><br>• The independent analysis of a test conducted by a different medical doctor or other licensed healthcare provider (not separately recorded).<br><br>**Category 3:** | additional diagnostic testing or treatment. |

| | | | |
|---|---|---|---|
| | | Discussion of management or test interpretation.<br><ul><li>Consulting with a competent healthcare professional, external doctor, or other suitable authority on management or test interpretation (not separately recorded).</li></ul> | |
| **High** | <ul><li>**1** (one) or more chronic illnesses with severe exacerbation, progression, or side effects of treatment.</li><li>**1** acute or chronic illness or injury threatens life or bodily function.</li></ul> | Extensive.<br><br>Must meet the requirement for at least 2 out of 3 categories:<br><br>**Category 1:** Tests, documents, and independent historian(s).<br><br>Any combination of 3 of the following:<br><ul><li>Review of prior external notes from each unique source.</li><li>Review of the results of each unique test.</li><li>Ordering of unique test.</li><li>Assessment</li></ul> | High risk of morbidity from additional diagnostic testing or treatment. |

| | | | |
|---|---|---|---|
| | | requiring independent historian.<br><br>**Category 2:** Independent interpretation of test.<br><br>• The independent analysis of a test conducted by a different medical doctor or other licensed healthcare provider (not separately recorded).<br><br>**Category 3:** Discussion of management or test interpretation.<br><br>• Consulting with a competent healthcare professional, external doctor, or other suitable authority on management or test interpretation (not separately recorded). | |

## Time-Based MDM Level Coding

When time is used as the criteria for coding, it includes the time spent by the physician or other qualified healthcare professionals in face-to-face interaction with the patient and/or relatives. It also includes the non-face-to-face time spent by the physician and/or other qualified healthcare professionals on the day of the encounter. The time included is that spent by the physician or other health care professional irrespective of their location. For services ≥ 55 minutes, the prolonged service code 99417 is used with CPT codes 99205 and 99215 for office or other outpatient services when the service provided exceeds the typical service time.

Only CPT code 99211 should be reported for office and outpatient services in which the duration spent by the physician or other qualified health care professional supervised by clinical staff evaluating the patient during the encounter.

Time is not a criterion for the emergency department. Emergency physicians may manage many patients simultaneously over an extended period. The fact that emergency physicians usually provide services on a variable intensity basis also renders time-based coding non-feasible.

## Service Locations

### Office and Outpatient Services

These services are those performed either in the office or on an outpatient basis. It is important to note that all patients are classified as outpatients UNTIL they are admitted into a healthcare facility when they transition to inpatient care. This could be a hospital or a nursing home.

These patients are usually stable, ambulatory (moving alone), or suffering from relatively minor health conditions. The service delivery is usually face-to-face with the physician and/or other qualified health professional. The office and outpatient services encounters are covered by CPT codes 99202–99215.

### Coding for Outpatient Services

In E/M coding for the above-stated services, there is a need for categorization of the patient into new or established, medically appropriate history and examination, leveled Medical Decision Making (MDM), and/or a document note stating the total time spent on the day of the encounter.

| | Code | Medical Decision-Making | Time |
|---|---|---|---|
| **New patient** | 99202 | Straightforward | 15–29 mins |
| | 99203 | Low | 30–44 mins |
| | 99204 | Moderate | 45–59 mins |
| | 99205 | High | 60–74 mins |
| **Established patient** | 99212 | Straightforward | 10–19 mins |
| | 99213 | Low | 20–29 mins |
| | 99214 | Moderate | 30–39 mins |
| | 99215 | High | 40–54 mins |

## Hospital Observation and Inpatient Services

A patient is placed in observation status within a hospital setting when the physician is uncertain whether this patient will need further care and management on admission or can be discharged home safely. According to CMS guidelines, observation status lasts less than 48 hours, but there are instances where observation can extend beyond 48 hours based on clinical judgment and the specifics of a patient's condition. The decision to admit a patient as an inpatient should be based on the medical necessity of hospitalization and not solely on the duration of the stay in observation. After this period, the patient can be discharged home or admitted for inpatient care.

Inpatient care refers to a patient's admission into a hospital or nursing home for treatment. Unlike the hospital observation admission status, inpatient care can last as long as needed for the patient. The initial coding for patients being observed or treated within a hospital requires detailed clinical history and examination, a level of medical decision-making, and/or a document note stating the total time spent to determine the appropriate code.

| | Code | Medical Decision-Making | Time |
|---|---|---|---|
| **Initial visit** | 99221 | Straightforward and Low | 40 mins |
| | 99222 | Moderate | 55 mins |
| | 99223 | High | 75 mins |
| **Subsequent visit** | 99231 | Straightforward and Low | 25 mins |
| | 99232 | Moderate | 35 mins |
| | 99233 | High | 50 mins |

When services for the first set of hospital inpatient or observation treatment are more than 90 minutes, and/or when services for the subsequent hospital inpatient or observation care are more than 65 minutes, use prolonged service code 99418 for each additional 15 minutes of the total time. This should be used in conjunction with CPT codes 99223 and 99233.

Certain factors may require you to change the inpatient code accounted for. Use CPT code 99477 for neonates (≤ 28 days) needing intensive observation or inpatient care. This includes intensive care.

CPT consultation codes 99241-99255 were no longer recognized by Medicare and many other payers for outpatient or inpatient consults. Healthcare providers should use the appropriate outpatient or inpatient service codes instead, depending on the encounter's specific circumstances. Use CPT codes·99231 to 99233 for subsequent hospital inpatient or observation care. Use the codes 99234 to 99236 for a patient admitted and discharged from inpatient or observation status on the same day.

## Discharge Service

Discharge codes are used when a patient is cleared to leave the hospital at the end of an observation period or treatment. The final code accounts for the final examination of the patient, the discussion of the hospital stay, preparation of necessary referral forms, discharge notes, and prescriptions. The determining factor of the code to use is the *amount of time* used for the procedure.

For inpatient or observation patient discharge day management on the day of discharge by the physician or other qualified healthcare professional offering discharge services, use CPT code 99238 if ≤ 30 minutes. Use CPT code 99239 if > 30 minutes. These do not apply if the patient was discharged on the same day. Address coding as discussed earlier in cases of same-day discharge.

## Consultation

A consult is a form of evaluation and management service that involves inviting another specialist, physician, or appropriate health practitioner to assist the initial service provider in optimal care for the patient. A consult is coded only if initiated by the physician or other appropriate source, not by the patient or their relatives. Consultation coding requires a medically appropriate history and examination, a Medical Decision-Making level, and the total duration of time to ensure proper coding.

| | Code | Medical Decision-Making | Time |
|---|---|---|---|
| **Office-based** | 99242 | Straightforward | 20 mins |
| | 99243 | Low | 30 mins |
| | 99244 | Moderate | 40 mins |
| | 99245 | High | 55 mins |
| **Inpatient** | 99252 | Straightforward | 35 mins |
| | 99253 | Low | 45 mins |
| | 99254 | Moderate | 60 mins |
| | 99255 | High | 80 mins |

## Emergency Department Services

The emergency department is an organized hospital-based facility that provides unscheduled, episodic services to patients who need immediate medical attention. The services of the emergency department must be available 24 hours a day.

The codes here report evaluation and management services implemented in the emergency department. Here, there is no distinction between new and established patients. Also, the total time spent is not considered in determining the level of service. The codes are as shown below.

| Code | Decision-Making |
|---|---|
| 99282 | Straightforward |
| 99283 | Low |
| 99284 | Moderate |
| 99285 | High |

**Critical Care Services**

Critical care provides patients who are seriously ill or wounded with direct medical treatment. A patient who has a critical disease or injury faces an immediate or potentially fatal deterioration in their physical condition due to an unexpected failure of the functioning of one or more organs. Highly complex and specialized decision-making is required in critical care to identify and address any life-threatening harm or worsening in the patient's clinical state.

In coding critical care services, the most important factor to consider is the duration of time. The primary code 99291 is used for the first 30–74 minutes. The code 99292 is used to report each additional 30 minutes after the first 74 minutes. This primary critical service code should be used only once daily. For a patient who received 110 minutes of critical care, the coding would be as follows:

First 74 minutes – 99291.

Remaining 36 minutes – 99292 X 1.

The appropriate code will then be: 99291 X 1 AND 99292 X 1.

## Nursing Facilities

These codes are used to evaluate and manage patients in inpatient care. This includes long-term care facilities, intermediate care facilities, and rehabilitative facilities. These services usually provide multidisciplinary patient care plans and are accessible 24 hours daily.

Use the codes 99238 or 99239 for a patient discharged from inpatient or observation care in a nursing facility on the same day. A patient might be admitted into a nursing facility during an encounter in another facility (hospital or non-hospital). In this case, all Evaluation and Management services on that admission are considered part of the initial nursing facility care if performed on the same day.

The nursing facility care codes require a medically appropriate history and examination, level of medical decision-making, and the duration of time on the encounter date. When using the total duration of the encounter, the time for each code must either be met or exceeded for it to be appropriate.

| | Code | Medical Decision-Making | Time |
|---|---|---|---|
| **Initial visit** | 99304 | Low | 25 mins |
| | 99305 | Moderate | 35 mins |
| | 99306 | High | 45 mins |
| **Subsequent visits** | 99307 | Straightforward | 10 mins |
| | 99308 | Low | 15 mins |
| | 99309 | Moderate | 30 mins |
| | 99310 | High | 45 mins |

For services ≥ 60 minutes, use prolonged service code 99418 with CPT codes 99306 and 99310 for each additional 15 minutes.

## Home or Residence Services

These codes report evaluation and management services provided in a home or residence. This may be a private residential home, temporary lodging, or short-term accommodation (hotels, hostels, cruise ships). This applies to assisted living accommodation, group homes, and custodian care facilities.

In the selection of code level based on time, the travel time is not considered. Also, the time for the code level must be met or exceeded.

The home and residence services require a medically appropriate history and/or examination with the proper medical decision level to ensure the correct code is used.

| | Code | Medical Decision Making | Time |
|---|---|---|---|
| **New patient** | 99341 | Straightforward | 15 mins |
| | 99342 | Low | 30 mins |
| | 99444 | Moderate | 60 mins |
| | 99345 | High | 75 mins |
| **Established patient** | 99347 | Straightforward | 20 mins |
| | 99348 | Low | 30 mins |
| | 99349 | Moderate | 40 mins |
| | 99350 | High | 60 mins |

Service time ≥ 90 minutes for a new patient or ≥ 75 minutes for an established patient is said to be prolonged. In this case, the prolonged service code 99417 should be used alongside CPT codes 99345 and 99350 for each additional 15 minutes of total time.

## Neonatal and Pediatric Care

This refers to evaluation and management codes that report services provided to newborns (≤ 28 days of life). E/M services for the newborn include fetal/newborn and maternal history, newborn physical examination, diagnostic tests and treatments, family meetings, and medical documentation. When additional intensive care or critical care service is received by a newborn on the same day as the normal newborn services were provided, report the appropriate E/M code for these services with modifier 25 alongside the newborn service code.

For E/M of a normal newborn infant in an initial hospital (or birthing center care), use the code 99460. For subsequent hospital care per day, use 99462. However, if the newborn infant service was received within one date with subsequent discharge on the same day, use the service code 99463.

## Delivery/Birthing Room Attendance and Resuscitation Services

This is also included in the newborn care services and includes the attendance of a physician or other qualified health care professional during the delivery to provide the initial stabilization of the newborn. The CPT code 99464 is used for this service. This code (99464) may be reported with 99221, 99222, 99460, 99468, and 99477.

Suppose the physician or healthcare professional is required to perform CPR on the newborn post-delivery as a result of respiratory or cardiac inadequacy. In that case, the CPT code 99465 is used. This code is intended to report the provision of CPR and should not be reported in conjunction with attendance at delivery (99464). If both delivery attendance and CPR are provided, only 99465 should be reported, as it encompasses the critical care nature of the service provided.

## Intensive Care

### Pediatric Critical Care Patient Transport

Usually, there might be a need for interfacility transportation of a critically ill or critically injured pediatric patient. CPT codes 99466 and 99467 are used to report the physical presence and face-to-face care during the interfacility transport of a critically ill or critically injured pediatric patient ≤ 24 months.

99466 is used to report the first 30–74 minutes of direct face-to-face time with the transport pediatric patient. Code 99467 is used for each additional 30 minutes on a given date. Pediatric transport services should be at least 30 minutes of face-to-face physician care to use CPT codes 99466 and 99467. Codes 99485 and 99486 are used to report the control physician's non-face-to-face supervision of the inter-facility transportation of a critically ill or critically injured pediatric patient ≤ 24 months.

### Inpatient Neonatal Intensive Care Services and Pediatric and Neonatal Critical Care Services

The neonatal intensive care services and pediatric and neonatal critical care services code are used when a critically ill neonate (≤ 28 days of life) or a pediatric patient (> 28 days up to 24 months) is admitted into the neonatal intensive care unit, or pediatric intensive care unit respectively. Pediatric critical care codes 99471–99476 apply to patients from 29 days to less than 18 years of age. The codes for these services are classified by age as below:

- ≤ 28 days.
- 29 days–24 months.
- 2 years–5 years.

The codes 99468 and 99469 report inpatient intensive care services for a critically ill neonate. Codes 99471–99476 are used to report the services of directing inpatient intensive care for a critically ill pediatric patient from 29 days of life up to 5 years of age.

For these patients, different codes are used based on different services and interventions offered during the admission. These could include the following:

- Vascular access procedures.
- Airway and ventilatory management.
- Monitoring or interpretation of blood gases and oxygen saturation.
- Oral or nasogastric tube placement.
- Transfusion of blood components.
- Car seat evaluation, lumbar puncture.
- Bladder catheterization.
- Suprapubic bladder aspiration.

Aside from those mentioned above, all other services must be reported separately.

## Continuing Intensive Care Services

This is used in the inpatient care of a child who is not critically ill but requires intensive observation, intervention, and continued care. Aside from the initial CPT code, the code for subsequent days depends on the child's weight. These codes are reported once per day unless there is an improvement in the condition of the neonate or infant to warrant discontinuing intensive care.

| | **Code** | **Weight** |
|---|---|---|
| **Initial care** | 99477 | |
| **Subsequent day(s) care** | 99478 | Very low birth weight (< 1500 grams) |
| | 99479 | Low birth weight (1500–2500 grams) |
| | 99480 | High birth weight (>2500 grams) |

## Care Management Evaluation and Management Services

Care management E/M services are management and support services provided to patients at home, rest home, domiciliary, or assisted living facility. These patients may have a single disease condition or multiple chronic conditions. Care management services help improve care coordination and patient engagement while decreasing care fragmentation.

The physician or other qualified health care professionals provide these coordination services. These include care plan monitoring, care coordination by other professionals and agencies, and patient/relative education about the condition, care plan, and prognosis.

There are three categories of care management services:

- Principal care management.
- Chronic care management.
- Complex chronic care management.

Chronic and complex chronic care management addresses the patient's medical conditions. This includes psychosocial needs and activities of daily living. Principal care management addresses only a single condition and is a disease-specific management service.

## Coding for Care Management Services

Principal care management codes are 99424–99427. Required elements for principal care management coding include the following:

- One complex condition is expected to last three months and puts the patient at significant risk of hospitalization, acute exacerbation/ decompensation, functional decline, or death.
- The condition requires the creation, observation, and revision of a disease-specific care plan.
- The condition requires frequent adjustment in the patient medication regimen.
- Continuous collaboration and communication between relevant practitioners involved in care.

The first 30 minutes of services are provided *personally* by a physician or other qualified health care practitioner (99424) or *directed* by a physician or other qualified health care practitioner (99426) each calendar month. 99425 and 99427 are add-on codes used for each additional 30 minutes by a physician or other health care professional per calendar month.

Required elements for chronic care management and complex chronic care management coding:

- Presence of multiple chronic conditions that last for 12 months or until the death of the patient.
- Chronic conditions that place a patient at significant risk of death, acute exacerbation, or functional decline.
- A detailed plan of care that is executed, updated, or monitored.

There is one additional element for complex care management, which is:

- Medical decision-making of moderate or high complexity.

Every calendar month, a doctor or other trained healthcare practitioner provides at least 20 minutes of chronic care management (99490). A doctor or other trained healthcare professional is responsible for the first 60 minutes of clinical staff time each calendar month for complex chronic care management (99487).

For every additional 30 minutes after the initial 30 minutes for chronic care services, use the add-on code 99437. For every additional 30 minutes after the initial 60 minutes for complex chronic care services, use the add-on code 99489.

## Preventive Medicine Services

This is used for described E/M services offered to patients without any complaint, clinical signs, or illness. An age-appropriate comprehensive exam is done here, which is different from the comprehensive exam obtainable with other E/M code categories, as the extent and focus of the services depend to a large extent on the age of the patient.

Preventive medical service codes are from 99381 through 99397. They are selected based on the patient's age and whether the patient is established or new.

There are two subcategories of Preventive Medicine which are:

- Counseling/Risk factor reduction interventions.
- Behavior change intervention.

### Counseling/Risk Factor Reduction Interventions

This is used for the services provided to the patient to prevent risky behavior they currently participate in from developing further or causing injury to them and others. The code selection depends on the duration of face-to-face interaction with the patient and whether this service is provided to only one person or a group.

**Behavior Change Interventions**

These are individual services provided to patients with established risky behavior. Some programs that could be offered here include smoking cessation and substance abuse counseling. The appropriate code to use here is determined by the substance and the time spent with the patient. The payment for preventive medical services depends on different payers' payment policies. Medicare provides coverage for specific preventive services under the Affordable Care Act, but it does not cover all services coded with Preventive Medicine CPT codes 99381 through 99397. Many commercial policies may cover a broader range of preventive visits than Medicare.

## Transitional Care

Transitional care management services are E/M services for patients whose medical or psychosocial problems require moderate or high-level medical decision-making. This decision-making is usually required during their transition from an inpatient setting (acute or long term), partial hospital, observation status, and skilled nursing facility to a community setting (patient's home, rest home, or assisted living).

Transition care management commences on the discharge date and continues till 29 days after. It comprises at least one face-to-face visit within the timeframe with subsequent non-face-to-face services performed by the physician, other qualified healthcare professionals, or other licensed clinical staff under their direction. CPT Codes 99495 and 99496 are used for reporting transitional care.

Some elements are required by the CPT guidelines to use the transitional care procedure coding:

- Communication via direct, electronic, or telephone contact with the patient or caregiver within two business days of discharge.
- Medical Decision-Making of moderate (code 99495) or high (code 99496) level within the service period.
- Face-to-face visit within seven days (code 99496) or 14 days (code 99495).

Note: To code 99496, the level of Medical Decision-Making must be high, and the face-to-face visit must be within seven days of the discharge. Otherwise, use 99495 if other elements are met.

## Case Management

Case management services are the E/ M procedures used when a physician or other qualified healthcare professional directly cares for a patient and coordinates other healthcare services as needed. This usually involves face-to-face or indirect conferences between the physician, their team of healthcare professionals, the patient, and their relatives. The codes used in this case separate non-physician qualified healthcare professionals from physicians.

# Chapter 20: Medicine

## Introduction

This chapter contains codes that describe therapeutic and diagnostic services in every specialty. These services are those confirmed not to be included in radiology and pathological services. Procedures listed under medicine are minimally invasive or non-invasive. The code range for medical services and procedures is found in the CPT codebook between 90281 and 99607.

## Immunoglobulins, Serum or Recombinant Products

90281–90399

Immunoglobulins are proteins produced by plasma cells of the body that perform an essential role in the immune system by attaching to foreign substances and enhancing their destruction. This section covers the codes for the products used in conferring immunity against specific disease conditions. The codes are listed as add-ons in conjunction with the service to be reported. An important example is the Rho D from healthy human volunteers who have undergone specified immunity against the rhesus antigen. Immunoglobulin is administered to women to prevent sensitization and development of hemolytic disease in newborns. When reporting the service, 90384 is the appropriate code to use.

## Immunization Administration for Vaccines/Toxoids

90460–90474

The code of a particular immunization administration should be reported alongside the code for the specific vaccine/toxoid. It is essential to consider factors that influence vaccine administration, such as the type of vaccine, the age of the patient, and the point of entry during the vaccine administration. A vaccine's entry point can be oral, intranasal, intramuscular, intradermal, subcutaneous, percutaneous, or intravesical. The appropriate description should be included while reporting the code.

## Vaccines/Toxoid (Substances)

90476–90759

The codes for vaccine/toxoid are reported to describe the substance of the vaccine/toxoid products only. The SARS-CoV-2 vaccines are described under a new category of codes 91304–91322 as vaccine products administered intramuscularly to prevent or reduce the risk of contracting COVID-19.

Other vaccines/toxoids are found under existing codes 90476–90759. An example is the meningococcal recombinant lipoprotein vaccine, administered into the intramuscular layer as a preventive intervention against meningococcal diseases such as *Neisseria meningitides* (coded 90621). This vaccine is part of a dose schedule and administered in children ten years and above and older adults at risk for the disease. The American Medical Association maintains this code set.

## Psychiatry

90785–90899

Psychiatric services such as psychotherapy, behavior modification, and addictive disease therapy are found in code set 90785–90899. The choice of code largely depends on the time spent with the patient, the type of psychotherapy carried out, and the location of the therapy.

If pharmacologic management is provided during the management of a psychiatric patient, the service is included in the primary psychotherapy or evaluation and management code and should not be reported separately with code 90863, as this code was deleted and is no longer used in the CPT code set. The medical code 90785 is used for interactive complexity psychiatry services and procedures. Diagnostic Evaluation Services are found in medical code 90791–90792 and depend on whether the medical provider renders additional medical services when making a diagnosis.

### Other Psychotherapy Procedures

Providing insight into an individual's unconscious motivations and conflict sources by use of technical analysis to cause a change in maladaptive techniques the individual has developed over time – 90845. Group psychotherapy (for a selected group of not more than 12 patients who do not belong to the same family in a group session that lasts 45–60 minutes) – 90853. Psychotherapy involving a group of patients' families – 90849.

Counseling of an individual patient alongside their family based on psychological issues that affect them to evaluate the treatment plan as well as the role of the family in treatment – 90847. Counseling of a patient's family without the patient in attendance to properly examine the psychological issues that affect them – 90846. Other psychiatric services or procedures are found in code set 90863–90899.

In a crisis where a patient is in a life-threatening situation that requires immediate attention, a medical provider may institute an intervention of psychotherapy that lasts between 30–74 minutes. A provider may perform an add-on service for 30 minutes following the psychotherapy intervention. Both services rendered during a crisis are between medical codes 90839 and 90840.

## Biofeedback

90901–90913

These codes are reported in cases where a medical provider trains a patient on control of involuntary functions of the body by altering brain activity and other parts of the body that would usually not require voluntary control.

This service is provided in conditions such as urinary or fecal incontinence or retraining muscle groups during physiotherapy. If a manometry or EMG is performed, it should be included in this service. Each additional 15 minutes of biofeedback training is reported in conjunction with the primary code as an add-on code.

## Dialysis

90935–90999

Dialysis is a renal replacement therapy instituted following the failure of the kidney to filter waste products and toxins using artificial equipment. Hemodialysis (90935–90940) is the drawing of blood into an artificial catheter and passing it through a semipermeable membrane to remove the toxins before transfusing the blood back into the body. The provider may also perform an E/M service related to the dialysis on the same day, and an appropriate code is assigned. The services for managing End-Stage Renal Disease are in code 90951–90970.

## Gastroenterology

91010–91322

Studies of the upper gastrointestinal tract motility are found in code set 91010–91022. These services include using a manometer to monitor the pressure and movement of esophageal, stomach, or duodenal muscles in a patient with gastroesophageal reflux disease or to diagnose abnormal stomach or small intestine function. Other procedures and services directly related to the gastrointestinal system are in code set 91030–91299.

## Ophthalmology

92002–92499

General ophthalmologic services and procedures are divided into those applicable to new patients (92002–92004) and established patients (92012–92014).

Contact lens services (92310–92326) are offered for patients who have had prior cataract surgery or require a change in their contact lens prescription by a provider or an independent technician that a medical provider may supervise.

Spectacles are offered in procedures under code set 92340–92371, which cover prostheses for aphakia. Eyeglasses fitting may be a bifocal, trifocal, or multifocal lens to correct visual defects. Implantation of prosthetic lenses in patients who undergo cataract surgery to remove the intraocular lens may be performed by a medical provider and reported under the code set as applicable.

## Otorhinolaryngology

92502–92700

This includes services rendered to diagnose or evaluate patients with primary diseases affecting the ear, nose, and throat or those resulting from secondary complications. Services related to otorhinolaryngology include:

- Audiologic Function Tests.
- Evaluative and Therapeutic Otorhinolaryngologic Services.
- Nasopharyngoscopy, Nasal Study, and Facial Nerve Study.
- Other Otorhinolaryngologic Services or Procedures.
- Otolaryngologic and Binocular Microscopy Procedure.
- Otorhinolaryngologic Evaluation and Procedures.
- Special Diagnostic Otorhinolaryngologic Procedures.
- Treatment of Auditory Processing Disorder.
- Vestibular Function Tests.

Special otorhinolaryngology services and procedures are in the code set 92640–92653.

## Cardiovascular

92920–93799

The cardiovascular system is coded into various subcategories based on the type of procedure being carried out. Therapeutic cardiovascular services and procedures are listed separately and cover procedures such as stenting using balloon-tipped catheters to treat partially stenosed or chronically blocked arteries supplying the heart. Cardiograph services (93000–93050) are also reported for records of electrical activities of the nature and interpretation of data generated by a provider.

A patient may require home and outpatient monitoring of their INR levels (International Normalized Ratio), and these services are listed under code set 93792–93793. They are reported differently from other home health procedures and services.

### Non-Invasive Vascular Diagnostic Studies

93880–93998

Diagnostic studies of the vascular system reported using this code set are those carried out non-invasively on the cerebrovascular arterial system, extremities, viscera, and penis. A provider may use an ultrasound machine to study the blood flow through vessels and take note of the presence of emboli or other masses clogging the vessel beds.

Non-invasive studies also include measuring the vessels' thickness to monitor the deposition of fatty materials that predispose to cardiovascular or cerebrovascular diseases. Patients with suspected compromised blood flow to the penis may require an ultrasound study of the vessels of the penis using duplex ultrasound which may be complete (93980) or limited (93981).

## Pulmonary

94002–94799

The CPT codes for the medical code are set for reporting ventilator management (94002–94005) and diagnostic testing and therapies (94010–94799).

## Allergy and Clinical Immunology

95004–95199

Patients with reported allergic reactions require further evaluation to confirm the substances that may trigger an allergic reaction in them. The review may be a percutaneous test with allergenic extracts applied under supervision by a medical provider to determine which allergen would trigger an allergic reaction in the patient – 95004.

A combination of allergy tests. This includes prick, puncture, scratch, or intradermal tests, which may be performed sequentially or otherwise. These tests may be carried out for immediate or delayed response to be reported by the provider. A patch test commonly conducted to determine a possible allergic reaction is reported using CPT code 95044. It is also important to note that allergic reactions can be tested on the eyes, nose, or airway, as seen in asthma. Those carried out by inhalation of test substances during diagnosis of asthma, such as methacholine, are also represented in this chapter.

## Endocrinology

95249–95251

CPT codes for this category are services offered for managing endocrinology disorders and are found in the chapter covering endocrinology.

## Neurology and Neuromuscular Procedures

95700–96020

This category covers procedures and services to evaluate and manage neurological and neuromuscular disorders.

## Medical Genetics and Genetic Counseling Services

96040

This CPT code is reported when a genetic counselor (not a physician) analyzes and discusses a patient's genetic disorder risk factors based on the available medical information.

## Central Nervous System Assessment/Tests

**(Neurocognitive, Mental Status, Speech Testing)**

96105–96146

This category includes the assessment of aphasia and cognitive performance testing (96105), developmental and behavioral screening and testing (96110–96113), and psychological and neurophysiological testing (96116–96146).

**Behavior Management Services**

96202–96203

A provider trains caregivers on creating an environment that supports patient care and improves quality of life despite the negative impact of a debilitating diagnosis. The CPT codes are applied according to the time spent with caregivers.

## Hydration, Therapeutic, Prophylactic, Diagnostic Injections and Infusions, and Chemotherapy and Other Highly Complex Drug or Highly Complex Biologic Agent Administration

96360–96549

This category extensively covers the administration of infusions in disease management protocols or chemotherapeutic interventions in cancer management.

## Photodynamic Therapy

96567–96574

Photosensitive drugs exposed to specific wavelengths can be applied to lesions to destroy pre-cancerous cells (96567). Other modalities of use of photodynamic therapy are also highlighted by the other CPT code subcategories in the category.

## Special Dermatological Procedures

96900–96999

These treat skin conditions with special procedures, such as applying rays of different wavelengths depending on the extent of the skin lesion.

## Physical Medicine and Rehabilitation Evaluation

97010–97799

The CPT codes for all physical medicine and rehabilitation modalities and therapeutic procedures, physical therapy evaluations, occupational therapy evaluations, athletic training, active wound care management, tests and measurements, and orthotic or prosthetic management and training are in this category.

## Adaptive Behavior Services

97151–97158

A provider interacts with a patient to identify adaptive or maladaptive behaviors using standard tests, which are interpreted, and a care plan instituted following discussion with the caregivers. The time spent during the interaction is also considered when making the report.

## Medical Nutrition Therapy

97802–97804

A provider's use of diet therapy is described using CPT codes in this category. Further classification is based on the number of minutes spent with a patient.

## Acupuncture

97810–97814

This category covers the age-long procedure where fine needles are used to pierce the skin and stimulate designated anatomical points through skilled hand manipulation by the provider to relieve pain or other health conditions. The subcategories are based on the amount of time spent during treatment. The initial 15 minutes of this therapeutic intervention is reported with code 97810. When electrical stimulation is applied, the CPT codes 97813 and 97814 are reported according to the extra 15 minutes each.

## Osteopathic Manipulative Treatment

98925–98929

This category describes the treatment of somatic and non-somatic disorders in a patient through controlled manual pressure in different body regions. The CPT codes are categorized based on the number of body regions on which the procedure is carried out.

## Chiropractic Manipulative Treatment

98940–98943

A chiropractor is a professional who manipulates joints to improve neurophysiological function using trained techniques. The CPT codes for this procedure are reported according to the number of spinal regions involved in a session carried out by the chiropractor.

## Education and Training for Patient

### Self-Management

98960–98962

A healthcare professional who is not a physician may educate patients on their disease condition and how to manage it effectively. A hypertensive patient can be educated on taking their medications and monitoring their blood pressure. The session lasted 30 minutes and was reported using CPT code 98960. Education of a group of two to four patients for 30 minutes is reported using code 98961. For a group of five to eight patients addressed and educated for thirty minutes on effective management of their disease condition, code 98962 is reported.

## Non-Face-to-Face Non-Physician Services

98966–98981

This chapter was previously limited to telephone services but expanded to include online digital assessment and management services by qualified healthcare professionals who are not physicians. The use of various communication technologies online to discuss and possibly initiate management with a patient is reported based on whether the patient is established or new, as well as the cumulative number of minutes spent in a session for days. It also includes remote therapeutic monitoring services (98975–98978) and treatment management services (98980–98981).

## Special Services and Reports

99000–99091

This chapter covers a report of all miscellaneous medical services. Preparation of a specimen for laboratory analysis in the office, as well as the transport of this specimen to an outside testing laboratory, is reported using CPT code 99000. When the specimen is collected from a patient at a location different from the medical provider's office to be sent to an outside laboratory for analysis, code 99001 is used. A physician may prescribe a medical device for patient care, and code 99002 is used to report all steps associated with providing the device to the patient, from measurement and selection to the final application of the device.

All emergency services carried out on a patient during the global surgery period are reported with code 99024. The availability of a medical provider for on-call services or as-needed services in a medical facility in fulfillment of a prior agreement is a service reported as code 99026. Other miscellaneous CPT codes for medicine services can be found in this chapter.

## Qualifying Circumstances for Anesthesia

99100–99140

Some add-on codes are used alongside the primary code for anesthesia. The direct anesthesia code can be found in the main chapter for anesthesia.

## Moderate (Conscious) Sedation

99151–99157

The use of medication to reduce the level of consciousness without causing the patient to become entirely unconscious is reported in this category. Also, note the time spent on correct reporting.

## Other Medicine Services and Procedures

99170–99199

This category covers all other medical services and procedures not listed in previously highlighted categories.

## Home Health Procedures and Services

99500–99602

Healthcare assistants may offer services at home for some patients or in assisted care facilities and voluntary group homes.

## Medication Therapy Management Services

99605–99607

These CPT codes are reported by a qualified pharmacist dispensing medication for patient evaluation or management. The codes examine the complications and interactions that may occur with some medicines. The appropriate code is selected based on the time spent during service and the patient's status as either new or established.

# Chapter 21: Compliance and Regulatory

## Brief Overview of the Significance of Compliance in Healthcare

Compliance in healthcare is important for maintaining ethical standards, patient trust, and legal integrity. It ensures that healthcare providers adhere to existing regulations, such as HIPAA, safeguard patient information, and uphold professional standards. Proper compliance with the existing protocols minimizes the risk of legal actions and protects patient confidentiality. It also enhances the overall quality of healthcare services. As the healthcare landscape evolves, the significance of compliance becomes increasingly vital in fostering a trustworthy and responsible healthcare environment.

## Introduction to AAPC and CPC Standards

The American Academy of Professional Coders (AAPC) plays a pivotal role in setting and upholding standards for medical coding professionals. The Certified Professional Coder (CPC) certification is offered by AAPC and signifies expertise in accurate and ethical medical coding. These standards ensure uniformity, accuracy, and integrity in medical coding practices, which contribute to the efficiency and reliability of healthcare systems.

## Understanding AAPC and CPC

Understanding AAPC (American Academy of Professional Coders) and CPC (Certified Professional Coder) is important for professionals in the healthcare coding domain. AAPC serves as the guiding force in setting the standards for medical coders. This ensures a uniform and ethical approach to coding practices. As a leading authority, AAPC provides a framework that emphasizes accuracy, integrity, and compliance with established regulations.

The core of AAPC's influence is the Certified Professional Coder (CPC) certification. This CPC certification, widely recognized in the coding industry, validates a coder's proficiency in accurate and ethical medical coding. CPC-certified professionals are equipped with the knowledge to navigate through complex coding scenarios. This ensures that medical records are coded precisely, which facilitates proper billing and reimbursement processes.

The relationship between AAPC and CPC is symbiotic, with AAPC acting as the standard-bearer and CPC as the tangible demonstration of individual expertise. The certification signifies a coder's competence and serves as a marker for employers seeking professionals committed to maintaining the highest standards of coding excellence. This interdependence reinforces the importance of ongoing education, adherence to industry best practices, and the cultivation of a compliance-oriented mindset. This ensures that healthcare coding professionals contribute to a robust and ethical healthcare ecosystem.

## Regulatory Landscape in Healthcare Coding

In the intricate web of the healthcare system, the Regulatory Landscape stands as a sentinel that shapes and safeguards the industry. This regulatory framework includes key regulations such as the Health Insurance Portability and Accountability Act (HIPAA) and the Health Information Technology for Economic and Clinical Health (HITECH) Act. Understanding their implications is vital for healthcare professionals and organizations to ensure compliance and maintain ethical practices.

*HIPAA*, enacted in 1996, is a cornerstone in healthcare regulation and mainly focuses on protecting patients' sensitive health information. AAPC (American Academy of Professional Coders) and its Certified Professional Coder (CPC) certification are integral in aligning with and supporting HIPAA. The CPC certification ensures that professionals are well-versed in the intricacies of HIPAA regulations and emphasizes the importance of maintaining the confidentiality and security of patient data in the coding process.

The *HITECH Act*, enacted in 2009, complements HIPAA by promoting the adoption of Electronic Health Records (EHRs) and strengthening the enforcement of confidentiality and security requirements. AAPC and CPC contribute significantly to compliance with the HITECH Act by emphasizing accurate coding practices for electronic health information. This ensures that the integration of EHRs is seamless and aligns with the highest possible standards of security and privacy.

The symbiotic relationship between AAPC and CPC strengthens the compliance fabric. AAPC, as a leading authority, regularly updates its standards to incorporate recent changes in regulations. This ensures that CPC professionals are equipped with the latest knowledge available. CPC certification, in turn, serves as a tangible demonstration of an individual's commitment to compliance, aligning seamlessly with industry regulations. Noncompliance with these regulations carries significant consequences for healthcare organizations and professionals.

## Legal Ramifications

This includes hefty fines and penalties, which are examples of the consequences of noncompliance. The impact of noncompliance on patient trust, reputational damage, and the overall stability of healthcare entities can be severe. The breach of patient confidentiality can cause a loss of faith in healthcare institutions, which erodes the foundation of the patient-provider relationship.

Professionals certified by CPC and guided by AAPC standards are the vanguard against noncompliance. Their comprehensive training ensures that medical coding practices meet regulatory requirements and exceed them, which minimizes the risk of breaches. This proactive approach safeguards healthcare organizations from legal consequences and fosters a culture of trust and integrity within the industry.

## Core Principles of AAPC and CPC Compliance

In the dynamic realm of healthcare coding, adherence to the Core Principles of AAPC and CPC Compliance is fundamental. These principles encompass AAPC's Code of Ethics and Standards. Along with CPC guidelines, they form the bedrock of ethical and accurate medical coding practices.

AAPC's commitment to excellence encapsulates its comprehensive Code of Ethics and Standards. This code establishes the ethical framework within which coding professionals must operate. It encompasses integrity, objectivity, confidentiality, and professional competence. Integrity ensures that professionals are honest and transparent in their dealings. Objectivity demands impartiality and avoids conflicts of interest. Confidentiality is a cornerstone and emphasizes the protection of patient information. Professional competence underscores the necessity for continuous learning and adherence to coding guidelines.

AAPC offers the CPC certification, a testament to a coder's proficiency in accurate and ethical medical coding. Understanding the guidelines set by CPC is imperative for professionals. This includes mastery of the Current Procedural Terminology (CPT), Healthcare Common Procedure Coding System (HCPCS), and International Classification of Diseases (ICD). CPC guidelines ensure that codes accurately reflect the services provided. This facilitates proper billing and reimbursement. The rigorous examination process for CPC certification ensures that certified professionals possess the knowledge and skills to navigate medical coding complexities.

The Current Procedural Terminology (CPT) is a standardized system of medical codes that describes medical, surgical, and diagnostic services healthcare professionals provide. It was developed and maintained by the American Medical Association (AMA). CPT codes are pivotal in billing, reimbursement, and data analysis within the healthcare industry.

These codes provide a common language for communication among healthcare providers, insurers, and regulatory entities. This ensures accuracy and consistency in describing medical procedures and services. CPT codes are regularly updated to reflect advancements in medical technology and evolving healthcare practices, which makes them an essential tool for coding professionals and healthcare organizations to document and categorize various medical interventions and services accurately.

The Healthcare Common Procedure Coding System (HCPCS) is a comprehensive set of codes used in the healthcare industry to identify and report medical services and supplies. It is maintained by the Centers for Medicare & Medicaid Services (CMS) and plays a vital role in billing, reimbursement, and data analysis. It consists of two levels:

- **Level I** of the Healthcare Common Procedure Coding System is based on the American Medical Association's CPT codes and is used for coding medical services and procedures provided by healthcare professionals. However, HCPCS Level I is not identical to CPT codes, as HCPCS also includes additional codes and modifiers that are not found in the CPT system.
- **Level II** includes alphanumeric codes for various healthcare products, supplies, and services not covered by CPT.

The International Classification of Diseases (ICD) is a globally recognized system for categorizing and coding diseases, injuries, and health conditions. It is managed by the World Health Organization (WHO) and provides a standardized framework for healthcare professionals to document and track diagnoses. The regularly updated system facilitates consistent data collection, statistical analysis, and billing processes worldwide.

ICD codes are alphanumeric and offer a universal language for reporting health issues. This aids in international collaboration, research, and resource allocation. This comprehensive classification system is a cornerstone in global health information management and contributes to improved healthcare delivery and policy development.

In addition to ICD (International Classification of Diseases), CPT (Current Procedural Terminology), and HCPCS (Healthcare Common Procedure Coding System), other bodies contribute to the realm of medical coding, examples of which include:

- The National Drug Code (NDC) system is managed by the FDA and assigns codes to identify medications.
- SNOMED CT (Systematized Nomenclature of Medicine Clinical Terms) facilitates the exchange of clinical health information.
- LOINC (Logical Observation Identifiers Names and Codes) standardizes laboratory test results.

These coding systems collectively contribute to comprehensive and standardized documentation, which enables effective communication and data exchange within the healthcare industry.

## Confidentiality and Security in Medical Coding

Confidentiality and security in medical coding are important considerations to safeguard sensitive patient information. The AAPC and its CPC certification play instrumental roles in addressing these concerns. AAPC emphasizes stringent guidelines within its Code of Ethics, which stresses the importance of protecting patient confidentiality.

CPC-certified professionals are trained to handle patient data with the utmost care. This ensures that privacy remains a top priority in the coding process. This includes the ethical handling of electronic health records (EHRs) and other medical documentation. The best practices for maintaining confidentiality in medical coding involve limiting access to patient information strictly to authorized personnel. This necessitates robust authentication measures, secure storage of physical records, and encryption of electronic data.

Privacy breaches in medical coding can have severe consequences and pose risks to patients and healthcare organizations. Unauthorized access to patient information may cause identity theft, compromised medical histories, and emotional distress for the individuals involved. Legal repercussions include fines and lawsuits, which can significantly impact healthcare entities' financial stability. Regulatory bodies may impose penalties for noncompliance, which exacerbates the consequences of privacy breaches.

## Challenges in Compliance

Healthcare professionals encounter challenges in maintaining compliance, which include the navigation of complex regulations, up-to-date standards, and resource constraints. Solutions to these challenges include ongoing training to stay updated with the latest guidelines, the implementation of robust technology for accurate documentation, and a culture of compliance within organizations.

Proactive measures involve regular audits to identify and rectify potential issues before they escalate. An organizational culture centered on compliance promotes transparency, accountability, and shared responsibility among staff, which reduces the likelihood of errors. Prioritizing compliance mitigates risks and enhances the overall quality of patient care, which fosters a trustworthy and reliable healthcare environment.

## Benefits of Compliance

Compliance with AAPC and CPC standards ensures the accuracy and integrity of coded medical records, which reduces billing errors and denials. This, in turn, causes improved financial outcomes for healthcare organizations. Additionally, compliance mitigates legal risks and promotes a proactive approach to evolving healthcare regulations.

Adherence also fosters a culture of ethical coding practices and enhances patient trust and satisfaction. Certified professionals with CPC credentials are recognized for their proficiency. This opens up career advancement opportunities.

## Staying Current: Updates and Changes

Staying current with updates and changes is imperative for coding professionals in the ever-evolving healthcare landscape. Healthcare regulations and coding practices are dynamic and subject to frequent revisions. To navigate these changes successfully, professionals must employ proactive strategies. These include regularly attending workshops, webinars, and conferences offered by reputable organizations.

Ongoing education plays a pivotal role in this process. Pursuing additional certifications and participating in continuous professional development programs enhances expertise and adaptability. Networking with other professionals and engaging in online forums fosters knowledge-sharing and provides insights into practical applications of updated coding practices.

Those who embrace the fluid nature of healthcare regulations and proactively seek knowledge are better equipped to provide accurate and compliant coding services. Coding professionals can navigate the complexities of the ever-changing healthcare landscape with confidence and competence by prioritizing ongoing education and remaining adaptable.

# Test 1: Questions

(1) Which insurance packages are not run by the government?

(A) Medicare Part A.

(B) Medicare Part B.

(C) Medicare Part C.

(D) Medicare Part D.

(2) Which act protects the rights of a patient in regard to the security and privacy of their health information?

(A) HIPAA.

(B) Social Security Act (SSA).

(C) HITECH Act.

(D) OIG.

(3) A patient presented to the doctor's clinic with tiredness and reduced appetite. There were no other complaints. Further review by the physician showed the patient was worried about their quality of life and a tumor in her brain. However, there was no history of headaches or blurry vision, and other assessments and physical examinations yielded no significant findings. Blood work and imaging were requested, and the results were all normal. The patient's diagnosis in the physician's notes was "worried well." What is the appropriate code for this visit?

(A) R53.83, R63.0, Z04.6.

(B) R53.83, R63.0, Z71.1.

(C) E89.1.

(D) L20.9.

(4) A forty-eight-year-old patient was admitted for an ophthalmology cataract surgery on both eyes. The patient was admitted the day before the procedure and had immediate sequential bilateral cataract surgery (ISBCS). The existing lens capsule was removed from both eyes, and an intraocular lens was inserted. What is the physician's report for this encounter?

(A) H26.0, 66983, H26.0, 66983.

(B) H26.0, 66983.

(C) H26.0, 66982.

(D) H26.0, 66982, H26.0, 66982.

(5) Which of the following is the medical term for the voice box?

(A) Trachea.

(B) Larynx.

(C) Pharynx.

(D) Bronchus.

(6) Which of the following best describes the purpose of a colonoscopy?

(A) To check heart function.

(B) To examine the large intestine.

(C) To assess kidney health.

(D) To study brain activity.

(7) The anatomical position indicates that the body be placed in which of the following arrangements?

(A) Standing upright with feet parallel.

(B) Bent forward at the waist.

(C) Lying on the back.

(D) Seated with crossed legs.

(8) In anatomical language, the term *superior* refers to which of the following?

(A) Closer to the midline.

(B) Farther from the midline.

(C) Above or higher.

(D) Below or lower.

(9) Which of the following actions is an example of a lateral movement?

(A) Flexion.

(B) Extension.

(C) Abduction.

(D) Circumduction.

(10) Which of the following best describes the term *pronation* in relation to anatomical movements?

(A) Turn the forearm palm down.

(B) Turn the forearm palm up.

(C) Move the limb toward the midline.

(D) Move the limb away from the midline.

(11) Which of the following describes the anatomical term for the front of the body?

(A) Posterior.

(B) Anterior.

(C) Superior.

(D) Inferior.

(12) Which of the following best describes abduction?

(A) To move a body part toward the midline.

(B) To straighten a joint.

(C) To move a body part away from the midline.

(D) To bend a joint.

(13) A group of friends brought a twenty-one-year-old man to the emergency room. He was involved in a fight where he sustained a knife injury to his right elbow. What is the ICD-10-CM code for this encounter?

(A) S51.09.

(B) S51.01.

(C) S51.02.

(D) S51.011A.

(14) A fifty-one-year-old man requested a transfer of care from his cardiologist following a diagnosis of long-standing persistent atrial fibrillation. What is the ICD-10-CM code assigned to his condition?

(A) I48.

(B) I48.11.

(C) I45.09.

(D) I48.32.

(15) A 58-year-old patient presents to the emergency department with severe abdominal pain, nausea, and vomiting. After a thorough examination and endoscopy, the patient is diagnosed with a bleeding gastric ulcer. The physician performs an endoscopic cauterization to stop the bleeding. How should this scenario be coded?

(A) 43235 - Upper gastrointestinal endoscopy including esophagus, stomach, and either the duodenum and/or jejunum as appropriate; diagnostic, with or without collection of specimens by brushing or washing.

(B) 43255 - Endoscopic thermal cautery for bleeding ulcer.

(C) 43239 - Upper gastrointestinal endoscopy including esophagus, stomach, and either the duodenum and/or jejunum as appropriate; with biopsy.

(D) 43251 - Upper gastrointestinal endoscopy including esophagus, stomach, and either the duodenum and/or jejunum as appropriate; with endoscopic mucosal resection.

(16) A thirty-four-year-old man is brought to the hospital following a road traffic accident that resulted in acute kidney injury due to massive blood loss. What ICD-10-CM code is assigned to acute kidney injury?

(A) N70.9.

(B) N17.9.

(C) N71.9.

(D) N17.

(17) Which of the following is the code for chronic right otitis media with effusion?

(A) H65.9.

(B) H65.21.

(C) H65.2.

(D) H64.9.

(18) A 45-year-old patient visits their primary care physician with complaints of sharp and localized pain in the right lower quadrant of the abdomen. After a detailed exam, the physician suspects appendicitis and orders further diagnostic tests. How should this abdominal pain, which is not generalized, be coded?

(A) R10.0 - Acute abdomen.

(B) R10.9 - Unspecified abdominal pain.

(C) R10.11 - Right upper quadrant pain.

(D) R10.31 - Pain localized to the right lower quadrant of the abdomen.

(19) A thirty-five-year-old woman was admitted for a scheduled hysterectomy because of some medical indication. What is the duration of the postoperative services this patient can access under the global package?

(A) Zero days.

(B) Ten days.

(C) Thirty days.

(D) Ninety days.

(20) A twenty-three-year-old man was brought in for a laparoscopic biopsy for diagnostic purposes. What is the duration of the postoperative services this patient can access under the global package?

(A) Zero days.

(B) Ten days.

(C) Thirty days.

(D) Ninety days.

(21) You are coding for Medicare outpatient hospital services, and you encounter a new and innovative procedure that does not have a permanent National Code. Which type of code should be used to report this procedure to ensure proper billing and reimbursement?

(A) HCPCS Level I Codes.

(B) HCPCS Level II Codes.

(C) CPT Category II Codes.

(D) HCPCS Level II C Codes (Temporary Codes).

(22) Which of the following is not included in the global package for surgery?

(A) Postoperative pain services provided by the surgeon.

(B) Intraoperative services that are normal and essential for the surgical procedure.

(C) A preoperative visit as covered by the respective classification of the surgery.

(D) Organ transplantation immunotherapy management.

(23) Which type of sweat gland is responsible for body odor?

(A) Eccrine gland.

(B) Apocrine gland.

(C) Sebaceous gland.

(D) Sudoriferous gland.

(24) What is the term for the natural shedding of dead skin cells?

(A) Desquamation.

(B) Exfoliation.

(C) Ecdysis.

(D) Ablation.

(25) Which of the following is the medical term for a blister?

(A) Papule.

(B) Vesicle.

(C) Pustule.

(D) Nodule.

(26) What is the ICD-10 code range for skin and subcutaneous tissue diseases?

(A) C00-C14.

(B) M00-M99.

(C) L00-L99.

(D) R00-R99.

(27) Which ICD-10 code is used for eczema?

(A) L25.

(B) L30.

(C) L40.

(D) L50.

(28) Which of the following is the ICD-10 code for psoriasis?

(A) L20.

(B) L30.

(C) L40.

(D) L50.

(29) Which of the following is the ICD-10 code range for disorders of the joints (arthropathies)?

(A) M00-M25.

(B) M40-M54.

(C) M60-M79.

(D) M80-M99.

(30) A 52-year-old patient with a history of autoimmune disease presents to their rheumatologist with joint swelling, stiffness, and pain that affects multiple joints, including hands, wrists, and knees. After a comprehensive evaluation, the patient is diagnosed with rheumatoid arthritis, which is an inflammatory polyarthropathy. Which ICD-10-CM code range should be used to accurately document this diagnosis?

(A) M05-M06 - Rheumatoid arthritis.

(B) M15-M19 – Osteoarthritis.

(C) M20-M25 - Other joint disorders.

(D) M45-M49 – Spondylopathies.

(31) The ICD-10 code M54.5 corresponds to which of the following?

(A) Low back pain.

(B) Osteoarthritis of the hip.

(C) Rheumatoid arthritis.

(D) Scoliosis.

(32) Codes in the M80-M85 range are related to which of the following?

(A) Osteoporosis with current pathological fracture.

(B) Rheumatoid arthritis.

(C) Fibromyalgia.

(D) Osteoarthritis of the knee.

(33) A patient reports to the physical therapy department complaining of severe back pain due to muscle spasms. The spasms are documented as being localized in the lumbar region. How should the muscle spasm be coded for accurate billing?

(A) M62.830 - Muscle spasm of the back.

(B) M54.5 - Low back pain.

(C) M62.40 - Contracture of muscle, unspecified site.

(D) M79.1 – Myalgia.

(34) The ICD-10 code M75.50 corresponds to which of the following?

(A) Bursitis of unspecified shoulder.

(B) Osteomyelitis of unspecified shoulder.

(C) Rotator cuff tear or rupture, unspecified shoulder.

(D) Tennis elbow.

(35) The ICD-10-CM code J44.9 represents which of the following?

(A) Chronic obstructive pulmonary disease, unspecified.

(B) Pneumonia, unspecified.

(C) Emphysema.

(D) Chronic respiratory failure, unspecified.

(36) The ICD-10-CM code D38.6 is associated with which of the following?

(A) Hodgkin's disease, unspecified.

(B) Lymphoma, unspecified.

(C) Mediastinal tumor, unspecified.

(D) Neoplasm of uncertain behavior of respiratory organ, unspecified.

(37) A 67-year-old female patient is diagnosed with chronic kidney disease stage 3. During her routine follow-up, her primary care physician notes that she has developed anemia as a complication of her CKD. How should this anemia be coded?

(A) D63.1 - Anemia in chronic kidney disease.

(B) D50.9 - Iron deficiency anemia, unspecified.

(C) D64.9 - Anemia, unspecified.

(D) D62 - Acute posthemorrhagic anemia.

(38) The ICD-10-CM code I27.89 is used for which of the following?

(A) Other specified secondary pulmonary hypertension.

(B) Primary pulmonary hypertension.

(C) Chronic thromboembolic pulmonary hypertension.

(D) Pulmonary embolism.

(39) Which of the following is the ICD-10-CM code for mediastinitis?

(A) K85.9.

(B) J98.51.

(C) I89.1.

(D) T81.1.

(40) The ICD-10-CM Code I70.0 is used for which of the following?

(A) Atherosclerosis of native arteries of the extremities.

(B) Atherosclerosis of aorta.

(C) Atherosclerosis of coronary arteries.

(D) Atherosclerosis of carotid artery.

(41) Which of these structures returns oxygen-depleted blood to the heart?

(A) Vein.

(B) Artery.

(C) Capillary.

(D) Valve.

(42) What is the term for the network of blood vessels that supply the heart muscle?

(A) Pulmonary circuit.

(B) Systemic circuit.

(C) Coronary circuit.

(D) Cardiac circuit.

(43) Which anatomical structure separates the left and right sides of the heart?

(A) Pulmonary valve.

(B) Interventricular septum.

(C) Aortic valve.

(D) Coronary sinus.

(44) Which term describes the contraction phase of the heart muscle?

(A) Diastole.

(B) Systole.

(C) Aneurysm.

(D) Bradycardia.

(45) In ICD-10-CM, which chapter is dedicated to diseases of the circulatory system?

(A) Chapter 1.

(B) Chapter 9.

(C) Chapter 10.

(D) Chapter 15.

(46) A 56-year-old patient visits their physician for a routine health check-up. After reviewing the patient's medical history and conducting a physical exam, the physician diagnoses the patient with primary (essential) hypertension. Which ICD-10-CM code should be used to accurately document this diagnosis?

(A) I10 - Essential (primary) hypertension.

(B) I12.9 - Hypertensive chronic kidney disease, without renal failure.

(C) I15.9 - Secondary hypertension, unspecified.

(D) I11.0 - Hypertensive heart disease without heart failure.

(47) Which of the following terms indicates the semi-liquid mixture of food and digestive juices in the stomach?

(A) Chyme.

(B) Bolus.

(C) Gastrin.

(D) Chyle.

(48) What digestive system component absorbs water and creates fecal matter?

(A) Stomach.

(B) Small intestine.

(C) Large intestine.

(D) Liver.

(49) What is the medical term for difficulty in swallowing?

(A) Dyspepsia.

(B) Dysphagia.

(C) Diarrhea.

(D) Dysentery.

(50) Which of the following hormones stimulates the release of digestive enzymes from the pancreas?

(A) Insulin.

(B) Glucagon.

(C) Somatostatin.

(D) Secretin.

(51) A patient presents to the emergency department with severe right lower quadrant pain, nausea, and fever. After a thorough evaluation, including an abdominal CT scan, the patient is diagnosed with acute appendicitis without perforation or abscess. How should this diagnosis be coded?

(A) K35.80 - Acute appendicitis without perforation or gangrene, unspecified.

(B) K35.89 - Other acute appendicitis.

(C) K35.2 - Acute appendicitis with generalized peritonitis.

(D) K37 - Unspecified appendicitis.

(52) Which of the following ICD-10-CM codes is used for gastroesophageal reflux disease (GERD)?

(A) K21.9.

(B) K21.0.

(C) K21.1.

(D) K21.2.

(53) A fourteen-year-old girl was admitted to the pediatrics unit with complaints of abdominal pain, vomiting, and a temperature of 106° F. There was positive right costovertebral tenderness. An ultrasound scan showed a collection in the perirenal space of the right kidney. Her parents were informed of the findings, and she was immediately prepared for drainage of the perirenal abscess. Report the CPT code for this procedure with the appropriate modifier.

(A) 35024, Modifier 50.

(B) 50020, Modifier 49.

(C) 50020, Modifier RT.

(D) 50120, Modifier 50.

(54) A thirty-four-year-old woman with left-sided nephrolithiasis is scheduled to undergo a lithotripsy procedure following the failure of pharmacological therapy and recurrent abdominal pain. What CPT codes are relevant to this procedure?

(A) 50590.

(B) 50082.

(C) 50135.

(D) 50421.

(55) A seventy-three-year-old man is brought to his urologist appointment by his son. He is concerned about his father's worsening lower urinary tract symptoms. The results of the prostate biopsy revealed a malignant neoplasm of the prostate with no evidence of metastasis. His father declined open surgery, and so a transurethral resection of the prostate is suggested. The patient agreed, and the surgeon reported the procedure to be scheduled for the next week. What CPT code is the surgeon required to report to prevent inaccurate billing of this procedure?

(A) 52630.

(B) 52730.

(C) 52410.

(D) 53403.

(56) A mother brought her fourteen-month-old boy to his pediatric appointment for a routine checkup. He had an abnormal urine stream some months ago. He underwent urethroplasty for repair of hypospadias at their local hospital three months ago. However, his mother reports that his urine stream has not improved, and she noticed a fibrous band between his penile shaft and scrotum. Further examination by the pediatric surgeon shows a fistula at the site of the surgical repair. The surgeon explained to the mother that her son would require surgery to correct the fistula. What is the CPT code for the correction?

(A) 54200.

(B) 54340.

(C) 54120.

(D) 54103.

(57) A twenty-day-old boy is scheduled for circumcision through surgical excision only. What is the CPT code for this procedure?

(A) 54521.

(B) 54120.

(C) 54830.

(D) 54160.

(58) An eleven-month-old boy is evaluated for bilateral undescended testes. He is being worked up for open exploration with abdominal exploration. What is the CPT code and modifier for this procedure?

(A) 54560, Modifier 50.

(B) 54500, Modifier RT.

(C) 54310, Modifier 75.

(D) 54560, Modifier 51.

(59) A young woman presents at her post-natal clinic two weeks after delivery of a healthy female neonate weighing 2.7 kg. She is worried as she has not been able to breastfeed her baby due to pain in her breasts whenever the baby attempts to latch onto her nipple. She is examined, and an area of erythema, which is painful to touch, is found around the nipple. She explains that it has gotten worse in the past few days. State the ICD-10-CM diagnosis code.

(A) O91.2.

(B) O90.3.

(C) O91.5.

(D) O91.0.

(60) A twenty-nine-year-old woman is thirty-four weeks pregnant with twins. She begins to feel lower abdominal cramps, which cause her to drain liquor. Her partner drives her to the hospital immediately, and the assessment reveals that she is in the active phase of labor. She delivers two live male neonates via spontaneous vaginal delivery, and the babies are stable with no complications reported. What are the ICD-10-CM diagnosis codes for both deliveries?

(A) O60.14X1, O60.14X2.

(B) O60.15X1, O60.14X1.

(C) O60.17X1, O60.14X2.

(D) O60.15X1, O61.14X2.

(61) A thirty-seven-week pregnant woman goes into labor, which a midwife supervises. She delivers a live neonate that cries immediately after birth. However, there is a layer of umbilical cord wrapped around the neck, which the midwife removes. The placenta is delivered without any adverse effects. Report the ICD-10-CM diagnosis code.

(A) O60.81X2.

(B) O68.82X1.

(C) O69.80X.

(D) O69.81X1.

(62) A thirty-eight-week pregnant woman goes into spontaneous labor and presents at the hospital for vaginal delivery. During close feto-maternal vital signs monitoring, the midwife observes that the fetal heart rate is persistently greater than 180 bpm. Report the ICD-10-CM diagnosis code.

(A) O76.

(B) O75.

(C) O76.3.

(D) O76.0.

(63) A patient experiences significant bleeding immediately after the delivery of her baby, which the attending physician diagnoses as postpartum hemorrhage. This condition requires immediate intervention to manage the bleeding. How should this diagnosis be coded?

(A) O72.0 - Third-stage hemorrhage.

(B) O72.1 - Other immediate postpartum hemorrhage.

(C) O90.2 - Postpartum hemorrhage.

(D) O72.3 - Delayed and secondary postpartum hemorrhage.

(64) A forty-week pregnant woman delivered a live male neonate via spontaneous vertex delivery by a midwife at home. Vaginal examination following delivery of the placenta shows a first-degree perineal laceration in the vagina wall. The midwife promptly repairs the tear. State the diagnosis code according to ICD-10-CM and the current procedural terminology for the repair.

(A) O70.0, 59300.

(B) O70.0, 59350.

(C) O70.0, 58300.

(D) O78.0, 59300.

(65) A newborn is diagnosed with congenital hypothyroidism during their initial screening. The condition is identified without the mention of goiter. Which code should be used to accurately document this diagnosis?

(A) E03.1 - Congenital hypothyroidism without goiter.

(B) E03.9 - Hypothyroidism, unspecified.

(C) P72.0 - Transient neonatal disorders of thyroid function, not elsewhere classified.

(D) E00.9 - Congenital iodine-deficiency syndrome, unspecified.

(66) A forty-three-year-old man comes for his endocrinology follow-up appointment. He was diagnosed with diabetes five years ago and prescribed metformin tablets for glycemic control. However, he has been non-compliant with his medications and appointments. A random blood sugar check at the clinic is 205 mg/dl. An examination reveals decreased tactile stimulation in both lower limbs and an ulcer on the right big toe. The patient says he sustained the injury six weeks ago while out in his yard. A biopsy of the ulcer is done, and a diagnosis of a diabetic foot ulcer is confirmed. Describe the diagnosis code according to the ICD-10-CM code index.

(A) E11.6.

(B) E11.62.

(C) E11.621.

(D) E11.620.

(67) A 63-year-old patient with a long-standing history of type 2 diabetes mellitus presents to the emergency department with confusion, excessive thirst, and high blood glucose readings. After evaluation, the patient is diagnosed with type 2 diabetes mellitus with hyperosmolarity, without mention of nonketotic hyperglycemic hyperosmolar coma (NKHH). Which code should be used to accurately document this diagnosis?

(A) E11.00 - Type 2 diabetes mellitus without complications.

(B) E11.65 - Type 2 diabetes mellitus with hyperglycemia.

(C) E11.69 - Type 2 diabetes mellitus with other specified complications.

(D) E11.00 - Type 2 diabetes mellitus with hyperosmolarity.

(68) A patient presents to their healthcare provider with symptoms including tremors, palpitations, sweating, noticeable swelling in the neck area, and laboratory tests confirm high thyroxine levels. What is the most appropriate code to document this diagnosis?

(A) E05.90 - Thyrotoxicosis, unspecified, without thyrotoxic crisis or storm.

(B) E04.0 - Nontoxic diffuse goiter.

(C) E07.9 - Disorder of thyroid, unspecified.

(D) R25.1 - Tremors, unspecified.

(69) A young woman comes for a follow-up after having a total thyroidectomy for a large multinodular goiter. She complains of perioral numbness. She is examined, and a slight tap of the jaw causes her facial muscles to twitch. Her serum calcium levels are low. She is informed by her surgeon that there appears to have been damage to her parathyroid glands during the procedure, which is the likely cause of her current symptoms. State the ICD-10-CM diagnosis code.

(A) E89.

(B) E89.2.

(C) E89.3.

(D) E89.1.

(70) A patient is seen with elevated blood pressure, acne, and purple striae on the neck and abdomen. Their body mass index is 36 kg/m, and their serum cortisol levels are elevated. A diagnosis of Cushing's syndrome is made. State the ICD-10-CM diagnosis code.

(A) E24.9.

(B) E24.

(C) E24.5.

(D) E24.3.

(71) What is the function of the semicircular canals?

(A) Balance.

(B) Reception.

(C) Hearing.

(D) Cleaning.

(72) A fifteen-year-old boy is referred to an ophthalmologist to evaluate excessive tearing in the right eye. It was noticed five weeks ago. He thought it was a simple allergic reaction and used multiple types of eyedrops. However, the tearing has gotten worse. The ophthalmologist examines both eyes and makes a preliminary assessment of epiphora. What is the appropriate ICD-10-CM code that the ophthalmologist would report?

(A) H06.211.

(B) H01.211.

(C) H04.210.

(D) H04.211.

(73) An older woman noticed a swelling on her right upper eyelid a week ago. She dismissed it as a minor issue. However, she found a similar swelling on the left lower eyelid yesterday. The swelling has remained the same size and is not painful. She presented at her GP for evaluation, and she was told she has bilateral chalazion of the eyes. What is the appropriate ICD-10-CM diagnosis for each of these swellings?

(A) H00.11, H00.15.

(B) H00.01, H00.15.

(C) H00.11, H00.16.

(D) H00.11, H00.11.

(74) A seven-year-old boy has been constantly itching his eyes for two days. Both eyes are red and watering. He also has nasal discharge. There is history of similar symptoms in his older brother, and their father is a known asthmatic. State the ICD-10-CM code for the diagnosis made for this patient.

(A) H10.19.

(B) H10.15.

(C) H10.12.

(D) H10.13.

(75) A 72-year-old male patient is diagnosed with cortical cataracts in both eyes after he experiences gradual vision loss and undergoes a comprehensive ophthalmologic exam. Which code should be used to accurately document this diagnosis?

(A) H25.89 - Other age-related cataract.

(B) H26.9 - Unspecified cataract.

(C) H25.9 - Unspecified age-related cataract.

(D) H25.013 - Bilateral age-related cortical cataracts.

(76) A young man comes to the clinic with a two-week history of pain in the left eye. It is associated with itching and a foreign body sensation in the affected eye. The left eye appears reddened and watery. An examination confirms the presence of an ulcer in the central part of the cornea. What is the correct diagnosis code according to ICD-10-CM?

(A) H16.012.

(B) H16.01.

(C) H16.0.

(D) H16.016.

(77) What code is used to report arterial catheterization?

(A) 36620.

(B) 36520.

(C) 36670.

(D) 36622.

(78) What HCPCS modifier is used when an anesthesiologist supervises a service?

(A) GA.

(B) AA.

(C) GY.

(D) AG.

(79) What is a patient's physical status with mild systemic disease?

(A) P1.

(B) P2.

(C) P3.

(D) P4.

(80) What is a patient's physical status with severe systemic disease?

(A) P5.

(B) P4.

(C) P3.

(D) P2.

(81) A young woman presents to her hospital with a week's history of recurrent headaches, fever, and neck pain. She had three episodes of vomiting in the past twenty-four hours. Her temperature is 38.9 C. Her pulse is 107 bpm, and her BP is 110/65 mm Hg. Kernig's and Brudzinski's signs are positive. An urgent MRI of the brain and brainstem without contrast confirms a diagnosis of meningitis. State the correct CPT code for this investigation. Also, state the ICD-10-CM code for the diagnosis made.

(A) 70551, G03.9.

(B) 70551, G03.8.

(C) 70550, G03.9.

(D) 70541, G03.9.

(82) A sixty-three-year-old man enters the clinic with a four-day cough, chest pain, and fever history. His temperature is 38.6 C. He is tachycardic with a pulse rate of 89 bpm, and his blood pressure is 105/56 mm Hg. A sputum culture is requested. Plain chest radiographs in anteroposterior and lateral views confirm the presence of infiltrate in the left lower lung and right lower lobe. What is the CPT code for the radiological investigation requested?

(A) 71045.

(B) 71046.

(C) 71036.

(D) 71044.

(83) A patient presents with chronic lower back pain, and the physician orders a radiographic exam of the lumbosacral spine to assess for possible causes. The radiology department performs a series of images and obtains a minimum of four views of the lumbosacral spine. Which CPT code should be used to accurately document this radiographic exam?

(A) 72100 - Radiologic exam, spine, lumbosacral; two or three views.

(B) 72110 - Radiologic exam, spine, lumbosacral; minimum of four views.

(C) 72120 - Radiologic exam, spine, lumbosacral; bending views only (2 or 3 views).

(D) 72131 - Computed tomography, lumbar spine; without contrast material.

(84) A young boy is evaluated for abnormal lateral curvature of the spine. A radiological image of the entire thoracic and lumbar spine has been requested for management. What is the CPT code to be reported by the physician?

(A) 72080.

(B) 72062.

(C) 72081.

(D) 72082.

(85) A young woman is referred for radiological investigation of her thyroid gland. It is to determine overactivity in the gland following a diagnosis of Graves' disease. She reports palpitations and tremors in both hands. Examination shows proptosis of the eyes, sweaty palms, and swelling in the neck. For the procedure, she ingested a small quantity of radioactive iodine I-131 and was asked to return within four to twenty-four hours to measure the radioactivity within the thyroid gland. She returns, and a probe is placed over the swelling in her neck caused by the thyroid gland. The radioactivity is measured, compared with the radioactivity of the original dose, and reported as a percentage of the initial amount. Report the CPT code for this procedure.

(A) 78012.

(B) 78010.

(C) 78001.

(D) 78112.

(86) A young woman with a family history of breast cancer presents at her primary care facility for a screening. She is worried that she might have undetected cancer in her breasts. Her physician requested a screening mammography for her. What is the CPT code for the procedure?

(A) 77057.

(B) 77067.

(C) 77066.

(D) A 77068.

(87) What does the acronym CAP stand for in pathology?

(A) Clinical assessment protocol.

(B) College of American Pathologists.

(C) Coding and analysis procedure.

(D) Cellular anatomy protocol.

(88) Which coding system is commonly used to identify medications and chemical substances?

(A) SNOMED CT.

(B) CPT.

(C) ICD-10-CM.

(D) RxNorm.

(89) What is the meaning of the acronym EHR in the context of medical coding?

(A) Electronic health record.

(B) Emergency hospital reporting.

(C) Epidemiological health registry.

(D) Enhanced healthcare resourcing.

(90) What does the acronym CLIA stand for in laboratory medicine?

(A) Clinical Laboratory Integration Act.

(B) Comprehensive laboratory information analysis.

(C) Clinical Laboratory Improvement Amendments.

(D) Cellular Lab Inspection Agency.

(91) What does the acronym PCR stand for in molecular pathology?

(A) Polymerization chain reaction.

(B) Pathological cell resolution.

(C) Protein coding regulation.

(D) Pathogen capture and recognition.

(92) What does a Kleihauer-Betke test refer to in laboratory medicine?

(A) A blood clotting assay.

(B) A test for fetal-maternal hemorrhage.

(C) A viral culture technique.

(D) An enzyme-linked immunosorbent assay.

(93) What does the CPT code 80061 represent?

(A) Complete blood count.

(B) Comprehensive metabolic panel.

(C) Coagulation profile.

(D) Lipid panel.

(94) A patient is admitted to the hospital for observation due to chest pain. The cause of the chest pain is not known. The admitting physician performs an evaluation that includes a detailed history, a detailed exam, and medical decision-making of low complexity. The patient's stay in the observation unit lasts less than 24 hours. Which CPT code should be used to accurately document the initial observation care provided by the physician?

(A) 99218 - Initial observation care, 30 minutes.

(B) 99219 - Initial observation care, 50 minutes.

(C) 99220 - Initial observation care, 70 minutes.

(D) 99217 - Observation care discharge.

(95) A young man was diagnosed with major depressive disorder a few months ago. He has been on antidepressants and is compliant with his medication. He has an appointment with his psychiatrist for a psychotherapy session lasting thirty minutes. State the appropriate CPT code to be reported.

(A) 91893.

(B) 90932.

(C) 90732.

(D) 90832.

(96) A forty-seven-year-old woman with a month's history of the involuntary passage of urine undergoes training by her medical provider to control her heart rate whenever she feels the urge to pass urine. She is educated on controlling her blood pressure and breathing pattern to prevent involuntary urine passage. The session lasts fifteen minutes. State the CPT code for this service.

(A) 90912.

(B) 90913.

(C) 90915.

(D) 90911.

(97) A patient with end-stage renal disease (ESRD) undergoes a dialysis session that includes comprehensive monitoring for acute changes of patient status, adjustment of dialysate composition, and a repeated assessment of intradialytic vital signs. This session also involves the provision of anticoagulation and the management of the extracorporeal circuit. Which CPT code accurately documents this procedure?

(A) 90935 - Hemodialysis procedure with single physician evaluation.

(B) 90937 - Hemodialysis procedure requiring repeated evaluations with or without a substantial revision of the dialysis prescription.

(C) 90945 - Dialysis procedure other than hemodialysis (e.g., peritoneal dialysis, hemofiltration), with single physician evaluation.

(D) 90947 - Dialysis procedure other than hemodialysis (e.g., peritoneal dialysis, hemofiltration), requiring repeated evaluations with or without a substantial revision of the dialysis prescription.

(98) A patient with suspected gastroesophageal reflux disease undergoes manometry analysis of the esophageal muscle pressure. What is the CPT code?

(A) 91101.

(B) 91012.

(C) 91013.

(D) 91010.

(99) An eighteen-month-old boy is brought into the hospital due to lethargy. The boy has been vomiting and passing loose, watery stools for a couple of days. He appears lethargic, with poor capillary refill and reduced skin turgor. An assessment of severe dehydration with hypovolemic shock secondary to diarrheal disease is made. An IV infusion is immediately set up, and an anti-shock regimen commenced for the next thirty minutes. Report this encounter using a CPT code.

(A) 96362.

(B) 96363.

(C) 96360.

(D) 96361.

(100) What is the role of a medical coder in ensuring healthcare compliance?

(A) To manage hospital finances.

(B) To ensure patient confidentiality.

(C) To conduct surgical procedures.

(D) To market healthcare services.

# Test 1: Answers and Explanations

(1) (C) Medicare Part C.

Private Medicare-approved insurers run Medicare Part C. It is usually a mix of services defined by the respective insurer. They include inpatient and outpatient care services and often prescription drug coverage.

(2) (A) HIPAA.

HIPAA is a critical piece of legislation that protects patient rights regarding a covered entity's electronic transfer of sensitive and private health information. The Social Security Act is not related to the security, privacy, and safety of healthcare information or the protection of patient rights.

(3) (B) R53.83, R63.0, Z71.1.

R53.83 is used to code for other fatigue. It signifies a marked lack of energy and mental alertness without a definite cause. R63.0 is used to code for a loss of appetite for food (anorexia) and may include insufficient intake of food and water, probably due to self-neglect. Z71.1 is used to code for a patient with health complaints without any medical observation or evidence to validate this condition.

(4) (B) H26.0, 66983.

H26.0 is used to code for infantile, juvenile, and presenile cataracts. Senile cataracts usually apply to cataracts in a patient at least fifty years old. 66983 is the code to report the ophthalmology procedure of cataract lenses and capsule removal and insertion of a lens prosthesis. 66982 is the code for the ophthalmology procedure of extracapsular cataract extraction and implanting lens prostheses using complex techniques and devices. The ICD-10-CM general guidelines do not allow the repetition of codes. Each unique code is to occur only once in each encounter.

(5) (B) Larynx.

The medical term for the voice box is the *larynx*. It is located in the neck. The larynx houses the vocal cords responsible for sound production during speech and singing. It also helps respiration. Conditions that affect the larynx can impact voice quality and respiratory function.

(6) (B) To examine the large intestine.

A colonoscopy is a medical procedure to inspect the colon and rectum (parts of the large intestine). A physician inserts a flexible tube with a camera, called a colonoscope, through the rectum to inspect the lining of the large intestine. This procedure helps detect abnormalities such as polyps, inflammation, or colon cancer. Colonoscopies are cardinal for diagnostic and preventive purposes. They allow for early detection and removal of potentially harmful growths in the colon.

(7) (A) Standing upright with feet parallel.

The anatomical position is a standard reference to characterize and find bodily structures. The patient stands upright in this posture, with their arms at their sides and their palms facing front. Their feet are parallel and level on the ground. The head and eyes are directed forward. This consistent posture provides a universal reference point for medical practitioners and anatomists. It facilitates precise communication about body structures and their relationships. It serves as the baseline for directional terms and anatomical descriptions and enables accurate communication between professionals.

(8) (C) Above or higher.

In anatomical literature, the term *superior* denotes a position or structure situated above another in relation to the axis of the body. For example, the head is superior to the neck. This directional term aids in precise communication about the location of body parts and structures. It also allows healthcare professionals to navigate the human body's three-dimensional complexity precisely and consistently.

(9) (C) Abduction.

In anatomical terms, lateral movement refers to motion away from the midline toward the side. Examples include lateral flexion, where the spine bends sideways, and lateral rotation, which involves the outward rotation of a limb or body part. In limb movement, the arm raised sideways is an instance of lateral abduction. Bringing it back toward the body is lateral adduction. Lateral movements are vital for overall body flexibility and functionality.

(10) (A) Turn the forearm palm down.

Pronation in anatomical movements refers to the rotation of a body part, usually a limb, in a way that brings it into a face-down or palm-down position. This term is commonly used in reference to the forearm and foot. In the forearm, pronation involves inward rotation, which positions the palm facing downward. In the foot, pronation occurs during the natural rolling motion, where the ankle and arch collapse inward.

(11) (B) Anterior.

The anatomical term for the front of the body is *anterior*. Anterior refers to structures or positions situated toward the front of the body, i.e., facing forward. This directional term is fundamental in anatomy. It provides a standardized reference point to describe the relative placement of body parts. For example, the chest is anterior to the spine.

(12) (C) To move a body part away from the midline.

In anatomical terms, abduction involves moving a body part away from the midline. The term derives from the Latin word *abducere*, which means "to lead away." This directional term provides a clear way to describe outward movements. It aids in precise communication about the positioning and motion of limbs or other body structures.

(13) (D) S51.011A.

The information provided specifies a laceration to the right elbow and does not mention a foreign body in the wound. This particular code includes a seventh character, which indicates whether this encounter was initial, subsequent, or sequala. The letter *A* is used for an initial encounter.

(14) (B) I48.11.

This listed medical condition involves the atrium of the heart. Look up atrial fibrillation as the keyword in the index of disease and injury. Further information is listed as a subcategory for persistent atrial fibrillation. Verify the code in the diagnoses set.

(15) (B) 43255 - Endoscopic thermal cautery for bleeding ulcer.

Code 43255 specifically describes an endoscopic procedure for controlling bleeding within the upper gastrointestinal tract through thermal cautery. This code is the most appropriate for the scenario given, as it directly addresses the action taken to stop the bleeding from the gastric ulcer. The description of code 43255 includes the use of thermal energy (e.g., heat) to cauterize, or burn, the bleeding vessel in the ulcer, which is exactly the procedure performed according to the scenario.

(16) (B) N17.9.

A principal diagnosis is made by selecting and locating injury from the index of disease and injury of ICD-10-CM. Renal disorders are category N, and the code for unspecified acute injury is N17.9.

(17) (B) H65.21.

Diseases of the ear are indexed in Category H, and infection of the middle ear with serous discharge is coded as H65.21.

(18) (D) R10.31 - Pain localized to the right lower quadrant of the abdomen.

R10.31, specifically addresses pain that is localized to the right lower quadrant of the abdomen. This code is part of the R10 series in the ICD-10, which deals with different types of abdominal and pelvic pain. The specific localization of the pain is important for accurate coding because it helps to diagnose potential causes of the pain, such as appendicitis in this case.

(19) (D) Ninety days.

Hysterectomy is classified as a major procedure. Under the CMS global package, postoperative services are available within ninety days of the procedure. This includes complications following surgery but without a need for repeat visits to the operating room.

(20) (A) Zero days.

For laparoscopic procedures, the patient comes in for the procedure and goes home on the same day.

(21) (D) HCPCS Level II C Codes (Temporary Codes).

HCPCS Level II C Codes are temporary codes specifically designed for outpatient hospital services and procedures that are not represented by the codes in the permanent HCPCS Level II set. These codes are intended to facilitate the processing of claims by providing a means to report and track the usage of emerging technologies, services, and procedures that are awaiting a more permanent coding solution.

(22) (D) Organ transplantation immunotherapy management.

The global package for surgery covers patients' procedures and services in the preoperative, intraoperative, and postoperative periods. Services include:

- Intraoperative services that are a normal and essential part of the surgical procedure.
- Postoperative pain management services provided by the surgeon.
- Care of complications following the surgery. This includes medical and surgical services provided in the postoperative period that do not require another visit to the operating room.
- Follow-up visits that are related to postop recovery.

Organ transplantation immunotherapy management is not one of the services included in the global package and will be billed separately.

(23) (B) Apocrine gland.

Body odor is mainly associated with the apocrine sweat glands. These glands are concentrated in specific areas like the armpits and groin. They produce a thicker, protein-rich sweat. Bacteria on the skin break down sweat and release by-products responsible for the unpleasant body odor. Unlike eccrine sweat glands, which are widespread and produce a watery sweat for temperature regulation, apocrine glands are more involved in scent production.

(24) (A) Desquamation.

The natural shedding of dead skin cells is termed desquamation. This continuous process is part of the skin's renewal mechanism, where older cells at the skin's surface are sloughed off and replaced by newer ones from the underlying layers. Desquamation helps to maintain skin integrity, eliminates damaged cells, and supports the regeneration of healthy skin. Proper exfoliation practices can promote this natural shedding, which contributes to a smoother and more vibrant complexion.

(25) (B) Vesicle.

The medical term for a blister is *vesicle*. A vesicle is a small, fluid-filled sac within or beneath the skin, usually caused by friction, burns, or other skin irritation. Vesicles can vary in size, and their contents may include serum, blood, or other bodily fluids. They serve as a protective mechanism for the damaged skin underneath and isolate the injured area to aid healing.

(26) (C) L00-L99.

The ICD-10 code range for diseases of the skin and subcutaneous tissue falls under L00-L99. This alphanumeric coding system, established by the World Health Organization, categorizes various skin conditions. It includes infections, dermatitis, neoplasms, and other disorders.

(27) (B) L30.

The ICD-10 code used for eczema, a group of inflammatory skin conditions, is mainly found within the L30 category. The code required may differ based on the type and location of the eczema. For example, common eczema codes include L30.0 for nummular eczema and L30.1 for dyshidrosis.

(28) (C) L40.

The ICD-10 code used for psoriasis is L40. Red, scaly plaques are the defining features of psoriasis, a skin condition that persists over time. Within the L40 category, specific codes further identify the type and location of psoriasis. For example, L40.0 is for psoriasis vulgaris, the most common form.

(29) (A) M00-M25.

The ICD-10 code range for disorders of the joints (arthropathies) is M00-M25. This category includes various conditions that affect the joints, such as osteoarthritis, rheumatoid arthritis, and other inflammatory joint disorders.

(30) (A) M05-M06 - Rheumatoid arthritis.

The correct ICD-10-CM code range for documenting a diagnosis of rheumatoid arthritis is M05-M06. This range specifically covers rheumatoid arthritis and includes codes for various manifestations of the disease as it allows for the detailed documentation of the patient's condition. Rheumatoid arthritis is characterized by inflammation of multiple joints, which causes swelling and pain.

(31) (A) Low back pain.

The ICD-10 code M54.5 corresponds to *low back pain*. This code specifically identifies and classifies non-specific lower back pain, a prevalent condition that affects individuals across various age groups.

(32) (A) Osteoporosis with current pathological fracture.

The ICD-10 codes in the M80-M85 range relate to *disorders of bone density and structure*. This category encompasses conditions such as osteoporosis, pathological fractures due to osteoporosis, and other disorders that affect bone density and structure.

(33) (A) M62.830 - Muscle spasm of the back.

This code is specifically designated for muscle spasms and provides a precise location (the back) for where the spasms are occurring. Muscle spasms are involuntary contractions of a muscle or group of muscles, which can cause a significant amount of pain and discomfort.

(34) (A) Bursitis of unspecified shoulder.

The ICD-10 code M75.50 corresponds to *bursitis of unspecified shoulder*. This code documents cases of inflammation that affect the bursa in the shoulder joint with unspecified laterality.

(35) (A) Chronic obstructive pulmonary disease, unspecified.

The ICD-10-CM code J44.9 is used for chronic obstructive pulmonary disease (COPD), unspecified. This code is assigned when the specific type of COPD is not further specified or identified. It serves as a diagnostic code to indicate the presence of a chronic respiratory condition that affects airflow in the lungs. Proper coding with J44.9 helps with precise medical documentation and management for patients with COPD.

(36) (D) Neoplasm of uncertain behavior of respiratory organ, unspecified.

The ICD-10-CM code D38.6 is associated with neoplasm of uncertain behavior of respiratory organ, unspecified. This code is used when the specific characteristics of a respiratory system neoplasm cannot be precisely determined, but its potential malignancy warrants attention.

(37) (A) D63.1 - Anemia in chronic kidney disease.

This code is used to accurately document the presence of anemia as a condition that directly results from the patient's chronic kidney disease. Anemia is a common complication of CKD. It occurs as a result of the kidneys' reduced ability to produce erythropoietin, which is a hormone needed for red blood cell production.

(38) (A) Other specified secondary pulmonary hypertension.

I27.89 is used for other specified types of secondary pulmonary hypertension, which refers to high blood pressure in the lungs due to another medical condition, other than those specifically classified under primary or chronic thromboembolic categories.

(39) (B) J98.51.

The ICD-10-CM code for mediastinitis is J98.51. This code is used to classify inflammation or infection of the mediastinum, the central compartment in the chest between the lungs.

(40) (B) Atherosclerosis of aorta.

The ICD-10-CM code I70.0 is used for atherosclerosis of the aorta. This code specifically denotes the presence of atherosclerotic plaques in the aorta that contribute to the narrowing or hardening of the aorta.

(41) (A) Vein.

Veins return deoxygenated blood to the heart after the body's tissues and cells have used the oxygen. After reoxygenation in the pulmonary circuit, it will be pushed back into the left heart for eventual delivery to the other parts of the body. This completes the deoxygenation-reoxygenation cycle within the cardiovascular system.

(42) (C) Coronary circuit.

The network of blood vessels that supply the heart muscle is called the coronary circuit. This network ensures that the heart receives an adequate supply of oxygen and nutrients to sustain its continuous pumping action. The coronary circuit includes arteries and veins specifically dedicated to nourishing the cardiac tissues, which are critical to the heart's function.

(43) (B) Interventricular septum.

The anatomical structure that separates the left and right sides of the heart is the interventricular septum. It is made up of muscular tissue and forms a barrier between the left and right ventricles. The septum prevents the mixing of oxygenated and deoxygenated blood. This division ensures the efficient circulation of blood and helps the heart maintain blood flow and oxygenation throughout the body.

(44) (B) Systole.

The contraction phase of the heart muscle is called *systole*. During systole, the heart contracts, which pumps blood into the arteries for circulation. This phase ensures the effective propulsion of oxygenated blood to various tissues and organs throughout the body.

(45) (B) Chapter 9.

In ICD-10-CM, Chapter 9 is dedicated to diseases of the circulatory system. This section encompasses a comprehensive range of codes specific to cardiovascular conditions. The codes facilitate precise documentation and classification of diseases such as hypertension, heart failure, and coronary artery disease.

(46) (A) I10 - Essential (primary) hypertension.

This code is specifically designated for cases where the hypertension has no identified secondary cause, such as kidney disease or endocrine disorders, making it "essential" or "primary" in nature. Primary hypertension is a common condition characterized by persistently high blood pressure levels without an identifiable secondary cause. It is a major risk factor for cardiovascular diseases.

(47) (A) Chyme.

The semi-liquid mixture of food and digestive juices in the stomach is called chyme. Once food enters the stomach, it undergoes mechanical and chemical digestion facilitated by stomach acid and enzymes. The result is a partially broken down, acidic fluid known as chyme. This mixture is then gradually released into the small intestine for further digestion and absorption of nutrients, which is an essential role in the digestive process.

(48) (C) Large intestine.

The large intestine, which includes the colon, absorbs water and forms feces. As partially digested food moves through the colon, water is reabsorbed. This action transforms it from a liquid state into a more solid form. This process ensures that the body retains essential water as it prepares the remaining waste for elimination. The formed feces are then stored in the rectum until they are ready to be expelled during a bowel movement.

(49) (B) Dysphagia.

Dysphagia can result from various causes, such as muscle or nerve disorders that affect the esophagus. Dysphagia may cause discomfort, choking, or aspiration.

(50) (D) Secretin.

Secretin is the hormone that stimulates the release of digestive enzymes from the pancreas. When acidic chyme enters the duodenum, secretin is released. This signals the pancreas to produce and release bicarbonate to neutralize the acidity. Additionally, secretin prompts the pancreas to release digestive enzymes. This includes amylase, lipase, and proteases. This coordinated response aids the optimal digestion of carbohydrates, fats, and proteins in the small intestine.

(51) (A) K35.80 - Acute appendicitis without perforation or gangrene, unspecified.

The correct ICD-10-CM code for a diagnosis of acute appendicitis without perforation or abscess is K35.80. The specificity of code K35.80 is important for coding because it provides clear information on the severity and nature of the appendicitis.

(52) (A) K21.9.

K21.9 is the ICD-10-CM code for gastroesophageal reflux disease (GERD) without esophagitis, unspecified. This code is commonly used to represent GERD in patients where there is no specified presence of esophagitis.

(53) (C) 50020, Modifier RT.

Modifier 50 is used for bilateral procedures, and RT can replace the modifier's numerical character to provide greater specificity.

(54) (A) 50590.

Lithotripsy is a procedure in which the physician breaks up a kidney stone by applying shock waves directly over the affected kidney through a liquid surrounding the patient. 50592 is the CPT code for a unilateral procedure.

(55) (A) 52630.

CPT code 52630 is used for a transurethral resection of the prostate (TURP). This procedure is indicated for patients with prostate problems, such as those described for the patient declining open surgery for malignant neoplasm of the prostate without evidence of metastasis.

(56) (B) 54340.

Repair of hypospadias complications such as fistula, strictures, or diverticular by closure, incision, or excision is coded with 54340 in the CPT codebook.

(57) (D) 54160.

Circumcision of a neonate less than twenty-eight days old through surgical excision is coded as 54160 by the certified personnel.

(58) (A) 54560, Modifier 50.

Exploration for undescended testes with abdominal exploration is coded with CPT 54560 and modifier 50 for the bilateral nature of the condition.

(59) (A) O91.2.

The infection of the nipple associated with the puerperium in this patient is found in subcategory O91.2

(60) (A) O60.14X1, O60.14X2.

The case reported is preterm labor with preterm delivery in the third trimester with twin delivery. Therefore, the diagnosis codes are to be reported separately.

(61) (D) O69.81X1.

The ICD-10-CM diagnosis code for labor and delivery complicated by the cord around the neck without compression is O69.81X1.

(62) (A) O76.

The diagnosis of an abnormality in fetal heart rate and rhythm complicating labor and delivery is reported with the ICD-10-CM code O76.

(63) (B) O72.1 - Other immediate postpartum hemorrhage.

This code is used for significant bleeding that occurs immediately after the delivery of a baby, which is not related to the third stage of labor (the delivery of the placenta). Immediate postpartum hemorrhage is a potentially life-threatening condition that requires prompt medical attention to manage the bleeding and stabilize the patient. The designation of "other" in the code O72.1 indicates that the hemorrhage is not classified under the more specific categories of postpartum hemorrhage, such as third-stage hemorrhage (O72.0) or delayed and secondary postpartum hemorrhage (O72.3).

(64) (A) O70.0, 59300.

The ICD-10-CM diagnosis for first-degree perineal laceration sustained during delivery is O70.0, and the CPT code for repair is 59300.

(65) (A) E03.1 - Congenital hypothyroidism without goiter.

This code addresses congenital hypothyroidism, which is a condition present at birth due to an underactive thyroid gland and results in the insufficient production of thyroid hormones. The specification "without goiter" indicates that there is no enlargement of the thyroid gland associated with this condition for the newborn.

(66) (C) E11.621.

This patient likely has type 2 diabetes, given the age of onset and the current medication regimen. Poor glycemic control in this patient has resulted in a foot ulcer, which is a complication of diabetes.

(67) (D) E11.00 - Type 2 diabetes mellitus with hyperosmolarity.

This code indicates a condition where a patient with type 2 diabetes mellitus experiences hyperosmolarity. It is a state characterized by high blood sugar levels that causes a high serum osmolality without progressing to nonketotic hyperglycemic hyperosmolar coma (NKHH). This condition is a serious and potentially life-threatening complication of diabetes that requires immediate medical attention to correct the osmotic imbalance and manage the high blood glucose levels.

(68) (A) E05.90 - Thyrotoxicosis, unspecified, without thyrotoxic crisis or storm

This code corresponds to thyrotoxicosis, which is a condition that arises from an excess of thyroid hormone. Thyrotoxicosis can manifest through various symptoms such as tremors, palpitations (heart beating rapidly or irregularly), sweating (increased perspiration), and swelling in the neck area due to thyroid enlargement or goiter, which are indicative of overactive thyroid function. The specification of "unspecified" with "without thyrotoxic crisis or storm" indicates that while the patient exhibits significant symptoms of thyrotoxicosis, they do not currently meet the criteria for a thyrotoxic crisis or storm, which would be a more severe and life-threatening condition.

(69) (B) E89.2.

This patient likely has postprocedural hypoparathyroidism. This complication is a common cause of hypocalcemia following thyroid surgery, as evidenced in this clinical scenario by perioral numbness and positive chopstick signs. The ICD-10-CM diagnosis code is listed under complications associated with endocrine procedures. The code is E89.2.

(70) (A) E24.9.

The clinical information provided correlates with the diagnosis made, and the ICD-10-CM diagnosis code for Cushing's syndrome with an unspecified cause is E24.9.

(71) (A) Balance.

The function of the semicircular canals is to maintain balance alongside the vestibule of the inner ear.

(72) (D) H04.211.

The proper diagnosis code for a diagnosis of epiphora limited to the right eye is H04.211.

(73) (A) H00.11, H00.15.

This patient has bilateral chalazion. This is a slowly enlarging inflammatory nodule of the eyelid. It is coded in category H00.1 for chalazion. However, the appropriate subcategory ICD code for chalazion of both eyes affected in this patient is the right upper eyelid: H00.11 and left lower eyelid: H00.15.

(74) (D) H10.13.

The associated family history and the symptoms listed for this patient are consistent with an atopy-related condition. The most likely diagnosis is allergic conjunctivitis, which affects both eyes, and the proper ICD-10-CM code is H10.13.

(75) (D) H25.013 - Bilateral age-related cortical cataracts.

This code identifies the type of cataract as cortical, which affects the lens's cortex and is characterized by white and wedge-like opacities that start in the periphery of the lens and work their way to the center in a spoke-like fashion. The designation of "bilateral" indicates that both eyes are affected.

(76) (A) H16.012.

The correct ICD-10-CM diagnosis code for a central corneal ulcer, which affects only the left eye, as seen in this patient, is H16.012.

(77) (A) 36620.

The correct CPT code used to report arterial catheterization done as a procedure by an anesthesiologist is 36620. The code is categorized under surgical procedures due to its peculiarity.

(78) (B) AA.

The correct HCPCS level modifier used for a service supervised directly by an anesthesiologist is AA.

(79) (B) P2.

A patient with mild systemic disease who receives anesthesia is coded P2.

(80) (C) P3.

The correct answer is P3. No other information is provided on whether the disease is a constant threat to the patient's life.

(81) (A) 70551, G03.9.

The correct CPT code for an MRI of the brain and brainstem without contrast, as described above, is 70551. The ICD-10-CM diagnosis code for meningitis due to an unspecified pathogen is G03.9.

(82) (B) 71046.

This patient had a plain chest radiograph for diagnosis in two views. This includes the anteroposterior and lateral views. The CPT code for a chest radiograph in two views is 71046.

(83) (B) 72110 - Radiologic exam, spine, lumbosacral; minimum of four views.

The correct CPT code for a radiographic exam of the lumbosacral spine with a minimum of four views is 72110. This code is designed to capture diagnostic radiographic imaging of the lumbosacral spine when at least four views are taken. The purpose of obtaining multiple views is to provide a comprehensive assessment of the spine, which allows for a detailed evaluation of the vertebrae, intervertebral disc spaces, and any potential abnormalities that could be contributing to the patient's symptoms, such as chronic lower back pain.

(84) (D) 72082.

The evaluation of scoliosis using an entire thoracic (upper and middle) and lumbar (lower) spine in two planes is reported as 72082.

(85) (A) 78012.

Radioiodine uptake of the thyroid gland within four to twenty-four hours following ingestion to determine overactivity in Graves' disease is coded as 78012.

(86) (B) 77067.

Bilateral screening mammography is coded as 77067.

(87) (B) College of American Pathologists.

The acronym CAP stands for the College of American Pathologists. CAP is a prominent organization that sets quality and performance standards in pathology and laboratory medicine. It accredits laboratories, promotes excellence in diagnostics, and advances the practice of pathology for improved patient care.

(88) (D) RxNorm.

RxNorm is the coding system commonly used to identify medications and chemical substances. Developed by the National Library of Medicine, RxNorm provides a standardized nomenclature for clinical drugs, which facilitates accurate and interoperable electronic communication in healthcare. This system aids in drug information exchange, prescription processing, and clinical decision support.

(89) (A) Electronic health record.

In the context of medical coding, EHR stands for electronic health record. The purpose of EHR is to store and manage patients' health information digitally. It provides a comprehensive, accessible, and secure platform for healthcare professionals to document, code, and share patient data, which improves overall healthcare delivery.

(90) (C) Clinical Laboratory Improvement Amendments.

In laboratory medicine, CLIA stands for Clinical Laboratory Improvement Amendments. CLIA regulations establish quality standards for laboratory testing to ensure accuracy, reliability, and proficiency in medical diagnostics. These amendments regulate and certify clinical laboratories and promote excellence in laboratory practices across healthcare settings.

(91) (A) Polymerization chain reaction.

In molecular pathology, PCR stands for polymerization chain reaction. This revolutionary technique amplifies and analyzes DNA, which enables the detection of specific genetic sequences. Widely used in diagnostics, research, and forensic science, PCR has transformed genetic analysis by producing millions of copies of DNA segments. Its precision and efficiency make PCR a cornerstone in molecular pathology, which contributes significantly to genomics, microbiology, and personalized medicine.

(92) (B) A test for fetal-maternal hemorrhage.

In laboratory medicine, the eponym Kleihauer-Betke test refers to a diagnostic assay for fetal-maternal hemorrhage. This test detects fetal hemoglobin in the maternal circulation. It helps assess the extent of fetal blood exposure and determines the appropriate dosage of Rh immune globulin. This prevents complications of Rh incompatibility during pregnancy and ensures the well-being of both mother and fetus.

(93) (D) Lipid panel.

CPT code 80061 represents a lipid panel, a diagnostic laboratory test. This code covers the analysis of various blood components, including cholesterol and triglycerides. It is essential for the assessment of a patient's risk of cardiovascular disease and to monitor various lifestyle changes. It provides valuable information for healthcare professionals to make informed decisions about patient care and treatment strategies.

(94) A) 99218 - Initial observation care, 30 minutes.

This code is designated for initial observation care when the service provided includes these key components and usually involves 30 minutes of face-to-face time with the patient. It is the most appropriate code for scenarios where the patient's condition requires observation, but the complexity of care and the duration of the physician's direct involvement are on the lower end of the spectrum for observation care services.

(95) (D) 90832.

The CPT code for a psychotherapy session for the treatment of a psychiatric disorder for thirty minutes is 90832.

(96) (A) 90912.

The service rendered in training a patient to control heart rate for urinary incontinence to alter brain activity in a session that lasts fifteen minutes is 90912.

(97) (D) 90947 - Dialysis procedure other than hemodialysis (e.g., peritoneal dialysis, hemofiltration), requiring repeated evaluations with or without substantial revision of the dialysis prescription.

This code is appropriate for sessions that involve comprehensive monitoring of the patient, adjustments to the dialysate, repeated assessments of vital signs during the dialysis, management of anticoagulation, and handling of the extracorporeal circuit.

(98) (D) 91010.

The code 91010 is used for the first analysis of esophageal muscle pressure in a patient with GERD using a manometer.

(99) (C) 96360.

IV infusion to treat severe dehydration for the first thirty minutes is reported as 96360.

(100) (B) To ensure patient confidentiality.

A medical coder ensures healthcare compliance by accurately translating medical procedures into standardized codes. These codes, such as those from the Current

Procedural Terminology (CPT) or the International Classification of Diseases (ICD), are essential for precise billing and adherence to regulatory standards.

## Test 2: Questions

(1) What agency runs the most popular government healthcare insurance plan?

(A) AMA.

(B) CPC.

(C) CMS.

(D) WHO.

(2) Which section of the Medicare program focuses on outpatient care and medically necessary physician services?

(A) Medicare Part A.

(B) Medicare Part B.

(C) Medicare Part C.

(D) Medicare Part D.

(3) A 47-year-old patient is diagnosed with stage III cervical cancer after undergoing a series of diagnostic tests, including a biopsy and imaging studies. Which ICD-10-CM code should be used to accurately document this diagnosis?

(A) C53.0 - Malignant neoplasm of endocervix.

(B) C53.1 - Malignant neoplasm of exocervix.

(C) C53.8 - Malignant neoplasm of overlapping sites of cervix.

(D) C53.9 - Malignant neoplasm of cervix uteri, unspecified, stage III.

(4) During a routine procedure to remove a benign skin lesion, a patient suffers an adverse effect directly related to the surgical operation. There was no misadventure during the surgery, and the adverse effect was an expected risk of the procedure. Which ICD-10-CM code accurately documents this scenario?

(A) Y84.2 - Radiological procedure and radiotherapy.

(B) Y83.0 - Surgical operation with implant of artificial internal device.

(C) Y83.2 - Surgical operation with anastomosis, bypass or graft.

(D) Y83.9 - Surgical operation and other surgical procedures as the cause of abnormal reaction of the patient, or of later complication, without mention of misadventure at the time of operation.

(5) Which organization is responsible for publishing the ICD-10-CM?

(A) World Health Organization.

(B) Center for Medicare and Medicaid Services.

(C) Centers for Disease Control and Prevention.

(D) United States Army Medical Research Institute of Infectious Diseases.

(6) A patient presents to the emergency department with fever, cough, and shortness of breath. After performing the necessary diagnostic tests, the patient is diagnosed with COVID-19. Which ICD-10-CM code should be used to accurately document this diagnosis?

(A) J12.9 - Viral pneumonia, unspecified.

(B) B34.2 - Coronavirus infection, unspecified.

(C) U07.1 - COVID-19.

(D) B97.29 - Other coronavirus as the cause of diseases classified elsewhere.

(7) The result of the COVID-19 PCR showed that a patient was positive for the infection, and a substantive diagnosis of COVID-19 infection was made. What is the appropriate code for this diagnosis?

(A) J10.0.

(B) U07.1.

(C) J15.3.

(D) Z20.828.

(8) What does the prefix hemo- refer to in medical terminology?

(A) Skin.

(B) Blood.

(C) Bone.

(D) Heart.

(9) Which suffix is commonly used to denote inflammation in medical terms?

(A) -itis.

(B) -emia.

(C) -ology.

(D) -osis.

(10) The term gastroenteritis specifically refers to which of the following?

(A) Inflammation of the liver.

(B) Inflammation of the stomach and intestines.

(C) Inflammation of the lungs.

(D) Inflammation of the kidneys.

(11) Which medical term is used for difficulty breathing?

(A) Dysphagia.

(B) Dyspnea.

(C) Dysuria.

(D) Dystrophy.

(12) What does the prefix neo-denote in medical terminology?

(A) Old.

(B) New.

(C) Large.

(D) Small.

(13) To which body system does ophthalmic refer?

(A) Respiratory.

(B) Vision.

(C) Cardiovascular.

(D) Muscular.

(14) What does the abbreviation CPR mean in medical practice?

(A) Cardiopulmonary resuscitation.

(B) Cardiovascular perfusion ratio.

(C) Continuous patient recovery.

(D) Cranial pressure reduction.

(15) The term hyperglycemia refers to which of the following?

(A) Low blood sugar.

(B) High blood sugar.

(C) No blood sugar.

(D) Normal blood sugar.

(16) A patient visits their primary care physician complaining of a persistent cough that has been troubling them for the past two weeks. After a thorough examination and ruling out more serious conditions, the physician diagnoses the patient with a simple cough. Which code should be used to accurately document this diagnosis?

(A) J20.9 - Acute bronchitis, unspecified.

(B) R05 – Cough.

(C) J18.9 - Pneumonia, unspecified.

(D) J45.909 - Unspecified asthma, uncomplicated.

(17) A middle-aged woman presented to an oncology clinic following a referral from a primary care physician. A diagnosis of hairy cell leukemia is made. What is the correct code reported by the oncologist under the current ICD-10-CM code set?

(A) C91.4.

(B) C91.420.

(C) B90.3.

(D) C90.XX6.

(18) A patient with a known diagnosis of sickle cell anemia presents to the clinic with symptoms of a vaso-occlusive crisis, including severe pain, swelling in the hands and feet, and fever. This is a recurrent issue for the patient, who has had multiple hospital admissions for similar episodes in the past. Which code should be used?

(A) D57.00 - Sickle-cell anemia with crisis, unspecified.

(B) D57.01 - Sickle-cell anemia with acute chest syndrome.

(C) D57.02 - Sickle-cell anemia with splenic sequestration.

(D) D57.419 - Sickle-cell thalassemia without crisis.

(19) What is the ICD-10-CM code for essential tremors?

(A) J31.44.

(B) G24.78.

(C) G25.

(D) G25.0.

(20) A seventy-eight-year-old man was brought in for a routine check-up by his son, who is visiting from South America. He noticed his father had developed a deep wound on his right heel, which had received poor care. Further assessment by the physician revealed a pressure ulcer on the right heel, stage 4. What ICD-10-CM code set is assigned to the diagnosis?

(A) L88.604.

(B) L89.614.

(C) L89.6.

(D) L89.61.

(21) A patient presents to the emergency department with symptoms of severe allergic reaction after a bee sting. The physician orders the administration of Rho(D) immune globulin intramuscularly to prevent complications. Which CPT code should be used to accurately document the administration of Rho(D) immune globulin?

(A) 90376 - Rho(D) immune globulin, human, for intravenous use.

(B) 90384 - Rho(D) immune globulin, human, for intramuscular use, not otherwise specified.

(C) 90386 - Rho(D) immune globulin (RhIG), human, full-dose, for intramuscular use.

(D) 90632 - Hepatitis A vaccine, adult dosage, for intramuscular use.

(22) According to the CPT surgery guidelines, which is not a component in the global package?

(A) Preoperative evaluation.

(B) Postoperative evaluation.

(C) Surgery for any procedure during the postoperative period.

(D) Services provided during the surgery.

(23) A patient complained of a fluid-filled lump in the neck region. The physician diagnosed a sebaceous cyst, and the patient was to have ultrasound-guided fine needle aspiration cytology. What is the appropriate CPT code for this procedure?

(A) 88182.

(B) 53855.

(C) 88173.

(D) 61680.

(24) The National Correct Coding Initiative (NCCI) is a US government initiative mainly controlled by which body?

(A) American Medical Association (AMA).

(B) Center for Disease Control and Prevention (CDC).

(C) Healthcare Common Procedure Coding System (HCPCS).

(D) Center for Medicare and Medicaid Services (CMS).

(25) Which statement about the CPT is correct?

(A) The CPT Category I code is a five-digit alphanumeric code for reporting and reimbursement.

(B) The CPT Category II code is a mandatory code set that must be included for reimbursement.

(C) CPT Category I codes are owned and updated yearly by the American Medical Association (AMA).

(D) The CPT Category III code is a temporary code assigned by the Center for Medicare and Medicaid Services (CMS) for experimental procedures and services.

(26) What is the largest organ in the human body?

(A) Liver.

(B) Heart.

(C) Skin.

(D) Lungs.

(27) Which layer of the skin helps insulate the body?

(A) Epidermis.

(B) Dermis.

(C) Subcutaneous tissue.

(D) Hypodermis.

(28) What type of tissue is the main component of the epidermis?

(A) Connective tissue.

(B) Nervous tissue.

(C) Epithelial tissue.

(D) Muscle tissue.

(29) What is the primary function of sweat glands?

(A) Temperature regulation.

(B) Vitamin synthesis.

(C) Protection from UV radiation.

(D) Sensation of touch.

(30) What is another term for the cuticle of the nail?

(A) Lunula.

(B) Matrix.

(C) Eponychium.

(D) Hyponychium.

(31) Which of the following is the outermost layer of the epidermis?

(A) Stratum corneum.

(B) Stratum basale.

(C) Stratum granulosum.

(D) Stratum spinosum.

(32) What is the primary function of the musculoskeletal system?

(A) Transportation of nutrients.

(B) Support and protection.

(C) Filtration of blood.

(D) Regulation of body temperature.

(33) Which term refers to the study of the structure and function of joints?

(A) Myology.

(B) Osteology.

(C) Arthrology.

(D) Chondrology.

(34) What anatomical term describes the outer covering of a bone?

(A) Epiphysis.

(B) Periosteum.

(C) Endosteum.

(D) Medullary cavity.

(35) Which of the following describes the movement of a body part toward the midline?

(A) Abduction.

(B) Adduction.

(C) Flexion.

(D) Extension.

(36) Which of the following is not a component of the axial skeleton?

(A) Skull.

(B) Vertebral column.

(C) Femur.

(D) Ribcage.

(37) Which ICD-10 category is designated for diseases of the musculoskeletal system?

(A) A00-B99.

(B) C00-D49.

(C) M00-M99.

(D) S00-T88.

(38) Which of the following terms refers to the space between the lungs in the chest cavity?

(A) Ventral.

(B) Dorsal.

(C) Mediastinum.

(D) Diaphragm.

(39) Which anatomical structure is associated with the term phrenic?

(A) Heart.

(B) Lungs.

(C) Diaphragm.

(D) Spleen.

(40) In anatomical terms, where is the thoracic cavity located in the body?

(A) Abdomen.

(B) Head.

(C) Chest.

(D) Pelvis.

(41) The suffix -emia in medical terminology refers to which of the following?

(A) Nervous system.

(B) Blood.

(C) Lymphatic system.

(D) Respiratory system.

(42) Which anatomical term describes the back or posterior side of the body?

(A) Anterior.

(B) Ventral.

(C) Dorsal.

(D) Superior.

(43) Which ICD-10-CM code range is used for diseases of the respiratory system?

(A) J00-J60.

(B) R00-R99.

(C) J00-J99.

(D) K20-K31.

(44) Which of the following is the primary function of the cardiovascular system?

(A) Digestion.

(B) Transportation of blood.

(C) Respiration.

(D) Immune response.

(45) Which of the following organs is the central pump of the cardiovascular system?

(A) Liver.

(B) Heart.

(C) Lungs.

(D) Kidneys.

(46) Which of the following best describes the role of arteries in the cardiovascular system?

(A) Carry deoxygenated blood to the heart.

(B) Pump blood to the body tissues.

(C) Exchange gasses in the lungs.

(D) Carry oxygenated blood away from the heart.

(47) Which chamber of the heart receives blood from the systemic circulation?

(A) Left atrium.

(B) Right atrium.

(C) Left ventricle.

(D) Right ventricle.

(48) What are the upper chambers of the heart called?

(A) Ventricles.

(B) Atria.

(C) Aorta.

(D) Coronary arteries.

(49) What term refers to the lower chambers of the heart?

(A) Ventricles.

(B) Atria.

(C) Aorta.

(D) Coronary arteries.

(50) Which of the following best describes the primary function of the digestive system?

(A) Respiration.

(B) Circulation.

(C) Digestion.

(D) Excretion.

(51) Which of the following organs produces bile to aid in the digestion of fats?

(A) Stomach.

(B) Pancreas.

(C) Liver.

(D) Gallbladder.

(52) What is the term for muscular contractions that move food through the digestive tract?

(A) Peristalsis.

(B) Digestion.

(C) Absorption.

(D) Segmentation.

(53) The process of nutrient absorption into the bloodstream is carried out by which part of the digestive system?

(A) Stomach.

(B) Small intestine.

(C) Large intestine.

(D) Esophagus.

(54) Which of the following is the gallbladder's central function?

(A) Produce insulin.

(B) Store bile.

(C) Absorb nutrients.

(D) Mix stomach contents.

(55) Which enzyme is produced by the salivary glands to begin the digestion of carbohydrates?

(A) Amylase.

(B) Lipase.

(C) Protease.

(D) Peptidase.

(56) A patient is diagnosed with congestive heart failure (CHF) after presenting with symptoms of shortness of breath, fatigue, and fluid retention. Echocardiography confirms the diagnosis and indicates reduced ejection fraction. Which code should be used to document this diagnosis of congestive heart failure?

(A) I50.9 - Heart failure, unspecified.

(B) I50.20 - Unspecified systolic (congestive) heart failure.

(C) I50.22 - Chronic systolic (congestive) heart failure.

(D) I50.43 - Acute on chronic combined systolic and diastolic heart failure.

(57) A patient undergoes a surgical procedure for the removal of a malignant neoplasm of the rectum. Which ICD-10-PCS code should be used for the surgical removal of the rectal tumor?

(A) 0DB78ZZ - Excision of rectum, via natural or artificial opening endoscopic.

(B) 0DB68ZZ - Excision of rectum, open.

(C) 0DTJ8ZZ - Resection of rectum, via natural or artificial opening endoscopic.

(D) 0DTJ0ZZ - Resection of rectum, open.

(58) A patient presents with severe left-sided flank pain and undergoes imaging, which reveals hydronephrosis of the left kidney due to an obstructing ureteral stone. Which ICD-10-CM code should be used to accurately document this diagnosis?

(A) N13.30 - Unspecified hydronephrosis.

(B) N20.0 - Calculus of kidney.

(C) N13.2 - Hydronephrosis with renal and ureteral calculous obstruction.

(D) N13.6 – Pyonephrosis.

(59) A patient undergoes a comprehensive metabolic panel (CMP) during a routine health examination. The CMP includes 14 different tests and covers electrolytes, kidney function, and liver function. Which CPT code should be used to accurately document this laboratory procedure?

(A) 80048 - Basic metabolic panel (BMP).

(B) 80053 - Comprehensive metabolic panel (CMP).

(C) 80069 - Renal function panel.

(D) 80076 - Hepatic function panel.

(60) A seventy-five-year-old man was previously diagnosed with benign prostatic hyperplasia. His urologist sees him for a review of his routine lab results. He currently has no symptoms. What is the ICD-10-CM code reported?

(A) N34.7.

(B) C23.H.

(C) C34.89.

(D) N40.0.

(61) A patient undergoes urodynamic testing to evaluate the capacity of the bladder due to complaints of frequent urination and urgency. The testing involves the measurement of bladder pressure and capacity, as well as flow rates. Which CPT code should be used for this urodynamic testing?

(A) 51725 - Simple cystometrogram (CMG).

(B) 51726 - Complex cystometrogram (CMG); without urethral pressure profile.

(C) 51728 - Complex cystometrogram (CMG); with urethral pressure profile (UPP).

(D) 51729 - Complex cystometrogram (CMG); with urethral pressure profile (UPP) and voiding pressure studies.

(62) In what part of the female reproductive system does normal fertilization occur?

(A) Fallopian tube.

(B) Cervix.

(C) Ovary.

(D) Fundus.

(63) A pap smear is used to screen for:

(A) Vaginal cancer.

(B) Cervical cancer.

(C) Ovarian cancer.

(D) Breast cancer.

(64) What is the ICD-10-CM code for endometrial cancer?

(A) C54.1.

(B) C57.1.

(C) C54.

(D) C53.0.

(65) A thirty-two-year-old woman sees her gynecologist for a routine check. At her previous appointment, she complained of heavy menstrual bleeding. This required a change of tampons five times a day, as opposed to her previous use of three tampons in a day. An examination of her abdomen finds a firm, mobile swelling in the suprapubic region, which extends toward the umbilicus. An abdominopelvic ultrasound is recommended, and the results confirm a diagnosis of uterine fibroids. What is the ICD-10-CM code to be reported by her gynecologist?

(A) D25.9.

(B) D24.4.

(C) D22.9.

(D) D25.8.

(66) A young woman presents at the emergency department a week after home delivery due to persistent fever, nausea, and malaise. She had no prophylactic antibiotics administered following vaginal delivery of her baby. Her temperature is 38.2° C, her blood pressure is 100/60 mm Hg, and her pulse rate is 110 bpm. A complete blood count reveals an elevated white blood cell count of 17,000 cells/mm3, with neutrophilia of eighty percent. The attending physician assesses puerperal sepsis and commences intravenous antibiotics. What is the diagnosis code according to ICD-10-CM?

(A) O83.0.

(B) O85.

(C) O842.

(D) O87.1.

(67) A thirty-eight-year-old pregnant woman complains of sudden chest pain while speaking to her husband earlier in the day. She is thirty-four weeks pregnant and weighs 110 kg. An examination of the lower extremities reveals bilateral pedal edema up to the knees, and she complains of occasional pain in the calf. She has mostly been at home for the past two months and requires help lifting herself from the bed for a few activities. Doppler ultrasound of the lower limb confirms the presence of deep vein thrombosis. She is admitted by her obstetrician for close monitoring and further care. State the ICD-10-CM diagnosis code.

(A) O88.223.

(B) O89.212.

(C) O88.213.

(D) O78.215.

(68) What endocrine organ produces insulin in the body?

(A) Heart.

(B) Pancreas.

(C) Kidneys.

(D) Duodenum.

(69) Where is the thyroid gland located?

(A) Abdomen.

(B) Neck.

(C) Chest.

(D) Brain.

(70) What level of the nervous system are neurotransmitters produced?

(A) Dendrites.

(B) Synapse.

(C) Axon.

(D) Nerves.

(71) The brainstem is composed of which of the following?

(A) Pons, cerebellum, medulla.

(B) Pons, medulla, globus pallidus.

(C) Pons, midbrain, medulla.

(D) Midbrain, cerebrum, putamen.

(72) The pituitary gland produces which of the following hormones?

(A) Insulin.

(B) Thymosin.

(C) Cortisol.

(D) Oxytocin.

(73) Hydrocephalus is caused by excess cerebrospinal fluid accumulation in what part of the brain?

(A) Ventricles.

(B) Cerebellum.

(C) Globus pallidus.

(D) Pons.

(74) What part of the eye allows light to enter?

(A) Iris.

(B) Pupil.

(C) Retina.

(D) Cornea.

(75) On what part of the eye are images formed?

(A) Pupil.

(B) Choroid.

(C) Retina.

(D) Cornea.

(76) The inner ear consists of which of the following?

(A) Semicircular canals.

(B) Pinna.

(C) Eustachian tube.

(D) Stapes.

(77) What is the colored part of the eye called?

(A) Iris.

(B) Choroid.

(C) Uvea.

(D) Retina.

(78) A patient presents with a laceration on the outer ear that requires surgical repair. The physician performs a complex closure of the wound. Which CPT code should be used for the surgical repair of the outer ear?

(A) 12031 - Repair, intermediate, wounds of scalp, axillae, trunk and/or extremities (excluding hands and feet); 2.5 cm or less.

(B) 12051 - Repair, intermediate, wounds of neck, hands, feet and/or external genitalia; 2.5 cm or less.

(C) 13120 - Repair, complex, scalp, arms, and/or legs; 2.5 cm or less.

(D) 13121 - Repair, complex, eyelids, nose, ears and/or lips; 2.5 cm or less.

(79) Which of the following are middle ear bones?

(A) Stapes, malleus, and incus.

(B) Choroid, incus, and stapes.

(C) Stylus, incus, and malleus.

(D) Stapes, malleus, and indole.

(80) What type of anesthesia is an epidural?

(A) Neuraxial anesthesia.

(B) General anesthesia.

(C) Local anesthesia.

(D) Block anesthesia.

(81) During an emergency situation, a patient requires intubation to secure the airway. The physician performs an endotracheal intubation in a critical setting. Which CPT code should be used?

(A) 31500 - Intubation, endotracheal, emergency procedure.

(B) 99291 - Critical care, evaluation and management of the critically ill or critically injured patient; first 30-74 minutes.

(C) 31600 - Tracheostomy, planned (separate procedure).

(D) 31605 - Tracheostomy, emergency procedure (separate procedure).

(82) A surgeon performs a surgical procedure to create an opening into the small intestine for a patient who needs nutritional support due to a non-functioning gastrointestinal tract. Which CPT code best describes this surgical procedure?

(A) 44120 - Enterectomy, resection of small intestine; single resection and anastomosis.

(B) 43659 - Unlisted laparoscopy procedure, stomach.

(C) 44310 - Ostomy, small intestine.

(D) 49491 - Repair, initial inguinal hernia, preterm infant (younger than 37 weeks gestation at birth), neonate.

(83) What is the term for studying the uterus and fallopian tube following dye injection?

(A) Hysteroscopy.

(B) Hysterosalpingography.

(C) Angiography.

(D) Mammography.

(84) A patient presents with severe headaches and a recent history of trauma to the head. The physician orders a radiographic exam of the skull to assess for possible fractures or other abnormalities. Which CPT code should be used?

(A) 70250 - Radiologic examination, skull; less than four views.

(B) 70260 - Radiologic examination, skull; minimum of four views.

(C) 70450 - CT scan, head or brain; without contrast material.

(D) 70540 - MRI, orbit, face, and/or neck; without contrast material.

(85) A sialogram is a plain X-ray used to examine which of the following structures?

(A) Salivary gland.

(B) Sella turcica.

(C) Adrenal gland.

(D) Pancreas.

(86) Dr. A orders a chest radiograph for a patient with chest pain, cough, and drenching night sweats. The chest radiograph is reported appropriately, and the patient is asked to return for follow-up. During a follow-up appointment, Dr. B carries out a different chest radiograph on the same patient. Another report is made based on the findings. What is the correct code for the procedures?

(A) 71045-26, 71045-76.

(B) 71045-26, 71044-77.

(C) 71045-26, 71055-77.

(D) 71045-26, 71045-77.

(87) A mammogram assesses which of the following parts of the body for cancer?

(A) Thyroid.

(B) Breast.

(C) Neck.

(D) Thorax.

(88) A patient visits their primary care physician for a routine follow-up on their hypertension management. During the visit, the physician performs a blood pressure check, reviews the patient's current medication regimen, discusses lifestyle modifications, and makes minor adjustments to the medication. The encounter lasts approximately 15 minutes. Which CPT code should be used?

(A) 99211 - Office or other outpatient visit for the evaluation and management of an established patient, that may not require the presence of a physician. Usually, the presenting problem(s) are minimal.

(B) 99212 - Office or other outpatient visit for the evaluation and management of an established patient, which requires a problem focused history, a problem focused exam, and straightforward medical decision making.

(C) 99213 - Office or other outpatient visit for the evaluation and management of an established patient, which requires an expanded problem focused history, an expanded problem focused exam, and medical decision making of low complexity.

(D) 99214 - Office or other outpatient visit for the evaluation and management of an established patient, which requires a detailed history, a detailed exam, and medical decision making of moderate complexity.

(89) What does the acronym CBC refer to in laboratory medicine coding?

(A) Complete blood count.

(B) Cardiovascular bypass control.

(C) Centralized billing code.

(D) Comprehensive biochemical chart.

(90) What does the acronym ICD-10-CM stand for in pathology coding?

(A) International Classification of Diseases, 10th Edition, Clinical Modification.

(B) Integrated Coding Database for Medical Conditions.

(C) Invasive Cardiovascular Diagnosis, 10th Module.

(D) Internal Control of Disease Management.

(91) What does the acronym CPT stand for in medical coding?

(A) Clinical Pathology Terminology.

(B) Current Procedural Terminology.

(C) Critical Patient Tracking.

(D) Chronic Pain Treatment.

(92) Which term describes the microscopic examination of tissues to diagnose diseases?

(A) Radiography.

(B) Histology.

(C) Serology.

(D) Hematology.

(93) What does the acronym SNOMED CT mean in medical terminologies?

(A) Surgical Nomenclature and Outcome Measurement in Electronic Documentation.

(B) Systemized Nomenclature of Medicine Clinical Terms.

(C) Standardized Numerical Order for Medical Conditions and Treatments.

(D) Scientific Notation for Organizational Medical Entities Database.

(94) What does LOINC refer to in laboratory medicine coding?

(A) Laboratory Order and Inventory Control.

(B) Logical Observation Identifiers Names and Codes.

(C) Low-Oxygen Incubation for Nutrient Cultures.

(D) Longitudinal Organ Index for Normalized Classification.

(95) A patient is admitted to the hospital with severe chest pain and shortness of breath. The admitting physician performs a detailed history and physical exam, spends 30 minutes at the patient's bedside, and determines the need for immediate diagnostic testing to rule out a myocardial infarction. Which CPT code should be used?

(A) 99217 - Observation care discharge.

(B) 99218 - Initial observation care, 30 minutes.

(C) 99221 - Initial hospital care, for the evaluation and management of a patient, which requires these 3 key components: a detailed or comprehensive history; a detailed or comprehensive examination; and medical decision making of straightforward or low complexity. Physicians spend 30 minutes at the bedside and on the patient's hospital floor or unit.

(D) 99238 - Hospital discharge day management, 30 minutes or less.

(96) A patient presents to a hospital with complaints of headache and chest pain. The chest pain was said to be recurrent, intermittent, and relieved by rest. A focused history and exam were done, and the MDM level was moderate. An ECG was done, and he was placed in observation care for about two hours. He was discharged on medications as he insisted on leaving for a meeting in another state later in the day. He presented at a hospital in another state on the same day and was placed in inpatient care for treatment due to the worsening of his symptoms. He was discharged the following morning. What is the appropriate CPT code for the last presentation in the hospital?

(A) 99221.

(B) 99238, 99416.

(C) 99213.

(D) 99233, 99418.

(97) Mr. Cook is a long-term patient who is at a follow-up visit for diabetes and hypertension management. When taking his blood pressure measurements, his physician reviews the results of the previous three glucose tests. The patient's blood pressure was normal, but his glucose level was still higher than normal. The physician adjusted Mr. Cook's insulin dosage. A physical exam was made, a comprehensive history was obtained, and somewhat complex medical decisions were made. What is the appropriate CPT code?

(A) 99213.

(B) 99232.

(C) 99214.

(D) 99202.

(98) An anesthesiologist is paged for an emergency cesarean section. After reporting the CPT code for the anesthesia given during the cesarean section, what add-on code should be included in the complete medical code reported?

(A) +99100.

(B) +99116.

(C) +99135.

(D) +99140.

(99) A patient visits their primary clinic for a COVID-19 vaccine. The patient receives a five mcg/ml dose in the left upper arm. Report the correct CPT code for this procedure and the code for the vaccine received.

(A) 90483, 91314.

(B) 90470, 91305.

(C) 90380, 90304.

(D) 90480, 91304.

(100) A twenty-four-year-old rhesus-negative woman recently delivered a healthy male neonate. She had no prenatal care. She is counseled on receiving Rhesus D immunoglobulin to prevent hemolytic disease in newborns. What is the CPT code for the immunoglobulin?

(A) 90386.

(B) 90296.

(C) 90486.

(D) 91296.

# Test 2: Answers and Explanations

(1) (C) CMS.

The Center for Medicare and Medicaid Services (CMS) is responsible for Medicare, the largest insurance scheme in the US. It also oversees other insurance schemes that cover different target population groups, such as Medicaid, Child's Health Insurance Program (CHIP), and other state and federal insurance packages.

(2) (B) Medicare Part B.

The Medicare Program has different and distinct parts, but their services are often bundled. Medicaid Part B covers outpatient care and necessary physician services.

(3) (D) C53.9 - Malignant neoplasm of cervix uteri, unspecified, stage III.

C53.9 is used to indicate a malignant neoplasm of the cervix uteri without specifying the part of the cervix (endocervix or exocervix) when the documentation does not distinctly identify the origin within the cervix or when the cancer affects multiple areas making it difficult to pinpoint a more specific site. The designation of "stage III" in the diagnosis highlights the extent of cancer spread, which in the context of cervical cancer means that the cancer has extended beyond the cervix to the pelvic wall and/or the lower portion of the vagina, without spreading to distant sites.

(4) (D) Y83.9 - Surgical operation and other surgical procedures as the cause of abnormal reaction of the patient, or of later complication, without mention of misadventure at the time of operation.

This code is part of the ICD-10-CM chapter that deals with external causes of morbidity. It indicates complications that arise from surgical operations and other surgical procedures that cause abnormal reactions or later complications in the patient.

(5) (C) Centers for Disease Control and Prevention.

The ICD-10-CM is published by the CDC's National Center for Health Statistics. The World Health Organization (WHO) is responsible for the ICD-10 document upon which the ICD-10-CM is based. The Center for Medicare and Medicaid Services is responsible for the ICD-10-PCS codes used in the US in 2024. The United States Army Medical Research Institute of Infectious Diseases (USAMRIID) is not responsible for any code set.

(6) (C) U07.1 - COVID-19.

The correct ICD-10-CM code for a diagnosis of COVID-19 is U07.1. This code was created to document cases of the Coronavirus Disease 2019 (COVID-19), caused by the novel coronavirus SARS-CoV-2. The code is used for confirmed diagnoses of COVID-19 as documented by the provider, a positive COVID-19 test result, or a presumptive positive COVID-19 test result.

(7) (B) U07.1.

U07.1 is the code used for a confirmed case of COVID-19. Z20.828 is used for contact with and suspected exposure to other viral communicable diseases. J15.3 is the code used for a diagnosis of pneumonia due to streptococcus, group B. J10.0 is the code used for a diagnosis of influenza due to seasonal influenza virus.

(8) (B) Blood.

Hemo- in medical terminology, relates to blood. This prefix is derived from the Greek word *haima*, meaning blood. It is commonly used in terms like hemoglobin (the protein in red blood cells), hematology (the study of blood), and hemorrhage (excessive bleeding).

(9) (A) -itis.

The suffix -itis is frequently employed in medical terminology to indicate inflammation. Derived from Greek, it is added to the end of various organ or tissue names to denote inflammatory conditions. Examples include tonsillitis (inflammation of the tonsils), arthritis (inflammation of joints), and dermatitis (inflammation of the skin).

(10) (B) Inflammation of the stomach and intestines.

Viral or bacterial infections commonly trigger inflammation of the stomach and intestines. This is known as gastroenteritis. This condition usually presents with symptoms such as diarrhea, abdominal cramps, nausea, and vomiting. The prefix gastro- refers to the stomach, and -enteritis is inflammation of the intestines. Commonly contracted through contaminated food or water, the regular activity of the digestive system is interrupted by gastroenteritis. Although usually self-limiting, severe cases may require medical attention to prevent complications.

(11) (B) Dyspnea.

*Dyspnea* is the medical term used to describe difficulty with breathing. It originates from Greek roots, where *dys* means difficult, and *pnea* refers to breathing. Dyspnea describes a range of sensations, from shortness of breath to labored breathing. It is a critical symptom seen in various respiratory and cardiovascular disorders.

(12) (B) New.

The prefix neo- in medical terminology indicates new or recent. This prefix originated from the Greek word *neos*. It is commonly used to describe modern, novel, or regenerated things. Examples of its application in medical literature include neoplasm (a new and abnormal growth, often referring to tumors) and neonatology (the branch of medicine focused on caring for newborns).

(13) (B) Vision.

The term ophthalmic relates to the visual system or the eyes. It is derived from the Greek word *ophthalmos*, meaning eye. This term is commonly used in medical contexts associated with eye care and vision. Ophthalmic medications and procedures are used to diagnose and treat eye-related conditions. An ophthalmologist is a medical professional who identifies and treats eye-related illnesses.

(14) (A) Cardiopulmonary resuscitation.

Cardiopulmonary Resuscitation can be abbreviated as CPR. When a patient's respiration or heartbeat stops, this emergency treatment is carried out to save their life. Rescue breathing is used in CPR to supply oxygen, while chest compressions are used to keep blood flowing to the brain.

(15) (B) High blood sugar.

Hyperglycemia refers to elevated levels of glucose (sugar) in the blood. It commonly occurs in diabetic patients when the body cannot effectively regulate blood sugar levels. Factors such as insulin deficiency or insulin resistance contribute to its development. Symptoms of hyperglycemia include polydipsia, polyuria, and fatigue. Hyperglycemia must be appropriately managed to prevent complications.

(16) (B) R05 – Cough.

This code is designated for cases where the patient's primary complaint is coughing without an associated diagnosis of a more specific respiratory condition. The R05 code is used when the cough is the symptom being treated or noted, and no further underlying condition has been diagnosed at the time of the encounter.

(17) (A) C91.4.

The information provided is listed under blood disorders in the index. Verify code accuracy in the ICD-10-CM code book.

(18) (A) D57.00 - Sickle-cell anemia with crisis, unspecified.

This code accurately reflects the patient's condition, capturing both the underlying disease (sickle cell anemia) and the acute exacerbation (crisis) without specifying the type of crisis. Vaso-occlusive crises are common in sickle cell disease and are characterized by severe pain due to the obstruction of blood flow by sickled red blood cells.

(19) (D) G25.0.

Tremors are categorized as neurological symptoms with varying classifications. Essential tremor is listed as code set G25.0.

(20) (B) L89.614.

Ulcers are skin conditions due to several underlying factors. Pressure ulcers are listed under subcategory L89.61. Further details of the stage of pressure ulcers cause the inclusion of a sixth character. The code set is L89.614.

(21) (C) 90386 - Rho(D) immune globulin (RhIG), human, full-dose, for intramuscular use.

This code is designated for the full-dose administration of human Rho(D) immune globulin (RhIG) by the intramuscular route. Rho(D) immune globulin is used in various clinical scenarios, including the prevention of Rh immunization in individuals exposed to Rh-positive blood.

(22) (C) Surgery for any procedure during the postoperative period.

The global package includes the materials and services considered essential components of a procedure. Depending on the classification of the surgical procedure, the services covered may consist of preoperative, intraoperative, and postoperative. The duration for which it is valid depends on the classification as a major procedure, minor procedure, or endoscopy. The services, however, only apply to the primary condition for which the patient was admitted and is to have the surgical procedure.

(23) (C) 88173.

This is the correct CPT code for an ultrasound-guided fine needle aspiration cytology procedure.

(24) (D) Center for Medicare and Medicaid Services (CMS).

The American Medical Association (AMA) manages and updates the CPT codebook. The National Correct Coding Initiative is an initiative of the Center for Medicare and Medicaid Services (CMS). The Healthcare Common Procedure Coding System (HCPCS) is an in-house coding system of the CMS. The Center for Disease Control (CDC) is unrelated to medical coding guidelines.

(25) (C) CPT Category I codes are owned and updated yearly by the American Medical Association (AMA).

CPT Category I code is a five-digit numerical code (for example, 12345) used for reporting and reimbursement. It is not alphanumerical. CPT Category II codes are optional performance tracking codes and are not mandatory. CPT Category III codes are assigned by the AMA and not CMS. CPT Category I codes are copyrighted and reviewed and have a yearly update by the American Medical Association.

(26) (C) Skin.

The human body's largest organ is the skin. It has several functions that include protecting against harmful environmental microbes and substances. The skin regulates body temperature, prevents dehydration, and serves sensory functions. It comprises the epidermis and dermis and is vital to overall health and wellness.

(27) (C) Subcutaneous tissue.

The subcutaneous tissue is located below the dermis and insulates the body. It consists of fat cells, which act as a thermal regulator. This prevents heat loss and protects against extreme temperatures. It is a type of adipose tissue that cushions organs and provides protection. The subcutaneous layer's insulation properties contribute significantly to maintaining internal temperature and homeostasis.

(28) (C) Epithelial tissue.

Epithelial cells are the primary component of the epidermis. They create a protective barrier against external elements. The epithelial cells' stratified arrangement in the epidermis forms a robust, durable, and nearly impervious protective barrier. Keratinocytes are specialized types of epithelial cells. They produce keratin, which enhances the structural resilience of the epidermis. This cellular organization ensures that the epidermis protects the body from environmental factors, infections, and dehydration.

(29) (A) Temperature regulation.

The production of sweat is essential for thermoregulation. Sweat glands have a significant role in controlling body temperature. Sweat evaporates from the skin's surface and dissipates heat, which cools the body. Eccrine sweat glands found throughout the body mainly regulate body temperature. Apocrine sweat glands are concentrated in specific areas and contribute to scent production. Sweating also helps eliminate waste products and maintain electrolyte balance.

(30) (C) Eponychium.

The nail cuticle can also be called the eponychium. This thin, protective layer of tissue covers the base of the nail and connects the nail plate to the surrounding skin. The eponychium provides a seal to protect the developing nail.

(31) (A) Stratum corneum.

The stratum corneum is the outermost layer of the epidermis. It comprises flattened, dead skin cells known as corneocytes and is a protective barrier. This layer prevents dehydration, shields against pathogens, and improves overall skin strength. As corneocytes gradually slough off, new cells from the underlying layers replace them. This action maintains the epidermis's continuous renewal and ensures its role in skin protection.

(32) (B) Support and protection.

The musculoskeletal system is the body's framework and enables movement, support, and stability. It comprises bones, muscles, tendons, and ligaments. It protects vital organs and maintains posture. Additionally, the bone marrow is essential in hematopoiesis (the production of blood cells).

(33) (C) Arthrology.

Arthrology is the study of the intricate mechanics and anatomy of joints. It examines how they enable movement, provide flexibility, and contribute to the overall functionality of the musculoskeletal system.

(34) (B) Periosteum.

The outer covering of the bone is known as the periosteum. This thin, fibrous membrane envelopes bones and provides protection and nourishment. It also serves as a ligament and tendon attachment site. The periosteum is central to bone production and repair. It contains blood vessels and osteoblasts for bone regeneration. Its sensitivity contributes to pain perception, which guides the body's responses to potential injuries or fractures within the skeletal system.

(35) (B) Adduction.

The anatomical term for the movement of a body part toward the midline is adduction. Adduction involves bringing a limb or structure closer to the body's central axis. This movement is important in various activities, such as drawing the arm back to the side or bringing the legs together.

(36) (C) Femur.

The femur is not part of the axial skeleton, which comprises the skull, vertebral column, and ribcage. The femur is a significant component of the appendicular skeleton. It is the longest and strongest bone in the human body. The femur is located in the thigh region and is essential for lower limb movement.

(37) (C) M00-M99.

The ICD-10 category designated for diseases of the musculoskeletal system is M00-M99. This coding range encompasses various conditions that affect bones, joints, muscles, and connective tissues. From arthritis and osteoporosis to injuries and congenital anomalies, the M00-M99 category provides a systematic framework to classify and code disorders within the musculoskeletal system.

(38) (C) Mediastinum.

The space between the lungs in the chest cavity is called the mediastinum. The mediastinum is a central compartment of the thoracic cavity that houses vital structures such as the heart, major blood vessels, thymus gland, and esophagus. It extends from the sternum anteriorly to the vertebral column posteriorly and from the first rib to the diaphragm. It protects and supports the enclosed essential organs.

(39) (C) Diaphragm.

The term phrenic is mainly associated with anatomical structures related to the diaphragm. Specifically, it refers to the phrenic nerves, which originate from the cervical spine (C3-C5) and innervate the diaphragm. These nerves play a vital role in respiratory function by transmitting signals to the diaphragm, which prompts muscle contractions for breathing. The term phrenic is often used in diaphragmatic anatomy and physiological processes associated with respiration.

(40) (C) Chest.

In anatomical terms, the thoracic cavity is located in the chest region. It is situated between the neck and the abdomen and bound by the rib cage and sternum. It houses vital organs, such as the heart and lungs. This anatomical compartment is important in respiratory and circulatory functions, which contribute to the overall physiological well-being of the body.

(41) (B) Blood.

The suffix -emia in medical terminology refers to conditions relating to the blood. It is commonly used to indicate the presence of a particular substance or condition in the bloodstream. Examples include anemia (a deficiency of red blood cells) and bacteremia (the presence of bacteria in the blood). This suffix helps precisely describe various blood-related disorders and their underlying causes within the realm of medical terminology.

(42) (C) Dorsal.

The anatomical term that describes the back or posterior side of the body is dorsal. It refers to the side or surface that faces away from the front or ventral side. In anatomical positions, the spine is usually considered the dorsal side. This provides a standardized reference for medical and anatomical descriptions.

(43) (C) J00-J99.

The ICD-10-CM code range used for diseases of the respiratory system is J00-J99. This range encompasses a variety of conditions that affect the respiratory tract. This includes infections, obstructive pulmonary diseases, and other respiratory disorders. Proper coding within this range allows healthcare professionals to accurately document and classify respiratory conditions, which facilitates effective communication and management of patient health information.

(44) (B) Transportation of blood.

The cardiovascular system's primary function is to transport blood throughout the body. This intricate network of vessels includes arteries, veins, and capillaries. It works in conjunction with the heart—the central pump. Blood carries vital oxygen, nutrients, and hormones to tissues. It also removes waste products. This continuous circulation ensures proper oxygenation, nutrient delivery, and waste elimination, which supports the metabolic processes essential for the body's health and function.

(45) (B) Heart.

The heart serves as the central pump of the cardiovascular system. It is located in the chest, and its rhythm of contraction and relaxation propels blood throughout the circulatory network. It comprises four chambers: atria and ventricles. The heart ensures the unidirectional flow of oxygenated blood to the body and deoxygenated blood to the lungs. This vital organ plays a fundamental role as it maintains circulation and provides tissues with the necessary oxygen and nutrients.

(46) (D) Carry oxygenated blood away from the heart.

With the exception of the pulmonary arteries, which transport deoxygenated blood to the lungs for oxygenation, arteries in the cardiovascular system transport oxygenated blood from the heart to different tissues and organs throughout the body. These thick-walled vessels withstand the high pressure generated by the heart's contractions. This ensures the efficient distribution of oxygen and nutrients. As blood moves through the arteries, it sustains the metabolic needs of tissues, which support cellular activities and maintain homeostasis.

(47) (B) Right atrium.

Blood from the systemic circulation returns to the heart in the right atrium. After delivering oxygen to tissues and organs, systemic veins transport deoxygenated blood back to the heart. The right atrium receives this blood via the superior and inferior vena cavae.

(48) (B) Atria.

The upper chambers of the heart are called atria. Both the left and right atrium receive blood returning to the heart. During the cardiac cycle, atria contract to push blood into the ventricles. This coordinated atrial activity ensures efficient filling of the ventricles, which contributes to the heart's overall function to maintain blood circulation throughout the body.

(49) (A) Ventricles.

The term that refers to the heart's lower chambers is ventricles. The ventricles are the muscular chambers that pump blood to the lungs (right ventricle) or throughout the entire body (left ventricle). This ensures the efficient flow of oxygenated blood to various tissues and organs, which support the overall function of the cardiovascular system.

(50) (C) Digestion.

The digestive system breaks down ingested food into smaller, absorbable pieces. The body then uses these components for energy, growth, and repair. This process involves mechanical and chemical digestion, which starts in the mouth. Here, enzymes initiate the breakdown of food, which is followed by gastric acid and digestive enzymes. Nutrient absorption occurs in the small intestine. This ensures essential substances enter the bloodstream for distribution to cells and tissues

(51) (C) Liver.

The liver produces bile, a vital digestive fluid. Bile emulsifies fats and breaks them into smaller droplets that enzymes can efficiently digest. Once created, bile is stored in the gallbladder until needed. During digestion, the gallbladder secretes bile into the small intestine, which helps absorb fats and fat-soluble vitamins, which facilitates their utilization within the body.

(52) (A) Peristalsis.

Peristalsis is the rhythmic muscular contractions that propel food through the digestive tract. These coordinated waves of muscle contractions occur along the walls of the esophagus, stomach, and intestines. It facilitates the movement of ingested material from one part of the digestive system to the next. Peristalsis ensures the proper mixing and progression of food, which allows for mechanical breakdown and optimal absorption of nutrients along the digestive journey.

(53) (B) Small intestine.

The small intestine is mainly responsible for the absorption of nutrients into the bloodstream. Its specialized structures, i.e., villi and microvilli, maximize the surface area for nutrient absorption. As partially digested food passes through the small intestine, nutrients such as sugars, amino acids, and fatty acids are absorbed into blood vessels and eventually reach the bloodstream. This process ensures that the body gains essential elements for energy production, growth, and maintenance of various physiological functions.

(54) (B) Store bile.

The gallbladder stores and concentrates bile, a golden-yellow fluid produced by the liver. It is released into the small intestine when needed, particularly during the digestion of fats. The gallbladder's role aids the breakdown of fats into smaller particles, which makes them more accessible for enzymes to digest further. This process enhances the digestive system's absorption of essential fatty acids and fat-soluble vitamins.

(55) (A) Amylase.

Amylase is an enzyme produced by the salivary glands. It breaks down complex starches and carbohydrates into simpler sugars like maltose. This process begins in the mouth during chewing, which prepares the ingested food for further digestion in the stomach and small intestine. Amylase helps convert starches into more easily absorbable forms, which facilitates nutrient absorption in subsequent digestive stages.

(56) (C) I50.22 - Chronic systolic (congestive) heart failure.

Systolic heart failure is characterized by a reduced ejection fraction, where the heart's ability to pump blood is decreased. The term "congestive" refers to the buildup of fluid in the body that can result from the heart's reduced pumping efficiency. This code is specific to chronic conditions, which implies that the heart failure is a long-standing issue rather than a new or acute occurrence.

(57) (D) 0DTJ0ZZ - Resection of rectum, open.

This code indicates a resection, which in ICD-10-PCS terminology means the cutting out or off, without replacement, of all of a body part. The "0DTJ0ZZ" code breaks down as follows: 0 indicates the medical and surgical section, DT indicates the body system (gastrointestinal system), J indicates the root operation (resection), 0 indicates the body part (rectum), ZZ indicates the qualifier that no device was left in place, and the approach is open (0), signifying that the procedure was not performed endoscopically.

(58) (C) N13.2 - Hydronephrosis with renal and ureteral calculous obstruction.

Hydronephrosis is the swelling of a kidney due to a build-up of urine caused by an obstruction, such as a kidney stone, in the urinary tract. The inclusion of "with renal and ureteral calculous obstruction" in the code's description clearly links the hydronephrosis to the presence of a stone that impedes urine flow.

(59) (B) 80053 - Comprehensive metabolic panel (CMP).

This code is used for a CMP, which is a blood test that measures your sugar (glucose) level, electrolyte and fluid balance, kidney function, and liver function. The CMP includes 14 different tests, making it more extensive than the basic metabolic panel (BMP), renal function panel, or hepatic function panel.

(60) (D) N40.0.

Benign prostatic hyperplasia is a non-malignant disordered growth of the prostate found listed under category N40. This patient has no lower urinary tract symptoms. Therefore, the further subcategory is N40.0.

(61) (D) 51729 - Complex cystometrogram (CMG); with urethral pressure profile (UPP) and voiding pressure studies.

This code represents a complex cystometrogram (CMG) that includes comprehensive evaluations of bladder function, including the urethral pressure profile and voiding pressure studies, which are critical for diagnosing the cause of urinary complaints such as frequent urination and urgency. The inclusion of both UPP and voiding pressure studies indicates a detailed assessment of the bladder's ability to store and expel urine.

(62) (A) Fallopian tube.

The fallopian tubes are also known as uterine tubes or oviducts. After ovulation, an egg is released from an ovary and enters the fallopian tube. If sperm are present in the fallopian tube, fertilization may occur here, where a sperm cell fuses with the egg to form a zygote. The zygote then begins to divide as it moves towards the uterus for implantation.

(63) (B) Cervical cancer.

Papanicolaou (Pap) smear is the screening test for cervical cancer. It is performed on women of reproductive age.

(64) (A) C54.1.

Neoplasms are generally categorized in the ICD-10-CM chapter 3. Endometrial cancer is a malignant neoplasm of the endometrial layer of the uterus, and the diagnosis code is C54.1.

(65) (A) D25.9.

Uterine fibroids are benign smooth muscle proliferation of the uterus. This causes symptoms like menorrhagia, dysmenorrhea, and progressively increasing abdominal swelling. The ICD-10-CM code for uterine fibroid can be found in categories D10–D36. For an unspecified location, the diagnosis code is D25.9.

(66) (B) O85.

The keyword diagnosis is puerperal sepsis, and the ICD-10-CM code is O85.

(67) (C) O88.213.

The diagnosis of obstetric thromboembolism in pregnancy is listed in chapter 15, category O88. For thromboembolism detected in the third trimester, the diagnosis is the six-character code O88.213.

(68) (B) Pancreas.

The pancreas produces insulin.

(69) (B) Neck.

The thyroid gland is located in the anterior part of the neck.

(70) (B) Synapse.

Neurotransmitters are chemical messengers found in synapses.

(71) (C) Pons, midbrain, medulla.

The brainstem comprises the pons, midbrain, and the medulla.

(72) (D) Oxytocin.

The posterior pituitary gland produces oxytocin.

(73) (A) Ventricles.

The choroid plexuses in the ventricles within the brain produce cerebrospinal fluid.

(74) (B) Pupil.

The pupil is the aperture through which light enters the eye.

(75) (C) Retina.

The retina is the light-sensitive part of the eye on which images are formed.

(76) (A) Semicircular canals.

The semicircular canals are located in the inner ear and maintain balance.

(77) (A) Iris.

The iris is the colored part of the eye.

(78) (D) 13121 - Repair, complex, eyelids, nose, ears and/or lips; 2.5 cm or less.

This code is for complex repair procedures on the eyelids, nose, ears, and/or lips, covering wounds that are 2.5 cm or less in length. Complex repair involves more than layered closure. It includes debridement, extensive undermining, or other techniques that are used to achieve a satisfactory cosmetic and functional result.

(79) (A) Stapes, malleus, and incus.

The middle ear contains three small bones. They are called ossicles and include the stapes, incus, and malleus.

(80) (A) Neuraxial anesthesia.

An epidural is a form of neuraxial anesthesia injected into the epidural space. It is given for pain relief or to produce a lack of feeling in the lower part of the body

(81) (A) 31500 - Intubation, endotracheal, emergency procedure.

This code refers to the procedure of inserting a tube through the mouth and then into the airway, which is performed as an emergency measure to ensure that the airway remains open and to provide a means of mechanical ventilation if necessary. This code is used regardless of the patient's physical status classification and is appropriate for emergency situations where securing the airway is critical.

(82) (C) 44310 - Ostomy, small intestine

This code is for the creation of a small intestine ostomy, which is a surgical procedure that allows the passage of intestinal contents from the small intestine to the outside of the body through an artificially created opening (stoma) in the abdominal wall. This procedure is necessary when the patient cannot obtain nutrition through the normal digestive process due to a non-functioning gastrointestinal tract.

(83) (B) Hysterosalpingography.

Hysterosalpingography is the radiographic study of the female reproductive tract. An injection of dye is used to investigate the uterus and the fallopian tubes.

(84) (A) 70250 - Radiologic examination, skull; less than four views.

This code is used for plain radiography of the skull when fewer than four views are required to evaluate the patient's condition. It is ordered to assess for fractures, bone abnormalities, or other structural issues within the skull after trauma or in the evaluation of headache and other symptoms related to the cranial bones. The choice of less than four views would be determined by the clinical indication and the specific areas of concern identified by the physician.

(85) (A) Salivary gland.

A sialogram is a plain radiograph of the salivary glands.

(86) (D) 71045-26, 71045-77.

The correct CPT codes for this case are 71045-26 and 71045-77. The modifiers are based on different medical providers' reports for the same procedure.

(87) (B) Breast.

Mammo- means breast or relating to the mammary organs.

(88) (C) 99213 - Office or other outpatient visit for the evaluation and management of an established patient, which requires an expanded problem focused history, an expanded problem focused exam, and medical decision making of low complexity.

The correct CPT code for documenting an office visit that includes an expanded problem-focused history and examination with low complexity medical decision making, like the routine follow-up for hypertension management described, is 99213. This code is appropriate for encounters lasting around 15 minutes where the physician evaluates an established patient's condition, reviews and potentially adjusts medication, and advises on lifestyle changes.

(89) (A) Complete blood count.

The acronym CBC in laboratory medicine coding stands for complete blood count. This diagnostic test analyzes the composition of blood components, which provides valuable information about a patient's overall health. It includes assessments of red and white blood cells, hemoglobin, platelets, and other parameters. This aids in disease detection and management.

(90) (A) International Classification of Diseases, 10th Edition, Clinical Modification.

In pathology coding, ICD-10-CM refers to the International Classification of Diseases, 10th Edition, Clinical Modification. This standardized coding system accurately documents and categorizes diseases and health conditions. ICD-10-CM plays a pivotal role in medical billing, statistical analysis, and facilitating effective healthcare management and research.

(91) (B) Current Procedural Terminology.

The CPT (Current Procedural Terminology) code set is used to identify and document medical procedures and services systematically. Developed by the American Medical Association, CPT codes ensure uniformity in reporting healthcare services. It facilitates accurate billing, insurance claims, and communication among healthcare providers, payers, and regulators.

(92) (B) Histology.

Histology is the term used to describe the microscopic examination of tissues to diagnose diseases. This essential branch of pathology studies cellular structures and tissue composition. It helps identify abnormalities and contributes significantly to the accurate diagnosis and treatment of various medical conditions.

(93) (B) Systemized Nomenclature of Medicine Clinical Terms.

The primary function of SNOMED CT (Systemized Nomenclature of Medicine Clinical Terms) in medical terminologies is to provide a comprehensive and standardized language for coding clinical information.

(94) (B) Logical Observation Identifiers Names and Codes.

LOINC is a standardized system that assigns unique codes to medical tests and observations, which enables interoperability in healthcare information systems. This coding system streamlines data exchange. It ensures consistency and facilitates effective communication among healthcare providers and systems.

(95) (C) 99221 - Initial hospital care, for the evaluation and management of a patient, which requires these 3 key components: a detailed or comprehensive history; a detailed or comprehensive exam; and medical decision making of straightforward or low complexity. Physicians spend 30 minutes at the bedside and on the patient's hospital floor or unit.

This code accurately reflects the level of care provided to a patient admitted with severe symptoms that require immediate and thorough evaluation to rule out serious conditions such as a myocardial infarction.

(96) (A) 99221.

This code is used for the initial hospital care provided by the physician. This code is appropriate for the patient's last presentation, where he was placed in inpatient care due to the worsening of his symptoms and discharged the following morning.

(97) (C) 99214.

99214 is used to code an established patient visit with moderate medical decision-making complexity. 99213 is used to code for an established outpatient visit with a low medical decision-making complexity. 99232 is used to code for subsequent visits for a patient either in hospital observation status or inpatient care, with a moderate medical decision-making complexity. 99202 is used to code for a new outpatient visit with a straightforward medical decision-making complexity.

(98) (D) +99140.

This code describes emergency conditions and is found under the qualifying circumstances CPT category in the chapter covering medicine. The add-on code and a primary anesthesia procedure code are used but only apply when the anesthesia given becomes complex due to an emergency. The medical coder needs to document the reason for the emergency in the patient's record when the anesthesia service is provided.

(99) (D) 90480, 91304.

Two codes are to be reported separately in this scenario. The first code is the CPT code for administering the COVID-19 vaccine single dose via IM route, i.e., 90480. The second is for the COVID-19 vaccine of five mcg/0.5ml, i.e., 91304.

(100) (A) 90386.

The proper CPT code for Rhesus D immunoglobulin to prevent hemolytic disease for newborns is 90386.

## Test 3: Questions

(1) A physician administers moderate sedation to a 45-year-old patient who is undergoing a complex and non-cardiac procedure in an outpatient setting. The sedation lasts for 30 minutes. Which CPT code should be used?

(A) 99151 - Moderate sedation services provided by the same physician or other qualified health care professional performing the diagnostic or therapeutic service that the sedation supports. There is a requirement for the presence of an independent trained observer to help monitor the patient's level of consciousness and physiological status. There is an initial 15 minutes of intraservice time and the patient is younger than 5 years of age.

(B) 99152 - Moderate sedation services provided by the same physician or other qualified health care professional performing the diagnostic or therapeutic service that the sedation supports. There is an initial 15 minutes of intraservice time and the patient is younger than 5 years of age.

(C) 99153 - Moderate sedation services provided by the same physician or other qualified health care professional performing the diagnostic or therapeutic service that the sedation supports.

(D) 99155 - Moderate sedation services provided by a physician or other qualified health care professional other than the one performing the diagnostic or therapeutic service that the sedation supports. There is an initial 15 minutes of intraservice time and the patient is younger than 5 years of age.

(2) The investigation of fraud and abuse in healthcare services lies within the purview of which government agency?

(A) HIPAA.

(B) Social Security Administration (SSA).

(C) OIG.

(D) HITECH.

(3) A 52-year-old patient with a history of type 1 diabetes mellitus presents to the cardiology clinic for an evaluation of suspected coronary artery disease. The cardiologist performs an intracoronary ultrasound during a diagnostic cardiac catheterization to assess the extent of arterial blockage. How should this scenario be documented with ICD-10-CM and CPT codes?

(A) E10.1 - Type 1 diabetes mellitus with ketoacidosis, and 93674 - Intravascular Doppler velocity and/or pressure derived coronary flow reserve measurement.

(B) E10.9 - Type 1 diabetes mellitus without complications, and 93458 - Coronary angiography including intraprocedural injections for coronary angiography, imaging supervision and interpretation.

(C) E10.9 - Type 1 diabetes mellitus without complications, and 93674 - Intravascular ultrasound of coronary arteries.

(D) E10.1 - Type 1 diabetes mellitus with ketoacidosis, and 93458 - Coronary angiography including intraprocedural injections for coronary angiography, imaging supervision and interpretation.

(4) Which of the following statements reflects a limitation of medical terminology in cross-cultural healthcare?

(A) It promotes cultural sensitivity.

(B) It may not be universally understood.

(C) It facilitates seamless cross-cultural communication.

(D) It has no impact on cultural competence.

(5) How does medical terminology contribute to efficient electronic health record (EHR) systems?

(A) It increases data entry errors.

(B) It slows down information retrieval.

(C) It provides standardized terms for accurate documentation.

(D) It limits interoperability between healthcare systems.

(6) Medical terminology is vital in research because it:

(A) Hinders collaboration between researchers.

(B) Facilitates precise and unambiguous communication of findings.

(C) Delays the publication of research outcomes.

(D) Excludes non-medical professionals from contributing to research.

(7) Which body system supports and protects the body and provides a framework for movement?

(A) Respiratory system.

(B) Skeletal system.

(C) Nervous system.

(D) Cardiovascular system.

(8) Which of the following describes the primary function of the circulatory system?

(A) Facilitates oxygen exchange in the lungs.

(B) Transports nutrients and oxygen to cells.

(C) Produces and stores hormones.

(D) Filters waste from the blood.

(9) Where does digestion mainly occur in the human body?

(A) Stomach.

(B) Liver.

(C) Small intestine.

(D) Large intestine.

(10) Which body system produces chemical messengers that regulate various physiological functions?

(A) Endocrine system.

(B) Lymphatic system.

(C) Muscular system.

(D) Integumentary system.

(11) Which of the following functions does the respiratory system perform?

(A) Pumps blood throughout the body.

(B) Breaks down food into nutrients.

(C) Exchanges gases, such as oxygen and carbon dioxide.

(D) Maintains body temperature.

(12) A fifteen-year-old girl is evaluated for recurrent fatigue. An examination demonstrates pallor, widespread purpura, and ecchymoses. She also complained of recurrent fever in the last four weeks, which was refractory to medication. Peripheral blood smear reveals normochromic normocytic anemia, with leukopenia and thrombocytopenia. A biopsy of the bone marrow confirms a diagnosis of aplastic anemia. What is the ICD-10 diagnosis code that the hematologist should report?

(A) J51.7.

(B) D61.81.

(C) D60.9.

(D) D61.9.

(13) A young man was diagnosed with Crohn's disease three years ago. His gastroenterologist sees him for a review of his medications. An evaluation shows that the condition is limited to the large intestine, and he has been passing bloody stools for the past two weeks. What is the diagnosis code that the gastroenterologist should report?

(A) K50.09.

(B) K50.111.

(C) K50.10.

(D) K51.01.

(14) A twenty-seven-year-old woman presents for her medication refill at her clinic. She complained of burning chest pain that gets worse following meals, with associated occasional regurgitation of meals. She has been diagnosed with gastroesophageal reflux disease in her previous clinic visit but has poor medication adherence. What is the appropriate code to be reported by her physician for her condition?

(A) G56.3.

(B) K21.9.

(C) K21.0.

(D) K21.

(15) A seventy-four-year-old woman was admitted following a fall three hours ago, with an inability to bear weight on the right lower limb. An X-ray is ordered, and osteoporosis is noted in the right femur with a displaced fracture line. What is the diagnosis code to be reported for this patient's condition?

(A) M80.051A.

(B) M80.9.

(C) M80.051.

(D) M80.05.

(16) A male patient is seen in the mental health clinic for ongoing emotional distress after the loss of a loved one three months ago. The psychologist conducts an evaluation and determines that the patient is experiencing significant symptoms of persistent complex bereavement disorder, which is impacting his daily life. Which ICD-10-CM code should be used?

(A) F43.10 - Post-traumatic stress disorder, unspecified.

(B) F43.21 - Adjustment disorder with depressed mood.

(C) F43.22 - Adjustment disorder with anxiety.

(D) F43.23 - Adjustment disorder with mixed anxiety and depressed mood.

(17) A five-year-old boy was admitted from the children's emergency unit with a history of neck stiffness and fever for about three days before presentation. Kernig's sign is positive. CSF analysis demonstrated leukocytosis with neutrophilia. A diagnosis of bacterial meningitis was made, and the patient was started on intravenous antibiotics. What is the diagnosis code to be reported?

(A) G53.4.

(B) G00.9.

(C) G01.

(D) G00.

(18) Which code represents a prefabricated adjustable orthopedic cane, quad or three-prong tip?

(A) E0100.

(B) E0105.

(C) E0120.

(D) E0130.

(19) What is the ICD-10 code for cellulitis, unspecified?

(A) L02.9.

(B) L03.90.

(C) L04.9.

(D) L08.9.

(20) Which CPT code range is used for excision of benign and malignant skin lesions?

(A) 10040-10180.

(B) 11000-11047.

(C) 11400-11646.

(D) 12001-13160.

(21) Mr. A needs a simple repair of the superficial injuries to his scalp and neck. Which CPT code is appropriate for this procedure?

(A) 12031.

(B) 12041.

(C) 12051.

(D) 12071.

(22) Which code range is the CPT code for the removal of a malignant lesion found?

(A) 11400-11446.

(B) 11600-11646.

(C) 12001-13160.

(D) 14000-14302.

(23) Which CPT code is used for the removal of skin tags?

(A) 11200.

(B) 11300.

(C) 11400.

(D) 11900.

(24) A patient presents with a suspicious lesion on the back, which measures 1.2 cm in diameter. The dermatologist decides to perform an excision of the lesion because she suspects it could be malignant. The lesion is excised with a 0.3 cm margin all around, which results in a total diameter of the excised lesion of 1.8 cm. Which CPT code should be used for the excision of this malignant lesion on the skin of the trunk?

(A) 11600 - Excision of malignant lesion including margins, trunk, arms, or legs; lesion diameter 0.5 cm or less.

(B) 11601 - Excision of malignant lesion including margins, trunk, arms, or legs; lesion diameter 0.6 to 1.0 cm.

(C) 11602 - Excision of malignant lesion including margins, trunk, arms, or legs; lesion diameter 1.1 to 2.0 cm.

(D) 11603 - Excision of malignant lesion including margins, trunk, arms, or legs; lesion diameter 2.1 to 3.0 cm.

(25) A patient with a small, superficial chemical burn on the forearm undergoes a treatment session where the physician applies chemical cauterization to the lesion. This is done to promote healing and prevent infection. Which CPT code should be used for the application of chemical cauterization of a superficial wound?

(A) 17250 - Chemical cauterization of granulation tissue (proud flesh, sinus or fistula).

(B) 11042 - Debridement, subcutaneous tissue (includes epidermis and dermis, if performed); first 20 sq cm or less.

(C) 12001 - Simple repair of superficial wounds of scalp, neck, axillae, external genitalia, trunk and/or extremities (including hands and feet); 2.5 cm or less.

(D) 17000 - Destruction (eg, laser surgery, electrosurgery, cryosurgery, chemosurgery, surgical curettement) of premalignant lesions (eg, actinic keratoses); first lesion.

(26) A dermatologist performs a biopsy on a suspicious lesion located on the patient's neck to determine the presence of dermatological disease. The procedure involves the removal of a single lesion for diagnostic examination. Which CPT code should be used for the biopsy of the skin lesion?

(A) 11100 - Biopsy of skin, subcutaneous tissue and/or mucous membrane (including simple closure), unless otherwise listed; single lesion

(B) 11101 - Biopsy of skin, subcutaneous tissue and/or mucous membrane (including simple closure), unless otherwise listed; each separate/additional lesion (List separately in addition to code for primary procedure).

(C) 11300 - Shaving of epidermal or dermal lesion, single lesion, trunk, arms or legs; lesion diameter 0.5 cm or less.

(D) 11400 - Excision, benign lesion including margins, except skin tag (unless listed elsewhere), trunk, arms or legs; lesion diameter 0.5 cm or less.

(27) A patient presents with a 2.3 cm malignant melanoma located on the upper arm. The dermatologist performs an excision of the malignant lesion, including margins, with a final excised diameter of 3.0 cm. Which CPT code should be used for the excision of this malignant lesion on the upper arm?

(A) 11603 - Excision of malignant lesion including margins, trunk, arms, or legs; lesion diameter 2.1 to 3.0 cm.

(B) 11604 - Excision of malignant lesion including margins, trunk, arms, or legs; lesion diameter 3.1 to 4.0 cm.

(C) 11606 - Excision of malignant lesion including margins, trunk, arms, or legs; lesion diameter over 4.0 cm.

(D) 11602 - Excision of malignant lesion including margins, trunk, arms, or legs; lesion diameter 1.1 to 2.0 cm.

(28) A patient visits the dermatology clinic with a basal cell carcinoma located on the face, measuring 0.8 cm in diameter. The dermatologist decides to perform destruction of the lesion using cryosurgery. Which CPT code should be used for the destruction of a malignant lesion on the face using cryosurgery?

(A) 17260 - Destruction of malignant lesion on the face (0.5 cm or less).

(B) 17261 - Destruction of malignant lesion on the face (0.6 to 1.0 cm).

(C) 17262 - Destruction of malignant lesion on the face (1.1 to 2.0 cm).

(D) 17263 - Destruction of malignant lesion on the face (2.1 to 3.0 cm).

(29) A patient presents to the dermatology clinic with a seborrheic keratosis lesion on the back of the hand, measuring 0.4 cm in diameter. The dermatologist performs a shaving of the epidermal lesion. Which CPT code should be used for the shaving of an epidermal lesion for a lesion measuring 0.4 cm on the back of the hand?

(A) 11310 - Shaving of epidermal or dermal lesion, single lesion, face, ears, eyelids, nose, lips, mucous membrane; lesion diameter 0.5 cm or less.

(B) 11300 - Shaving of epidermal or dermal lesion, single lesion, trunk, arms or legs; lesion diameter 0.5 cm or less.

(C) 11311 - Shaving of epidermal or dermal lesion, single lesion, face, ears, eyelids, nose, lips, mucous membrane; lesion diameter 0.6 to 1.0 cm.

(D) 11301 - Shaving of epidermal or dermal lesion, single lesion, trunk, arms or legs; lesion diameter 0.6 to 1.0 cm.

(30) During a complex reconstructive surgery, a plastic surgeon uses a skin graft preparation technique to prepare a recipient site on a patient's lower leg for a future grafting procedure. This preparation involves the creation of a vascular bed to ensure the graft will have a high chance of successful integration. Which CPT code should be used for the recipient site for a skin graft on the lower leg?

(A) 15000 - Preparation of the recipient site for a skin graft.

(B) 15002 - Preparation for split-thickness skin graft, trunk, arms, legs; first 100 sq cm or less, or 1% of body area of infants and children.

(C) 15004 - Preparation for full-thickness skin graft, trunk, arms, legs; first 100 sq cm or less, or 1% of body area of infants and children.

(D) 15220 - Split-thickness skin graft, trunk, arms, legs; first 100 sq cm or less, or 1% of body area of infants and children.

(31) A patient undergoes a surgical procedure on the right knee due to a severe injury. Which modifier should be appended to the CPT code for the surgical procedure?

(A) LT - Left side.

(B) RT - Right side.

(C) 50 - Bilateral procedure.

(D) 59 - Distinct procedural service.

(32) What does the modifier RT signify in musculoskeletal system coding?

(A) Right side.

(B) Left side.

(C) Bilateral.

(D) Staged procedure.

(33) Which modifier is used to report a procedure done on both sides of a person's body in the same encounter?

(A) LT.

(B) 50.

(C) RT.

(D) 59.

(34) What does the modifier LT indicate in musculoskeletal coding?

(A) Left side.

(B) Right side.

(C) Bilateral.

(D) Distinct procedural service.

(35) When should the modifier 59 be used in musculoskeletal coding?

(A) To indicate a bilateral procedure.

(B) To denote multiple procedures during the same session.

(C) To signify distinct procedural service.

(D) To represent a staged or related procedure.

(36) HCPCS Level II code A6530 is associated with which of the following?

(A) Lymphedema garment.

(B) Lymphangiography contrast material.

(C) Thromboembolic deterrent stockings.

(D) Diaphragmatic hernia belt.

(37) During a single outpatient visit, a patient undergoes two separate and unrelated procedures by the same physician: a removal of a benign skin lesion on the forearm and a diagnostic endoscopy of the stomach. To accurately document that these are distinct and independent procedures performed during the same session, which modifier should be appended to the CPT code for the lesser-valued or secondary procedure?

(A) 51 - Multiple procedures.

(B) 59 - Distinct procedural service.

(C) 76 - Repeat procedure by the same physician.

(D) 24 - Unrelated evaluation and management service by the same physician during a postoperative period.

(38) A patient undergoes a bilateral carpal tunnel release surgery performed during the same operative session. Which modifier should be appended to the CPT code for the carpal tunnel release surgery?

(A) 50 - Bilateral procedure.

(B) LT - Left side.

(C) RT - Right side.

(D) 59 - Distinct procedural service.

(39) During a single outpatient visit, a patient receives multiple injections for chronic pain management. The injections are administered in different anatomical sites, including a trigger point injection in the left shoulder and a steroid injection in the right knee. To ensure accurate billing and demonstrate that these injections are distinct and separate services, which modifier should be appended to the CPT code for the second procedure?

(A) 59 - Distinct procedural service.

(B) 51 - Multiple procedures.

(C) LT - Left side.

(D) RT - Right side.

(40) Modifier 26 signifies which of the following?

(A) Right side.

(B) Left side.

(C) Professional component.

(D) Distinct procedural service.

(41) Modifier 76 indicates which of the following?

(A) Repeated procedure by the initial physician.

(B) Unrelated evaluation and management service during a postoperative period.

(C) Increased procedural services.

(D) Distinct procedural service.

(42) A surgeon performs a bilateral mastectomy on a patient diagnosed with breast cancer. Which modifier should be appended to the CPT code for the mastectomy?

(A) 50 - Bilateral procedure.

(B) 59 - Distinct procedural service.

(C) LT - Left side.

(D) RT - Right side.

(43) A patient undergoes two different surgical procedures during the same operative session: a cholecystectomy and a laparoscopic appendectomy. To document these procedures on the claim and indicate that multiple procedures were performed during the same operative session, which modifier should be appended to the CPT code for the procedure with the lower relative value unit?

(A) 51 - Multiple procedures.

(B) 59 - Distinct procedural service.

(C) 25 - Significant, separately identifiable evaluation and management service by the same physician on the same day of the procedure or other service.

(D) 50 - Bilateral procedure.

(44) A patient presents with a diagnosis of unspecified priapism and undergoes a penile injection procedure for diagnostic and therapeutic purposes. Which ICD-10-CM and CPT code combination should be used for this scenario?

(A) N48.30 - Unspecified priapism and 54220 - Injection procedure for Peyronie's disease.

(B) N48.30 - Unspecified priapism and 54235 - Injection procedure into the corpora cavernosa for priapism.

(C) N48.9 - Disorder of penis, unspecified and 54220 - Injection procedure for Peyronie's disease.

(D) N48.9 - Disorder of penis, unspecified and 54235 - Injection procedure into the corpora cavernosa for priapism.

(45) Which modifier signifies a staged or related procedure during the postoperative period?

(A) 24.

(B) 58.

(C) 78.

(D) 9.

(46) Which of the following modifiers indicates a discontinued procedure after anesthesia has been administered?

(A) 73.

(B) 74.

(C) 76.

(D) 77.

(47) Which modifier is applied when a laboratory service is repeated on the same day in different sessions?

(A) 32.

(B) 50.

(C) 76.

(D) 91.

(48) What HCPCS Level II code is assigned for the injection of glucagon hydrochloride per 1.0 mg for subcutaneous or intramuscular use?

(A) G0459.

(B) J1620.

(C) J1610.

(D) G0462.

(49) Which of the following modifiers indicates a procedure was discontinued due to a threat to the patient's health?

(A) 22.

(B) 52.

(C) 53.

(D) 59.

(50) What modifier is used when providing a separately identifiable evaluation and management (E/M) service during the postoperative period?

(A) 24.

(B) 25.

(C) 32.

(D) 57.

(51) A patient presents with symptoms of urinary retention and is diagnosed with urethral stricture. The urologist decides to perform a urethral dilation procedure to treat the stricture. Which CPT code should be used?

(A) 53060 - Bladder drainage, percutaneous, with insertion of suprapubic catheter.

(B) 53200 - Urethral dilation, initial.

(C) 53215 - Urethrotomy, internal, without optical urethrotomy; with or without dilation.

(D) 53430 - Urethroplasty, reconstruction of the male urethra.

(52) Which of the following modifiers is used for a repeat procedure by the same physician on the same day?

(A) 76.

(B) 77.

(C) 78.

(D) 79.

(53) Which modifier is applied for a service provided in the outpatient hospital setting that is not an emergency?

(A) AS.

(B) PO.

(C) 52.

(D) 73.

(54) A patient diagnosed with endometrial cancer undergoes a total abdominal hysterectomy, including the removal of the uterus, cervix, upper vagina, and surrounding tissues. Which CPT code should be used?

(A) 58150 - Total abdominal hysterectomy (corpus and cervix), with or without removal of tube(s), with or without removal of ovary(s).

(B) 58200 - Complete radical hysterectomy, with bilateral total pelvic lymphadenectomy, including para-aortic lymph node sampling (biopsy), or dissection, when performed.

(C) 58180 - Supracervical hysterectomy (subtotal hysterectomy), abdominal approach.

(D) 58210 - Radical hysterectomy with pelvic lymphadenectomy and para-aortic lymphadenectomy.

(55) A fifty-eight-year-old man presents to the urology clinic. He has had difficulty passing urine for the past seven months, which has progressively worsened. Further history reveals that he was treated for a complicated sexually transmitted infection, and examination confirms that he has developed a urethral stricture. The urologist informs the patient of a procedure that involves the dilation of the stricture with a urethral dilator. The patient explains that this procedure was performed on him several weeks ago with temporary relief of symptoms. However, he consents to a repeat of the procedure. What is the ICD-10-CM code of his diagnosis and the CPT code of the subsequent procedure?

(A) N37.1; 53600, Modifier 71.

(B) N35.21; 53510, Modifier 77.

(C) N45.11; 53500; Modifier 71.

(D) N35.11; 53600, Modifier 77.

(56) A three-year-old boy is rushed into the pediatric emergency room following sudden onset pain in the scrotum while he was playing with his older brother. Examination reveals swelling and worsening pain when the doctor tries to examine the testes further. A diagnosis of testicular torsion is made. What is the ICD-10-CM code of the diagnosis?

(A) N45.34.

(B) N44.00.

(C) N47.44.

(D) N43.00.

(57) A patient presents at the nephrology clinic due to excessive urination and thirst. He has previously been screened for diabetes mellitus, but his blood sugar levels are normal. Further serum analysis shows that the patient has hypokalemia, hypotonic urine, and reduced sensitivity of the kidneys to antidiuretic hormone due to a mutation of genes encoding the vasopressin receptors. A diagnosis of nephrogenic diabetic insipidus is made. What is the ICD-10-CM code?

(A) N51.2.

(B) N25.1.

(C) N24.2.

(D) N24.1.

(58) A patient undergoes an artificial insemination procedure as part of fertility treatment. The procedure involves the direct insertion of sperm into the uterus. Which CPT code should be used?

(A) 58321 - Artificial insemination; intracervical.

(B) 58322 - Artificial insemination; intrauterine.

(C) 58323 - Donor insemination procedure.

(D) 58340 - Catheterization for sperm injection.

(59) A seventy-two-year-old man reports difficulty in passing urine for the past six years, for which he has been placed on medications. However, he has been unable to pass urine for the last eighteen hours, with significant abdominal pain and a suprapubic fullness. All attempts to drain the urine using a urethral catheter have proven abortive. He is immediately scheduled for an urgent suprapubic catheterization to relieve the acute urinary retention. What is the CPT code for this procedure?

(A) 50142.

(B) 51102.

(C) 51111.

(D) 52105.

(60) A pregnant patient presents with symptoms indicating a potential complication, and the obstetrician decides to perform an amniocentesis to assess fetal health and diagnose any chromosomal abnormalities. Which CPT code should be used?

(A) 59000 - Amniocentesis; diagnostic.

(B) 59001 - Amniocentesis; therapeutic for reduction of amniotic fluid.

(C) 59025 - Fetal non-stress test.

(D) 59020 - Fetal contraction stress test.

(61) A twenty-seven-year-old woman comes to the reproductive health clinic for insertion of an intrauterine device. State the appropriate CPT code to be reported for this procedure by the healthcare professional.

(A) 58300.

(B) 57400.

(C) 58500.

(D) 58890.

(62) A patient undergoes an IVF procedure where eggs are retrieved from the ovaries to be fertilized in the lab before being transferred back into the uterus. Which CPT code should be used?

(A) 58970 - Follicle puncture for oocyte retrieval, any method.

(B) 58974 - Embryo transfer, intrauterine.

(C) 58976 - Gamete, zygote, or embryo intrafallopian transfer, any method.

(D) 89250 - Culture of oocyte(s)/embryo(s), less than 4 days.

(63) State the CPT code for a cesarean delivery.

(A) 59514.

(B) 49515.

(C) 48514.

(D) 59011.

(64) A patient undergoes a vaginal delivery without any complications. The obstetrician performs the delivery, including postpartum care of the mother. Which CPT code should be used?

(A) 59400 - Routine obstetric care including antepartum care, vaginal delivery (with or without episiotomy, and/or forceps) and postpartum care.

(B) 59409 - Vaginal delivery only (with or without episiotomy and/or forceps).

(C) 59410 - Vaginal delivery only (with or without episiotomy and/or forceps) including postpartum care.

(D) 59510 - Routine obstetric care including antepartum care, cesarean delivery, and postpartum care.

(65) A forty-three-year-old woman is evaluated for features suggestive of right ovarian malignancy. Her gynecologist schedules her for a biopsy of the right ovary. Report the CPT code and appropriate modifier for the procedure.

(A) 58912, Modifier RT.

(B) 57800, Modifier RT.

(C) 58900, Modifier RT.

(D) 57501, Modifier RT.

(66) A patient undergoes a laparoscopic adrenalectomy due to a diagnosis of an adrenal gland tumor. Which CPT code should be used?

(A) 60650 - Laparoscopy, surgical; adrenalectomy.

(B) 60500 - Parathyroidectomy or exploration of parathyroid(s).

(C) 49505 - Repair of inguinal hernia, patient age 5 years or older; reducible.

(D) 50545 - Laparoscopy, surgical; nephrectomy.

(67) A patient with increased intracranial pressure undergoes a procedure for the insertion of a ventricular catheter for external drainage. Which CPT code should be used?

(A) 61000 - Shunt; ventricular to external drainage.

(B) 61105 - Twist drill hole for subdural or ventricular puncture; for implanting ventricular catheter, reservoir, EEG electrode(s), or pressure recording device.

(C) 61210 - Burr hole(s) for ventricular shunt; for implanting ventricular catheter, reservoir, or pressure recording device.

(D) 62223 - Craniectomy for evacuation of hematoma; subdural.

(68) A patient is diagnosed with a brain tumor located at the base of the skull. The neurosurgeon performs a complex surgical procedure involving a craniotomy with excision of the tumor. The operation requires an approach through the base of the skull to access and remove the tumor. Which CPT code should be used?

(A) 61522 - Craniectomy or craniotomy for excision of brain tumor, infratentorial or posterior fossa; extradural, including dural repair, if performed.

(B) 61524 - Craniectomy or craniotomy for excision of brain tumor, infratentorial or posterior fossa; intradural, including dural repair, if performed.

(C) 61526 - Craniectomy or craniotomy for excision of brain tumor; transcortical approach.

(D) 61530 - Craniectomy, trephination, bone flap craniotomy for implantation of neurostimulator electrodes; cerebral, cortical.

(69) A patient presents with symptoms indicative of an acute subdural hematoma following a head injury. The neurosurgeon performs a craniectomy to evacuate the hematoma. Which CPT code should be used?

(A) 61154 - Burr hole(s); with drainage of hematoma, subdural.

(B) 61210 - Burr hole(s) for ventricular shunt; for implanting ventricular catheter, reservoir, or pressure recording device.

(C) 62223 - Craniectomy for evacuation of hematoma; subdural.

(D) 62225 - Craniectomy for evacuation of hematoma; epidural.

(70) A patient suffers bilateral acute subdural hematomas as a result of a severe head injury. The neurosurgeon performs bilateral burr hole surgery to drain the hematomas. Which CPT code and modifier combination should be used?

(A) 61154 - Burr hole(s); with drainage of hematoma, subdural, without modifier

(B) 61154 - Burr hole(s); with drainage of hematoma, subdural, with modifier 59 (Distinct procedural service)

(C) 61154 with modifier 50 - Burr hole(s); with drainage of hematoma, subdural, indicating a bilateral procedure

(D) 61154 with modifier LT and RT - Burr hole(s); with drainage of hematoma, subdural, indicating left and right side procedures.

(71) A patient with proliferative diabetic retinopathy in both eyes undergoes panretinal photocoagulation, a laser treatment performed to reduce the risk of blindness. Which CPT code and modifier combination should be used?

(A) 67228 - Treatment of extensive or progressive retinopathy (e.g., diabetic retinopathy), photocoagulation; without modifier

(B) 67228 with modifier 59 - Distinct procedural service

(C) 67228 with modifier 50 - Treatment of extensive or progressive retinopathy (e.g., diabetic retinopathy), photocoagulation; indicating a bilateral procedure

(D) 67228 with modifiers LT and RT - Treatment of extensive or progressive retinopathy, photocoagulation; indicating procedures on the left and right eyes

(72) A patient undergoes a retinal detachment repair with a scleral buckle on the left eye. Which CPT code and modifier combination should be used?

(A) 67107 - Repair of retinal detachment; with scleral buckle.

(B) 67107 with modifier 50 - Repair of retinal detachment; with scleral buckle, indicating a bilateral procedure.

(C) 67107 with modifier LT - Repair of retinal detachment; with scleral buckle, indicating the procedure was performed on the left eye.

(D) 67107 with modifiers LT and RT - Repair of retinal detachment; with scleral buckle, indicating procedures on both the left and right eyes.

(73) A patient presents with a cholesteatoma in the left ear that requires surgical removal. The otolaryngologist performs an excision of the cholesteatoma through an incision in the external auditory canal. Which CPT code and modifier combination should be used?

(A) 69000 - Excision external ear; cholesteatoma.

(B) 69000 with modifier 50 - Excision external ear; cholesteatoma, indicating a bilateral procedure.

(C) 69000 with modifier LT - Excision external ear; cholesteatoma, indicating the procedure was performed on the left ear.

(D) 69000 with modifiers LT and RT - Excision external ear; cholesteatoma, indicating procedures on both the left and right ears.

(74) A patient undergoes a surgical procedure under general anesthesia that lasts for 2 hours. The anesthesia base unit value for the procedure is 4, and the anesthesia practice in this region assigns a time unit value of 1 unit per 15 minutes. Considering these factors, what is the total unit value for the anesthesia service provided for this procedure?

(A) 12 units - Calculated by adding the base unit value (4 units) to the time units for the duration of the procedure (8 units for 2 hours).

(B) 8 units - Calculated solely based on the time the anesthesia was administered (2 hours).

(C) 16 units - Calculated by doubling the base unit value due to the complexity of the procedure.

(D) 20 units - Calculated by adding a modifier for the complexity of the procedure to the base and time units.

(75) An eight-year-old boy is brought to the emergency room after he puts a little plastic toy cap into his right ear while playing with his friends. The plastic cap is visible in the external ear, and the boy remains still while the doctor removes it. He is given analgesics and scheduled for a follow-up appointment. No anesthesia was administered for the procedure. What is the CPT code?

(A) 69210, Modifier RT.

(B) 69200, Modifier RT.

(C) 69211, Modifier RT.

(D) 69201, Modifier RT.

(76) A female toddler is assessed to have bilateral hearing loss at birth. Following numerous assessments, cochlear device implantation will occur for both ears. State the CPT code.

(A) 68890, Modifier 50.

(B) 69930, Modifier 50.

(C) 69730, Modifier 51.

(D) 69920, Modifier 50.

(77) A patient undergoes a procedure requiring anesthesia services. During the anesthesia, the patient is administered an agent to induce hypothermia as a special circumstance to protect the brain during the procedure. Which CPT code should be used?

(A) 99116 - Anesthesia complicated by utilization of total body hypothermia.

(B) 99135 - Anesthesia complicated by utilization of controlled hypotension.

(C) 99100 - Anesthesia for patient of extreme age, under one year and over seventy (List separately in addition to code for primary anesthesia procedure).

(D) 99140 - Anesthesia complicated by emergency conditions (List separately in addition to code for primary anesthesia procedure).

(78) A fifteen-year-old girl presents at a clinic due to constant ringing in her left ear, with associated pain and reduced hearing. An otoscopy reveals the presence of impacted wax in the left ear. Subsequently, she undergoes irrigation of the left ear to remove the impacted wax and relieve symptoms. State the correct ICD-10-CM diagnosis and CPT codes with correctly applied modifiers.

(A) H61.22; 69209, Modifier LT.

(B) H61.22; 69109, Modifier 50.

(C) H61.22; 69200, Modifier LT.

(D) H61.72; 69208, Modifier 50.

(79) Which is the correct choice for calculating the unit value of anesthesia service provided?

(A) Only the unit for the highest value.

(B) The unit for the highest value and lowest value.

(C) The unit for the highest value and modifier.

(D) Only the unit for the lowest value.

(80) An eighteen-month-old girl is scheduled for a repair of cleft lip and palate. About eight months before the current presentation, she had a repair of the cleft lip and palate but developed an infection following the procedure. Wound healing was compromised, and the outcome of the procedure was poor. She finally undergoes a definitive repair by a different surgeon and is placed under general anesthesia. The patient is otherwise healthy. Report the anesthesia code for this repeat procedure.

(A) 00102, 00172, P1, Modifier 77.

(B) 00102, 00172, Q1, Modifier 78.

(C) 00102, 00172, P2, Modifier 65.

(D) 00102, 00272, P1, Modifier 68.

(81) State the correct add-on code for a six-month-old who undergoes anesthesia.

(A) 99100.

(B) 99116.

(C) 99135.

(D) 99140.

(82) Select the appropriate add-on code for a patient induced with controlled hypotension while under anesthesia.

(A) 99100.

(B) 99116.

(C) 99135.

(D) 99140.

(83) A patient is scheduled for central venous access that uses ultrasound guidance. What is the CPT code?

(A) 76935.

(B) 76987.

(C) 76837.

(D) 76937.

(84) A pregnant woman undergoes amniocentesis under ultrasound guidance for an alpha-fetoprotein assay. What is the CPT code?

(A) 76946.

(B) 76948.

(C) 76956.

(D) 76976.

(85) An older man presents with an inability to bear weight on the right hip following a fall. A fracture is suspected, and a plain X-ray of the hip is requested. What is the correct CPT code?

(A) 73802, RT.

(B) 73502, RT.

(C) 73501, RT.

(D) 73510, RT.

(86) A fifty-four-year-old woman has had bilateral knee pain for the past four months. There is no previous history of falls. However, there is a family history of osteoarthritis. She is moderately obese and lives a sedentary lifestyle. The medical provider requests an X-ray of both knees. State the CPT code.

(A) 73580, 50.

(B) 73660, 50.

(C) 73560, 50.

(D) 73569, 50.

(87) A patient undergoes a dual-energy X-ray absorptiometry (DXA) of bony areas on the trunk to determine bone mineral density and screen for osteoporosis. Report the appropriate CPT code for the professional component of this procedure.

(A) 77080, 25.

(B) 77090, 26.

(C) 77080, 36.

(D) 77080, 26.

(88) A patient is evaluated for difficulty swallowing. A barium contrast study is scheduled to outline the esophagus bird beak appearance that is noted. Diagnosis of achalasia is made following careful evaluation of symptoms. A report on the imaging has been made available. State the correct code for the professional component of the procedure and the ICD-10-CM diagnosis code.

(A) 74240, 26; K21.0.

(B) 74240, 26; K22.0.

(C) 74250, 26; K22.0.

(D) 74240, 25; K22.0.

(89) What is the CPT imaging code of the left kidney?

(A) 76776, LT.

(B) 76745, LT.

(C) 76775, LT.

(D) 76475, LT.

(90) A patient with suspected pancreatic cancer undergoes a biopsy of the pancreas under fluoroscopic guidance. The tissue is collected and sent for histopathology. What is the code for this reported procedure and the ICD-10-CM diagnosis code for the suspected diagnosis?

(A) C25.9; 48102, 77082, 26.

(B) C25.9; 48402, 77002, 26.

(C) C25.9; 48102, 77002, 26.

(D) C25.8; 48102, 77002, 26.

(91) A provider carries out an echocardiogram on a two-year-old patient. He needs to visualize the heart chambers, valves, blood flow, and cardiac activity using transducers to obtain 2D images of the heart through the chest wall. State the CPT code for the professional component of this service.

(A) 93305, Modifier 26.

(B) 93304, Modifier 26.

(C) 93302, Modifier 26.

(D) 93307, Modifier 26.

(92) LOINC (Logical Observation Identifiers Names and Codes) is commonly associated with which of the following?

(A) Disease classification.

(B) Laboratory test codes.

(C) Surgical procedure codes.

(D) Diagnostic imaging codes.

(93) Which regulatory act safeguards the confidentiality and integrity of individually identifiable health information?

(A) HIPAA (Health Insurance Portability and Accountability Act).

(B) HITECH Act.

(C) Affordable Care Act.

(D) Medicare Access and CHIP Reauthorization Act (MACRA).

(94) What does NDC stand for in the context of medical coding?

(A) National Data Consortium.

(B) Numeric Drug Code.

(C) National Drug Code.

(D) Non-disclosure compliance.

(95) In medical coding, modifiers do which of the following?

(A) Indicate the patient's age.

(B) Specify the provider's specialty.

(C) Provide additional information about a service or procedure.

(D) Identify the patient's gender.

(96) What is the correct CPT code for a limited study duplex ultrasound imaging of the penile blood vessels for abnormalities carried out during a follow-up visit?

(A) 93981.

(B) 93980.

(C) 93983.

(D) 93982.

(97) A seventy-two-year-old woman with chronic obstructive pulmonary disease is scheduled for a routine spirometry test to assess her respiratory function. She is required to exhale rapidly over twelve to fifteen seconds after deep breathing. The report is recorded on a graph. What is the ICD-10-CM diagnosis code for her disease and the CPT code for the test?

(A) J44.9; 94010.

(B) J44.8; 98010.

(C) J45; 94245.

(D) J47; 94318.

(98) What is the structure of an ICD-10-CM code?

(A) Numeric with three to seven characters.

(B) Alphanumeric with three to seven characters.

(C) Alphabetic with two to five characters.

(D) Numeric with two to five characters.

(99) Which modifier indicates that two physicians worked together to perform a service?

(A) 32.

(B) 53.

(C) QW.

(D) 62.

(100) A seventy-eight-year-old female presents to a family physician with shortness of breath, cough, and diaphoresis. It has been two years since her last visit. She has a history of hypertension, diabetes, and congestive heart failure, which are still present. Her sister recently died of heart failure. An extended history of the present illness is documented. The physician reviews the systems related to the problems alongside a review of all other systems. A general multisystem examination is performed, as well as some investigations. This includes an EKG, chest X-ray, and blood work. The physician also orders for her records to be sent from her cardiologist. The medical decision-making is high. She is diagnosed with acute exacerbation of congestive heart failure. What is the correct code for the evaluation and management service for this encounter?

(A) 99205.

(B) 99215.

(C) 99204.

(D) 99214.

# Test 3: Answers and Explanations

(1) (B) 99152 - Moderate sedation services provided by the same physician or other qualified health care professional performing the diagnostic or therapeutic service that the sedation supports. There is an initial 15 minutes of intraservice time and the patient is younger than 5 years of age.

This code is used when the same physician or qualified health care professional provides both the moderate sedation and the primary diagnostic or therapeutic service. It applies to patients who are 5 years of age or older. For moderate sedation that lasts 30 minutes, 99152 would be used for the first 15 minutes, and code 99153 (which is for each additional 15 minutes of intraservice time) would be used to document the total duration of sedation accurately. However, since the question asks specifically for the initial documentation of moderate sedation, the correct answer is 99152, not including the additional time which would be captured separately with 99153.

(2) (C) OIG.

The OIG investigates fraud and abuse in healthcare services. The Office of Inspector General (OIG) for the US Department of Health and Human Services also educates physicians and healthcare service providers about Medicare and Medicaid programs and federal laws to prevent fraud and abuse.

(3) (C) E10.9 - Type 1 diabetes mellitus without complications, and 93674 - Intravascular ultrasound of coronary arteries.

This code should be used to document the patient's chronic condition of type 1 diabetes when no specific complications are mentioned in the scenario provided. The CPT code for the intravascular ultrasound of the coronary arteries is 93674. IVUS is a catheter-based procedure that provides detailed images of the inside of the coronary arteries and helps to assess the severity of coronary artery disease.

(4) (B) It may not be universally understood.

A limitation of medical terminology in cross-cultural healthcare is the potential for miscommunication due to linguistic and cultural differences. Patients from diverse backgrounds may struggle with terminology, which impacts effective communication.

(5) (C) It provides standardized terms for accurate documentation.

Medical terminology contributes to efficient electronic health record (EHR) systems as it provides standardized language. It ensures consistency and accuracy when recording patient information, which facilitates interoperability and streamlined communication among healthcare professionals. This results in improved coordination and quality of care.

(6) (B) Facilitates precise and unambiguous communication of findings.

Medical terminology facilitates precise communication as it provides a standardized language for findings. This makes it easier to communicate research findings among medical professionals.

(7) (B) Skeletal system.

The musculoskeletal system supports and protects the body. It provides a framework for movement through bones, muscles, and joints.

(8) (B) Transports nutrients and oxygen to cells.

The circulatory system's primary function is to transport blood, which carries oxygen, nutrients, and waste products. This ensures vital support for bodily functions.

(9) (C) Small intestine.

Digestion mainly occurs in the small intestine. It is where enzymes break down food, which facilitates nutrient absorption into the bloodstream.

(10) (A) Endocrine system.

The endocrine system produces chemical messengers (hormones) that regulate physiological functions. This ensures communication and coordination between different body systems.

(11) (C) Exchanges gases, such as oxygen and carbon dioxide.

The respiratory system facilitates gaseous exchange, which is important for cellular function and metabolism.

(12) (D) D61.9.

The keyword is anemia, and the diagnosis is pancytopenia due to aplastic anemia. Locate the code for anemia in the index of disease and injury. The appropriate code is D61.9.

(13) (B) K50.111.

Locate the index category for disorders of the digestive system. The diagnosis is Crohn's disease. However, further details given regarding this patient's condition require additional characters. A six-character code is generated for this reported condition.

(14) (B) K21.9.

Gastroesophageal reflux disease, as listed in this question, is categorized as unspecified due to the lack of detail given.

(15) (A) M80.051A.

The diagnosis for this patient is a pathological fracture of the right femur, initial encounter. It is important to note that as this is the initial encounter for this patient, a seventh character is needed to code for the diagnosis fully.

(16) (B) F43.21 - Adjustment disorder with depressed mood.

This code is used to describe a psychological response to an identifiable stressor (in this case, the loss of a loved one) that results in significant emotional or behavioral symptoms. The designation of an adjustment disorder with depressed mood accurately captures the clinical presentation of the patient, who is experiencing difficulty adjusting to a significant life change.

(17) (B) G00.9.

Bacterial meningitis is an inflammatory condition that affects the central nervous system. This diagnosis code is located in the subcategory G00. Further review of the information provided requires the fourth character of the code set.

(18) (B) E0105.

HCPCS Level II code E0105 represents a prefabricated adjustable orthopedic cane with a quad or three-prong tip. This code is utilized for billing and documentation purposes.

(19) (B) L03.90.

The ICD-10 code for unspecified cellulitis is L03.90. This code is used when medical documentation does not specify the location or cause of cellulitis. L03.90 falls within the L03 category. This provides a broad classification for billing and medical record purposes when details about the cellulitis are not specified.

(20) (C) 11400-11646.

The CPT code range 11400-11646 is used for excision of benign and malignant lesions. This includes skin cancers in various anatomical regions. These codes cover a spectrum of excision procedures, from simple to complex. Each specific code within this range corresponds to different factors, such as lesion size, location, and complexity. Accurate utilization of these codes ensures precise documentation and billing for excision procedures performed by healthcare providers.

(21) (A) 12031.

The CPT code 12031 indicates the simple repair of a superficial wound on the scalp, neck, axillae, external genitalia, trunk, or extremities. This code specifically applies to wound closure that involves the deeper layers of tissue beyond the subcutaneous tissue and may require more complex suturing techniques.

(22) (B) 11600-11646.

The CPT code range 11600-11646 is used for excision of malignant skin lesions. This includes carcinomas and melanomas. Each code within this range corresponds to specific factors such as lesion size, location, and complexity. These codes enable healthcare providers to accurately document and bill for excision procedures based on the details of skin cancer removal.

(23) (A) 11200.

The CPT code 11200 indicates the removal of benign skin lesions, such as tags, moles, or warts, with a diameter of less than four mm. This code is specific to simple lesion excision and is part of the range used for coding minor skin procedures.

(24) (C) 11602 - Excision of malignant lesion including margins, trunk, arms, or legs; lesion diameter 1.1 to 2.0 cm.

This code is used for lesions that measure between 1.1 to 2.0 cm in total diameter after including the margins required for complete excision. In this scenario, the original lesion measured 1.2 cm in diameter, and with a 0.3 cm margin all around, the total diameter of the excised area became 1.8 cm. This falls within the size range specified by CPT code 11602.

(25) (A) 17250 - Chemical cauterization of granulation tissue (proud flesh, sinus or fistula).

This code is designated for the chemical cauterization of granulation tissue, which can include the treatment of proud flesh, sinus, fistula, or similar conditions where cauterization is used to promote healing and prevent infection. While the description primarily mentions granulation tissue, in practice, this code can be applied to situations where chemical cauterization is performed on superficial lesions to achieve a therapeutic outcome.

(26) (A) 11100 - Biopsy of skin, subcutaneous tissue and/or mucous membrane (including simple closure), unless otherwise listed; single lesion.

This code is designated for the biopsy of skin, including subcutaneous tissue and/or mucous membrane, and includes simple closure if performed. It is used when a single lesion is biopsied.

(27) (A) 11603 - Excision of malignant lesion including margins, trunk, arms, or legs; lesion diameter 2.1 to 3.0 cm.

This code is designated for the excision of malignant lesions, including the margins, on the trunk, arms, or legs when the lesion's diameter after including margins measures between 2.1 and 3.0 cm. The final excised diameter reflects the original size of the lesion plus the margin taken to ensure clear margins around the malignant tissue, which in this case totals 3.0 cm.

(28) (B) 17261 - Destruction of malignant lesion on the face (0.6 to 1.0 cm).

This code is designated for the cryosurgical destruction of malignant lesions on the face that are within the size range of 0.6 to 1.0 cm. Cryosurgery is a technique that uses extreme cold to destroy abnormal or diseased tissue, including skin cancers such as basal cell carcinoma.

(29) (B) 11300 - Shaving of epidermal or dermal lesion, single lesion, trunk, arms or legs; lesion diameter 0.5 cm or less.

This code is designated for the shaving of epidermal or dermal lesions located on the trunk, arms, or legs, with a lesion diameter of 0.5 cm or less. The back of the hand is considered part of the arms for coding purposes.

(30) (B) 15002 - Preparation for split-thickness skin graft, trunk, arms, legs; first 100 sq cm or less, or 1% of body area of infants and children.

This code is specifically designated for the preparation of a site to receive a split-thickness skin graft on the trunk, arms, or legs and covers the initial 100 square centimeters or less, or 1% of the body area of infants and children. The preparation process includes creating a vascular bed to ensure the graft will have a high chance of successful integration.

(31) (B) RT - Right side.

This modifier is used to specify when a procedure is performed on the right side of the body. It indicates the side of the body on which procedures are performed, especially for bilateral body parts.

(32) (A) Right side.

The modifier RT in musculoskeletal system coding indicates that a procedure was performed on the right side of the body. It provides additional information about the location or side of a surgical or medical service.

(33) (B) 50.

The modifier 50 indicates that a procedure was performed bilaterally. This modifier is applied to certain CPT codes to communicate that the procedure was carried out on both the left and right sides concurrently.

(34) (A) Left side.

The modifier LT in musculoskeletal coding signifies that a procedure was performed on the left side of the body. This modifier provides additional information about the location or side of a surgical or medical service when appended to a CPT code.

(35) (C) To signify distinct procedural service.

The modifier 59 in musculoskeletal coding indicates that a procedure is a distinct procedural service. It is applied when a provider performs multiple procedures during the same session or on the same day, and each procedure is significant, separately identifiable, and not considered a component of another. Modifier 59 helps avoid claim denials for bundled services and ensures accurate coding and reimbursement for distinct and separate procedures.

(36) (C) Thromboembolic deterrent stockings.

HCPCS Level II code A6530 is associated with thromboembolic deterrent stockings. This code is used to report the provision of compression stockings designed to prevent or manage blood clot formation (thromboembolism). Accurate utilization of HCPCS code A6530 ensures proper documentation and billing for thromboembolic deterrent stockings. These stockings help patients with conditions that require compression therapy to reduce the risk of deep vein thrombosis or other vascular issues.

(37) (B) 59 - Distinct procedural service.

Modifier 59 is used to indicate that a procedure or service was distinct or independent from other services performed on the same day. This modifier helps to differentiate services that are not normally reported together but are appropriate under the circumstances. It signals to payers that two or more procedures were performed for different and unrelated reasons, and it supports the medical necessity of performing both procedures during the same session.

(38) (A) 50 - Bilateral procedure.

Modifier 50 is used to indicate procedures that are performed on both sides of the body during the same operative session. This modifier is applied to the procedure code to signify that the surgery was executed bilaterally on both the left and right sides.

(39) (A) 59 - Distinct procedural service.

Modifier 59 is used to indicate that a procedure or service was distinct or separate from other services performed on the same day. This modifier is particularly useful in situations where procedures performed during the same visit are not normally reported together, but are appropriate under the circumstances. The coder is specifying that the steroid injection in the right knee is a distinct service from the trigger point injection in the left shoulder.

(40) (C) Professional component.

The modifier 26 in medical coding signifies the professional component of a service. It indicates that a physician or qualified healthcare professional performed the interpretation or supervision of a diagnostic test or procedure. Modifier 26 is particularly relevant for procedures where both a technical component, e.g., conducting the test, and a professional component, e.g., interpreting the results, exist. Its use ensures accurate documentation and appropriate reimbursement for professional services rendered.

(41) (A) Repeated procedure by the initial physician.

In medical coding, the modifier 76 indicates a repeat procedure or service by the same physician or qualified healthcare professional. It denotes that a procedure or service was performed again on the same patient on the same day. Proper use of Modifier 76 ensures accurate documentation and billing for subsequent instances of a particular service, which assists in communication and reimbursement for additional procedures performed within the same encounter.

(42) (A) 50 - Bilateral procedure.

Modifier 50 is used to indicate that a procedure was performed on both sides of the body during the same operative session. This modifier accurately communicates to insurers that the surgical removal of both breasts was performed as part of the patient's treatment for breast cancer.

(43) (A) 51 - Multiple procedures.

Modifier 51 is used to indicate that multiple procedures were performed during the same operative session. This modifier helps to identify the secondary or tertiary procedures that are performed in addition to the primary procedure, which allows for appropriate adjustment and reimbursement by payers. It is designed to be used when reporting more than one procedure performed on the same day by the same physician or health care provider.

(44) (B) N48.30 - Unspecified priapism and 54235 - Injection procedure into the corpora cavernosa for priapism.

N48.30 is the ICD-10-CM code for unspecified priapism, which is a condition characterized by a persistent and often painful erection that is not related to sexual arousal. The correct CPT code for an injection procedure into the corpora cavernosa to relieve priapism is one that accurately reflects the procedure's direct treatment of the condition.

(45) (B) 58.

Modifier 58 signifies a staged or related procedure during the postoperative period. This modifier is used when a subsequent procedure is planned or anticipated during the global surgical period of the initial surgery. Applying Modifier 58 ensures proper documentation, billing, and reimbursement.

(46) (B) 74.

Modifier 74 indicates a discontinued procedure after anesthesia administration due to extenuating circumstances. It is applied when a procedure is halted before completion due to unforeseen reasons. This modifier communicates that the provider deliberately stopped the procedure for the patient's well-being.

(47) (D) 91.

Modifier 91 is used to code for a repeated lab test on the same day. This modifier distinguishes between multiple instances of the same procedure or service performed on the same day but during separate sessions.

(48) (C) J1610.

The HCPCS Level II code assigned for the injection of glucagon hydrochloride for subcutaneous or intramuscular use is J1610. This code specifically represents glucagon administration. Glucagon is a hormone used in emergencies such as severe hypoglycemia.

(49) (C) 53.

The modifier 53 indicates that a procedure was discontinued due to extenuating circumstances. This modifier is applied when the provider initiates a procedure but cannot complete it due to unforeseen factors or complications. It communicates the unique circumstances surrounding the discontinuation of the procedure for accurate billing and documentation.

(50) (B) 25.

If a separately identifiable evaluation and management (E/M) service is provided during the postoperative period, Modifier 25 is applied. It indicates that the E/M service is distinct and unrelated to the previous surgery, which allows for proper reimbursement and documentation of additional, necessary services during the postoperative phase.

(51) (B) 53200 - Urethral dilation, initial.

This code is designated for the initial procedure of dilating the urethra, which is a therapeutic approach to treating urethral strictures. Urethral dilation involves the stretching of the narrowed section of the urethra to relieve symptoms such as urinary retention.

(52) (A) 76.

The modifier 76 is used for a repeat procedure by the same physician on the same day. This modifier indicates that a procedure previously performed by the same physician for the same patient earlier in the day is being repeated. It aids in precise healthcare documentation, billing, and reimbursement. This provides a standardized way to convey the repetition of a specific procedure within the coding system.

(53) (B) PO.

The modifier PO is applied for a service provided in an off-campus outpatient department in a hospital setting that is not an emergency. It indicates services rendered in an ambulatory surgery center (ASC) distinct from emergency care.

(54) (A) 58150 - Total abdominal hysterectomy (corpus and cervix), with or without removal of tube(s), with or without removal of ovary(s).

This procedure is commonly performed for patients diagnosed with endometrial cancer to remove the primary site of cancerous growth and potentially involved adjacent structures. A total abdominal hysterectomy may involve the removal of additional reproductive organs depending on the extent of the cancer and the surgical plan determined by the physician.

(55) (D) N35.11; 53600, Modifier 77.

N35.11 indicates a diagnosis of post-infective urethral stricture in a male, not elsewhere classified. 53600 is used to describe a manipulation procedure on the urethra. Modifier 77 indicates that a different provider repeated a service after another provider performed the initial procedure.

(56) (B) N44.00

N44.00 is the diagnosis code for testicular torsion, unspecified.

(57) (B) N25.1.

Nephrogenic diabetic insipidus is a disorder that results from impaired renal tubular function listed in the ICD-10-CM codebook in category N25.

(58) (B) 58322 - Artificial insemination; intrauterine.

This code refers to intrauterine insemination, which is a fertility treatment that involves placing sperm inside a woman's uterus to facilitate fertilization. The key distinction of IUI is the placement of sperm directly into the uterus, which increases the chances of fertilization by reducing the distance sperm have to travel to reach the fallopian tubes.

(59) (B) 51102.

The CPT code for drainage of urine from the bladder through a suprapubic approach with the insertion of a catheter is listed as 51102 in the CPT code book under procedures for the urinary system.

(60) (A) 59000 - Amniocentesis; diagnostic.

This code is designated for amniocentesis procedures performed for diagnostic purposes, such as assessing fetal health or diagnosing chromosomal abnormalities. Diagnostic amniocentesis involves the extraction of a small amount of amniotic fluid from the amniotic sac surrounding the fetus, which can provide valuable information about the fetus's condition and the presence of any potential issues.

(61) (A) 58300.

The appropriate CPT code for intrauterine device insertion is reported as 58300.

(62) (A) 58970 - Follicle puncture for oocyte retrieval, any method.

This code refers to the follicle puncture for oocyte (egg) retrieval, regardless of the method used to perform the retrieval. The process involves the extraction of eggs from the ovaries, which are then fertilized in the laboratory setting.

(63) (A) 59514.

According to the Current Procedural Terminology, cesarean delivery is coded as 59514.

(64) (C) 59410 - Vaginal delivery only (with or without episiotomy and/or forceps) including postpartum care.

This code refers to vaginal delivery only, with or without the use of episiotomy and/or forceps, and includes the provision of postpartum care.

(65) (C) 58900, Modifier RT.

The CPT code for biopsy of the right ovary is 58900, Modifier RT.

(66) (A) 60650 - Laparoscopy, surgical; adrenalectomy.

This code refers to the laparoscopic surgical procedure for adrenalectomy, indicating that the surgery was performed using laparoscopic instruments and techniques, which result in smaller incisions, reduced pain, and quicker recovery times compared to traditional open surgery.

(67) (A) 61000 - Shunt; ventricular to external drainage.

This code refers to the establishment of a shunt from the ventricular space within the brain to external drainage. This procedure is critical for patients experiencing conditions that lead to increased intracranial pressure, as it allows for the controlled drainage of cerebrospinal fluid to relieve pressure.

(68) (B) 61524 - Craniectomy or craniotomy for excision of brain tumor, infratentorial or posterior fossa; intradural, including dural repair, if performed.

This code refers to intradural procedures, which involve operating within the dura mater (the tough outer layer of the meninges that surround the brain and spinal cord). The description of the procedure as involving an approach through the base of the skull to access and remove a tumor aligns with the infratentorial or posterior fossa approach.

(69) (C) 62223 - Craniectomy for evacuation of hematoma; subdural.

This code is designated for a craniectomy, which involves the surgical removal of a portion of the skull to access the brain and evacuate a hematoma located beneath the dura mater (subdural). This procedure is indicated in cases of acute subdural hematomas that pose a threat to the patient's health due to increased intracranial pressure or other complications that result from the hematoma.

(70) (C) 61154 with modifier 50 - Burr hole(s); with drainage of hematoma, subdural, indicating a bilateral procedure.

This combination accurately reflects that the procedure was performed bilaterally, on both sides of the head, to address bilateral subdural hematomas. The CPT code 61154 specifies the surgical procedure of creating burr holes with drainage of a subdural hematoma. When appended with modifier 50, it explicitly indicates that the procedure was performed on both the left and right sides during the same surgical session, which is essential for correct billing and reimbursement for bilateral procedures.

(71) (C) 67228 with modifier 50 - Treatment of extensive or progressive retinopathy (e.g., diabetic retinopathy), photocoagulation; indicating a bilateral procedure.

This combination reflects that the laser treatment was performed on both eyes to address extensive or progressive retinopathy, such as diabetic retinopathy, which can lead to blindness if not treated. The CPT code 67228 specifies the procedure of photocoagulation for extensive or progressive retinopathy, and when appended with modifier 50, it explicitly indicates that the procedure was performed bilaterally.

(72) (C) 67107 with modifier LT - Repair of retinal detachment; with scleral buckle, indicating the procedure was performed on the left eye.

This combination accurately reflects that the surgical procedure, which involves placing a silicone band (scleral buckle) around the eye to repair the detached retina, was performed specifically on the left eye. The CPT code 67107 specifies the procedure of repairing a retinal detachment with a scleral buckle. When appended with modifier LT, it indicates that the procedure was performed on the left side.

(73) (C) 69000 with modifier LT - Excision external ear; cholesteatoma, indicating the procedure was performed on the left ear.

This combination reflects that the surgical procedure, specifically the removal of a cholesteatoma, was performed on the left ear. The CPT code 69000 specifies the excision of an external ear condition, such as a cholesteatoma, which is a type of skin growth that can occur in the middle ear and mastoid bone. When appended with modifier LT, it indicates that the procedure was carried out on the left side, ensuring precise documentation for billing and medical records.

(74) (A) 12 units - Calculated by adding the base unit value (4 units) to the time units for the duration of the procedure (8 units for 2 hours).

This total is derived by adding the base unit value for the procedure, which is 4 units, to the time units accumulated during the procedure. Given that the anesthesia was administered for 2 hours and the practice assigns a time unit value of 1 unit per 15 minutes, the total time units amount to 8 (since 2 hours equal 120 minutes, and 120 divided by 15 equals 8).

(75) (B) 69200, Modifier RT.

The correct CPT code for removing a foreign body from the external ear without general anesthesia is 69200. The applicable modifier is Modifier RT.

(76) (B) 69930, Modifier 50.

Cochlear device implantation bilaterally is coded as 69930, Modifier 50

(77) (A) 99116 - Anesthesia complicated by utilization of total body hypothermia.

This code addresses situations where anesthesia is administered alongside induced hypothermia, which is a deliberate reduction of the patient's body temperature to lower metabolic demand and protect the brain and other vital organs during certain surgical procedures.

(78) (A) H61.22; 69209, Modifier LT.

The diagnosis in this case is impacted cerumen of the left ear, coded as H61.22 according to ICD-10-CM. The associated CPT code for removal by irrigation is 69209, Modifier LT.

(79) (A) Only the unit for the highest value.

The unit value of the anesthesia service is calculated by only the unit for the highest value.

(80) (A) 00102, 00172, P1, Modifier 77.

The appropriate code for anesthesia for a repeat procedure of a patient with cleft lip and palate in good health with a previous unsuccessful attempt at repair and presents for definitive repair is 00102, 00172, P1, Modifier 77.

(81) (B) 99116.

CPT code 99116 is used for anesthesia complicated by utilization of total body hypothermia. However, for a six-month-old undergoing anesthesia, the more appropriate code might be 99100 (Anesthesia for patient of extreme age, under one year and over 70), which addresses age as a complicating factor for anesthesia, not 99116 as initially indicated. This misinterpretation was due to an incorrect focus on age-specific anesthesia complications.

(82) (C) 99135.

99135 is an add-on code that describes the use of controlled hypotension alongside a primary anesthesia procedure by the anesthesiologist or other medical provider. This complicates the administration of anesthesia.

(83) (D) 76937.

The use of ultrasound guidance for central venous access is coded as 76937.

(84) (A) 76946.

The code for an ultrasound-guided amniocentesis is 76946.

(85) (B) 73502, RT.

The correct CPT code for an X-ray of one hip is 73502. The appropriate modifier for the right hip is Modifier RT.

(86) (C) 73560, 50.

The correct CPT code for an X-ray of one knee is 73560. The modifier for bilateral procedures is 50.

(87) (D) 77080, 26.

The correct CPT code for professional services for bone density studies of the hips, spine, and pelvis is 77080, 26.

(88) (B) 74240, 26; K22.0.

74240 is the appropriate code for an imaging series of the upper gastrointestinal tract. This includes the esophagus, stomach, and duodenum and uses barium sulfate contrast. The complete code is 74240, 26; K22.0.

(89) (C) 76775, LT.

The correct CPT code for imaging of just one kidney is 76775. The modifier is LT.

(90) (C) C25.9; 48102, 77002, 26.

The ICD-10-CM diagnosis code for an unspecified category of pancreatic cancer is C25.9. Biopsy of the pancreas is an excision procedure found under the surgical procedures category of CPT codes. Percutaneous pancreas biopsy with tissue collection to be sent for pathological analysis is coded 48102. The fluoroscopic guidance aspect of the procedure is coded 77002.

(91) (D) 93307, Modifier 26.

The correct CPT code for this service is 93307. The professional component is reported with Modifier 26.

(92) (B) Laboratory test codes.

LOINC (Logical Observation Identifiers Names and Codes) helps standardize laboratory test codes within the healthcare system. It is specifically designed to identify and exchange information related to laboratory observations. LOINC provides a universal coding system for various tests and measurements. Laboratories globally use LOINC codes to report results consistently, which streamlines communication among healthcare professionals and institutions. This standardized approach facilitates interoperability and enhances data exchange accuracy, which contributes to better patient care and more effective research. By serving as a common language for laboratory test codes, LOINC promotes efficiency, reduces errors, and fosters a cohesive environment for the interpretation and utilization of vital health information.

(93) (A) HIPAA (Health Insurance Portability and Accountability Act).

HIPAA ensures the confidentiality and integrity of individually identifiable health information in the United States. Enacted in 1996, HIPAA introduced comprehensive regulations to address the evolving healthcare landscape. It emphasizes the protection of sensitive patient data.

(94) (C) National Drug Code.

In the context of medical coding, NDC stands for the National Drug Code. This unique numeric code identifies and classifies prescription and over-the-counter medications. The NDC system is maintained by the US Food and Drug Administration (FDA). It helps streamline drug information and facilitates accurate billing and reimbursement processes in healthcare.

(95) (C) Provide additional information about a service or procedure.

Modifiers in medical coding provide additional information about a service or procedure performed. These two-digit codes, appended to the main procedure code, help convey specific circumstances or alterations in the service provided.

(96) (A) 93981.

The correct CPT code for a limited study is 93981.

(97) (A) J44.9; 94010.

The correct CPT code is 94010. The ICD-10-CM diagnosis code for COPD is J44.9 because there is no information specified for the subtype of COPD in this patient.

(98) (B) Alphanumeric with three to seven characters.

The structure of an ICD-10-CM code is alphanumeric, with three to seven characters. These codes are organized into categories and subcategories, which allows for a detailed classification of diseases, conditions, and health-related issues. The first character indicates the chapter or category. It is followed by additional characters that provide more specific details. The structure ensures a standardized and systematic approach to coding, which facilitates accurate communication of medical information for billing, statistical analysis, and healthcare management.

(99) (D) 62.

The modifier used to indicate that a different physician performed a service is 62. This modifier is applied when two physicians jointly perform a procedure or surgery as a team. It communicates shared responsibility for the service and ensures appropriate reimbursement. Modifier 62 emphasizes collaborative efforts in healthcare, which allows for accurate billing and documentation and fosters transparency in medical coding.

(100) (B) 99215.

This patient is established and seen in the outpatient setting with an MDM of high complexity. 99215 is the appropriate code.

## Test 4: Questions

(1) The development of a framework for medical necessity was based on what legislation?

(A) SSA.

(B) Medicaid.

(C) HITECH.

(D) OIG.

(2) In ICD-10 coding, what does the abbreviation NEC stand for, and how should it be applied?

(A) Not Elsewhere Classified - Used when a specific code does not exist for a condition and indicates that the information is not available for more specific coding.

(B) No Existing Code - Used to indicate that coding for a specific condition does not exist in the ICD-10 manual.

(C) Not Entirely Clear - Used when the coder is uncertain about the specific details of a condition.

(D) Non-Essential Coding - Used for supplementary codes that are not critical for the primary diagnosis.

(3) What procedure does the CPT code 59525 represent?

(A) Cesarean delivery only.

(B) Cesarean hysterectomy including removal of the uterus at the time of cesarean delivery.

(C) Vaginal delivery only.

(D) Repair of a third-degree obstetric laceration.

(4) As per CPT guidelines, which of the following cannot be reported as a stand-alone code?

(A) +59525.

(B) 56420.

(C) +99292.

(D) 78215.

(5) A 53-year-old man presents at the clinic with complaints of excessive thirst, weight loss, and fatigue. He has a history of nocturia and polyphagia. He had a pancreatectomy for a pancreatic tumor six months before the onset of his symptoms. The physician documents a diagnosis of post-pancreatectomy diabetes mellitus. What is the appropriate code for this patient?

(A) E11.

(B) O24.4.

(C) E89.1.

(D) Y84.2.

(6) Which condition does the ICD-10 code P91.6 represent?

(A) Neonatal cerebral ischemia.

(B) Neonatal cerebral hemorrhage.

(C) Neonatal jaundice.

(D) Neonatal sepsis.

(7) If a body part is located close to the surface, it is described as:

(A) Deep.

(B) Superficial.

(C) Proximal.

(D) Distal.

(8) Which of the following best describes the ICD-10 code M05.709?

(A) Seropositive rheumatoid arthritis with rheumatoid factor of the unspecified wrist without organ or systems involvement.

(B) Seronegative rheumatoid arthritis of the left knee.

(C) Seropositive rheumatoid arthritis with rheumatoid factor of unspecified wrist with organ or systems involvement.

(D) Osteoarthritis of the unspecified wrist.

(9) What does the HCPCS code L1682 describe?

(A) Knee orthosis, double upright, thigh and calf, with adjustable flexion and extension joint, medial-lateral and rotation control.

(B) Ankle-foot orthosis, spiral, fabricated.

(C) Knee orthosis, single upright, thigh and calf, with adjustable flexion and extension joint, medial-lateral and rotation control.

(D) Knee orthosis, suspension sleeve, prefabricated, includes fitting and adjustment.

(10) Which CPT code is most appropriate for billing a simple nebulizer treatment administered in a physician's office?

(A) 94640.

(B) 94010.

(C) 94760.

(D) 99213.

(11) What does the CPT code 39599 represent in medical coding?

(A) Unlisted procedure, spleen.

(B) Unlisted procedure, stomach.

(C) Unlisted procedure, diaphragm.

(D) Unlisted procedure, respiratory system.

(12) One of the advantages of medical terminology is its ability to:

(A) Limit healthcare information accessibility to the general public.

(B) Facilitate global communication in healthcare.

(C) Hinder research and medical advancements by nonprofessionals.

(D) Impede accurate diagnoses.

(13) Which CPT code should be used to bill for the use of an airway clearance system in a clinical setting?

(A) 94667.

(B) 94668.

(C) E0483.

(D) 94799.

(14) What does the CPT code 93325 represent in medical coding?

(A) Doppler echocardiography color flow velocity mapping.

(B) Transthoracic echocardiography for congenital cardiac anomalies; complete.

(C) Transesophageal echocardiography for congenital cardiac anomalies including probe placement, image acquisition, interpretation, and report.

(D) Cardiac catheterization for coronary artery imaging.

(15) What is the appropriate use of CPT code 33206?

(A) Insertion of a temporary transvenous single chamber cardiac electrode or pacemaker catheter.

(B) Implantation of a permanent pacemaker with transvenous electrode(s); single chamber, atrial or ventricular.

(C) Repair of a single chamber pacemaker system.

(D) Removal of a permanent pacemaker pulse generator.

(16) A 45-year-old woman is seen in the outpatient clinic with a two-day history of right iliac fossa pain, fever, and three episodes of non-projectile, non-bilious vomiting. Labs show an elevated white cell count with neutrophilia. An abdominal CT is carried out, and a diagnosis of acute appendicitis is made. What is the ICD-10-CM code for the diagnosis?

(A) K35.80.

(B) K35.7.

(C) K35.83.

(D) K35.46.

(17) A four-year-old boy presents with a swollen abdomen, which has progressively worsened over six months. Investigations reveal an abdominal mass with findings consistent with Wilms tumor. What is the appropriate code for this diagnosis?

(A) C64.5.

(B) C64.9.

(C) C68.7.

(D) C64.8.

(18) A 69-year-old man presents at the surgical outpatient clinic with swelling in the right inguinal region. He previously had surgery to correct this. The surgeon books him for a mesh repair of the recurrent inguinal hernia. What is the ICD-10-CM code?

(A) K40.7.

(B) K40.8.

(C) K41.91.

(D) K40.91.

(19) Which of the following best describes the range of CPT codes C1900-C1942?

(A) Implantable neurostimulator electrodes.

(B) Cardiac valve and other major cardiothoracic procedures with cardiac catheterization.

(C) Angioplasty or stenting procedures.

(D) Leadless pacemaker systems.

(20) A surgeon performs a surgical procedure for a patient in the early morning hours. Later in the evening of the same day, a second surgeon repeats the procedure due to complications. What is the appropriate modifier the second surgeon should use?

(A) 22.

(B) 25.

(C) 77.

(D) 76.

(21) A patient presents to the hospital for an X-ray of her leg after an injury sustained in a soccer game. The X-ray is taken by the technician and reviewed by the physician. What is the appropriate modifier for this service?

(A) 32.

(B) 47.

(C) 26.

(D) 24.

(22) How often does the AMA release updates for the Category I CPT code?

(A) Quarterly.

(B) Monthly.

(C) Annually.

(D) Biennially.

(23) A patient is admitted to the ER for extensive second- and third-degree burns after a gas explosion. The plastic surgery team is invited to review, and a plan is created for a skin flap and a multi-stage skin graft. The patient has the first surgery days after admission and then has the skin graft done three weeks later. What code should be reported by the surgeon after the second surgery?

(A) 15273–62.

(B) 15273–76.

(C) 15273–82.

(D) 15273–58.

(24) Which CPT code is used for the open treatment of an olecranon fracture with internal fixation?

(A) 24650.

(B) 24685.

(C) 24666.

(D) 24675.

(25) What is the CPT code for an arthroscopic meniscectomy of the knee, medial or lateral?

(A) 29874.

(B) 29877.

(C) 29880.

(D) 29881.

(26) Which CPT code represents an open treatment of a tibial shaft fracture with the insertion of an intramedullary nail?

(A) 27750.

(B) 27758.

(C) 27759.

(D) 27766.

(27) What HCPCS Level II code is used for a prefabricated wrist-hand-finger orthosis without joints? This includes fitting and adjustment.

(A) L3908.

(B) L3923.

(C) L3900.

(D) L3925.

(28) Which code represents a custom-fabricated knee orthosis with adjustable knee joints? This includes soft interface material.

(A) L1832.

(B) L1845.

(C) L1847.

(D) L1836.

(29) What is the purpose of establishing “medical necessity”?

(A) To ensure that healthcare services and procedures billed to insurance are for cosmetic purposes only.

(B) To confirm that the healthcare services and procedures billed are reasonable and necessary for the diagnosis or treatment of illness or injury.

(C) To guarantee that the most expensive treatment options are utilized for patient care.

(D) To validate that healthcare services are provided based on the healthcare provider’s preference.

(30) When coding for a stroke in the ICD-10-CM, which of the following codes would be most appropriate for an acute ischemic stroke?

(A) I60.9.

(B) I61.9.

(C) I63.9.

(D) I64.

(31) Which ICD-10-CM code should be used for a non-specified injury to the right index finger without mention of a foreign body?

(A) S60.501A.

(B) S61.201A.

(C) S65.501A.

(D) S69.90XA.

(32) When coding for a patient who was brought into the emergency department unconscious, which ICD-10-CM code is most appropriate to indicate the state of unconsciousness?

(A) R40.20.

(B) R40.2110.

(C) R40.3.

(D) R40.4.

(33) Which HCPCS Level II code is associated with a home ventilator?

(A) E0424.

(B) E0601.

(C) E0465.

(D) E0562.

(34) What is HCPCS Level II code E0570 used for?

(A) A nebulizer with a compressor.

(B) An oxygen concentrator.

(C) A positive airway pressure device.

(D) An incentive spirometer.

(35) Which HCPCS Level II code is associated with a lymphedema pump?

(A) E0601.

(B) E0650.

(C) E0676.

(D) E0652.

(36) Which ICD-10-CM code is most appropriate for a patient diagnosed with a generalized tonic-clonic seizure without mention of epilepsy or a recurrent condition?

(A) G40.909.

(B) R56.9.

(C) G41.9.

(D) R25.9.

(37) What is the appropriate application of modifier 23 for CPT coding?

(A) To indicate that a procedure was performed on an outpatient basis.

(B) To indicate that unusual anesthesia was used for a procedure that does not usually require any anesthesia.

(C) To indicate that multiple procedures were performed during the same surgical session.

(D) To indicate that a procedure was more complex than usual.

(38) What does the application of modifier 28 indicate in CPT coding?

(A) To signify a service performed bilaterally.

(B) To indicate a service was provided to a newborn patient.

(C) To denote services provided outside of regular office hours.

(D) To designate a repeat procedure by another physician.

(39) What condition does the ICD-10-CM code E11.9 represent?

(A) Type 1 diabetes mellitus without complications.

(B) Type 2 diabetes mellitus without complications.

(C) Gestational diabetes mellitus without complications.

(D) Secondary diabetes mellitus without complications.

(40) Which HCPCS Level II code is used for the insertion of a cardiovascular stent?

(A) C9600.

(B) C1888.

(C) C2610.

(D) C1752.

(41) Which HCPCS Level II code range is usually associated with cardiac rehabilitation services?

(A) G0422–G0424.

(B) G0237–G0239.

(C) G0250–G0251.

(D) G0299–G0301.

(42) What does the HCPCS code K0606 represent?

(A) Automatic external defibrillator, with integrated electrocardiogram analysis.

(B) Replacement battery for an implanted pacemaker defibrillator.

(C) Replacement battery for an external defibrillator.

(D) Automated external defibrillator, without integrated electrocardiogram analysis.

(43) What procedure does CPT code 43215 represent?

A) Esophagogastroduodenoscopy (EGD) with removal of a foreign body.

B) Esophageal dilation without fluoroscopic guidance.

C) Esophagogastroduodenoscopy with biopsy.

D) Endoscopic retrograde cholangiopancreatography (ERCP).

(44) What does CPT code 43246 represent?

(A) Esophagogastroduodenoscopy (EGD) with the insertion of a guide wire.

(B) Esophagogastroduodenoscopy with the injection(s) for esophageal varices.

(C) Esophagogastroduodenoscopy (EGD) with the placement of an endoscopic stent.

(D) Esophagogastroduodenoscopy (EGD) with the transoral placement of an intragastric balloon.

(45) What does the HCPCS code G0342 represent?

(A) Low dose rate (LDR) prostate brachytherapy using stranded seeds.

(B) Percutaneous skeletal fixation of the posterior pelvic bone.

(C) Transcatheter placement of an intravascular stent(s), except coronary, carotid, vertebral, iliac, and femoropopliteal arteries.

(D) Initial placement of a low-profile gastrostomy device.

(46) What does the HCPCS code B4162 represent?

(A) Enteral formula, for adults, soy based, lactose-free, with intact nutrients.

(B) Enteral formula, for pediatrics, amino acid based.

(C) Enteral formula, for pediatrics, soy based, lactose-free, with intact nutrients.

(D) Parenteral nutrition solution, amino acid based.

(47) When a patient presents with acute kidney failure (N17.0) and undergoes bladder catheterization (51702), which scenario best describes the appropriate use of these codes?

(A) N17.0 is used to indicate the catheterization procedure, and 51702 is used to diagnose acute kidney failure.

(B) 51702 is the CPT code for the insertion of a temporary bladder catheter, and N17.0 is the ICD-10-CM code for acute kidney failure.

(C) N17.0 is the HCPCS code for bladder catheterization supplies, and 51702 describes the diagnosis of acute kidney failure.

(D) 51702 is used to code for acute kidney failure, and N17.0 is used for the insertion of a non-indwelling bladder catheter.

(48) What condition does the ICD-10-CM code N14.8 represent?

(A) Chronic kidney disease, stage 4.

(B) Drug- and heavy metal-induced tubulo-interstitial and tubular conditions.

(C) Nephrotic syndrome.

(D) Unspecified urinary incontinence.

(49) In a scenario where a patient is diagnosed with other specified hydrocele (N43.8) and undergoes a hydrocelectomy on the left side (55040-LT), which statement best describes the correct coding?

(A) N43.8 is the CPT code for hydrocelectomy, and 55040-LT is the ICD-10-CM code for left-sided hydrocele.

(B) 55040-LT is the CPT code for hydrocelectomy of the left testis, and N43.8 is the ICD-10-CM code for other specified hydrocele.

(C) N43.8 is used to indicate the hydrocelectomy procedure, and 55040-LT specifies the diagnosis of hydrocele on the left side.

(D) 55040-LT represents the diagnosis of other specified hydrocele, while N43.8 codes for the surgical procedure on the left side.

(50) An elderly man is seen by his urologist for evaluation of erectile dysfunction for the past seven months. He was diagnosed with a malignant neoplasm of the prostate with metastasis one year ago and has since undergone numerous treatments. He started radiation therapy nine months ago with good results since onset. However, he complains of an inability to maintain an erection. He has tried multiple over-the-counter medications without success. What is the ICD-10-CM code for the primary condition and subsequent complication of therapy that this patient has developed?

(A) C61, N52.

(B) C51, N54.52.

(C) C61, N52.35.

(D) C62, N53.2.

(51) A young woman is diagnosed with a urinary tract infection. What is the ICD-10-CM code?

(A) N38.5.

(B) N39.0.

(C) N21.3.

(D) N35.3.

(52) An elderly woman comes to the urology clinic because of an inability to hold her urine when she laughs or coughs. She is examined, and the Valsalva maneuver is carried out. Urine is seen extravasating from the urethral orifice. Subsequently, the patient is scheduled to undergo corrective surgery. What is the ICD-10-CM code for the diagnosis made?

(A) N39.3.

(B) N25.7.

(C) M24.45.

(D) N39.0.

(53) What condition is represented by the ICD-10-CM code N97.2?

(A) Female infertility of uterine origin.

(B) Female infertility of ovarian origin.

(C) Female infertility of tubal origin.

(D) Female infertility, unspecified.

(54) What procedure is represented by the CPT code 58150?

(A) Total abdominal hysterectomy, including partial vaginectomy.

(B) Laparoscopic ovarian cystectomy.

(C) Dilation and curettage, diagnostic and therapeutic.

(D) Endometrial ablation.

(55) What condition is indicated by the ICD-10-CM code G91.0?

(A) Communicating hydrocephalus.

(B) Non-communicating hydrocephalus.

(C) Normal pressure hydrocephalus.

(D) Post-traumatic hydrocephalus.

(56) What condition is represented by the ICD-10-CM code G40.309?

(A) Generalized idiopathic epilepsy and epileptic syndromes, not intractable, without status epilepticus.

(B) Localization-related (focal) (partial) epilepsy and epileptic syndromes with simple partial seizures, not intractable, without status epilepticus.

(C) Generalized idiopathic epilepsy and epileptic syndromes, intractable, with status epilepticus.

(D) Localization-related (focal) (partial) epilepsy and epileptic syndromes with complex partial seizures, not intractable, without status epilepticus.

(57) What is the ICD-10-CM diagnosis code for female pelvic inflammatory disease?

(A) N73.9.

(B) N72.9.

(C) N71.0.

(D) N73.

(58) What condition is indicated by the ICD-10-CM code G20?

(A) Essential tremor.

(B) Parkinson's disease.

(C) Multiple sclerosis.

(D) Alzheimer's disease.

(59) An older woman is scheduled for incision and drainage of a Bartholin's gland abscess. What is the CPT code for this procedure?

(A) 55421.

(B) 54420.

(C) 56420.

(D) 57523.

(60) What procedure is represented by the CPT code 60257?

(A) Excision of lesion of thyroid, without radical dissection.

(B) Parathyroidectomy.

(C) Thyroid lobectomy, including isthmusectomy; with or without substernal thyroid.

(D) Total thyroidectomy, including substernal thyroid; with or without lymph node dissection.

(61) When CPT code 65111 is used with modifier RT, what procedure is being indicated?

(A) Enucleation of the eye, without implant; left eye.

(B) Enucleation of the eye, with implant; right eye.

(C) Enucleation of the eye, without implant; right eye.

(D) Enucleation of the eye, with implant; left eye.

(62) A young woman is referred to a neurologist. She has had unilateral pulsatile headaches for several months. Her current medications include sumatriptan, propranolol, and ibuprofen. She tells the neurologist that she recently started experiencing an odd sensation before the onset of her headaches. Her headaches are worsened by bright lights and noise. What is the ICD-10-CM diagnosis code?

(A) G43.

(B) G43.3.

(C) G43.5.

(D) G43.1.

(63) What does the CPT code 00810 represent?

(A) Anesthesia for lower intestinal endoscopic procedures, endoscope introduced distal to duodenum.

(B) Anesthesia for upper gastrointestinal endoscopic procedures, endoscope introduced proximal to duodenum.

(C) Anesthesia for intraperitoneal procedures in the lower abdomen including laparoscopy.

(D) Anesthesia for procedures on the integumentary system on the extremities, anterior trunk and perineum.

(64) A patient comes in with complaints of excessive daytime sleepiness. A preliminary review is consistent with a diagnosis of narcolepsy. What is the ICD-10-CM diagnosis code for this condition?

(A) G47.41.

(B) G47.39.

(C) G47.40.

(D) G47.93.

(65) What procedure is represented by the CPT code 00734?

(A) Anesthesia for upper gastrointestinal endoscopic procedures, endoscope introduced proximal to duodenum.

(B) Anesthesia for interventional radiologic procedures on the lower extremities.

(C) Anesthesia for magnetic resonance imaging (MRI).

(D) Anesthesia for percutaneous image-guided procedures on the spine and spinal cord.

(66) What procedure does the CPT code 00109 represent?

(A) Anesthesia for procedures on the eye; not otherwise specified.

(B) Anesthesia for procedures on the integumentary system, including subcutaneous tissues of the head and neck.

(C) Anesthesia for procedures on the auditory system, not otherwise specified.

(D) Anesthesia for diagnostic or therapeutic nerve blocks and injections.

(67) After a hearing test, a patient is confirmed to have conductive hearing loss in the left ear with preserved hearing in the right ear. What is the ICD-10-CM diagnosis code?

(A) H90.10.

(B) H90.1.

(C) H90.

(D) H90.12.

(68) An older man undergoes cataract removal for bilateral age-related cataracts. The ophthalmologist removes extracapsular cataracts through the insertion of an intraocular lens prosthesis with phacoemulsification. No cyclophotocoagulation is performed for the procedure. What is the appropriate CPT code and modifier?

(A) 68084, modifier 51.

(B) 67084, modifier 50.

(C) 66984, modifier 50.

(D) 66974, modifier 51.

(69) What is the CPT code for excision of a pterygium of the left eye without graft?

(A) 65420, modifier LT.

(B) 75420, modifier LT.

(C) 65620, modifier LT.

(D) 65429, modifier LT.

(70) Which of the following procedures does the CPT code 99100 represent?

(A) Moderate sedation services.

(B) Special anesthesia service for a patient of extreme age, younger than 1 year and older than 70.

(C) Anesthesia for extensive spine and spinal cord procedures.

(D) Anesthesia for open heart surgery.

(71) A young man is trapped in a fire at a lumber factory. He is found by paramedics and noticed to have multiple splinter injuries to his body. He also sustained wood splinter injuries to both eyes. A tiny piece of wood is sticking out of his right eye. The injury is packed with a sterile covering, and the patient is transported to the healthcare facility.

Further eye examination reveals the presence of a wood splinter in the right superficial conjunctiva. The left eye has a splinter that extends into the anterior chamber of the eye. What is the CPT code for the removal of the foreign body in each eye?

(A) 65215, modifier RT; 65260, modifier RT.

(B) 65345, modifier RT; 65345, modifier LT.

(C) 65105, modifier LT; 65235, modifier RT.

(D) 65205, modifier RT; 65235, modifier LT.

(72) What is the primary purpose of a compliance program in a healthcare setting?

(A) Maximize profits.

(B) Ensure patient safety and integrity.

(C) Market the healthcare facility.

(D) Reduce staff workload.

(73) What is the CPT code for the reparation of a partial thickness laceration of the left eyelid margin?

(A) 67930, modifier LT.

(B) 67689, modifier LT.

(C) 68930, modifier LT.

(D) 65030, modifier LT.

(74) Which of the following CPT codes represents flow cytometry services?

(A) 88184.

(B) 88305.

(C) 85025.

(D) 87210.

(75) Which of the following best describes the use of modifier -76?

(A) Indicates multiple procedures were performed on the same day.

(B) Identifies repeat procedures by the same physician.

(C) Denotes services performed bilaterally.

(D) Indicates a procedure was reduced or eliminated at the physician's discretion.

(76) What service does the CPT code 99238 represent?

(A) Prolonged outpatient service.

(B) Hospital discharge day management, 30 minutes or less.

(C) Initial hospital care.

(D) Critical care service.

(77) What does the term MUE in medical coding refer to?

(A) Maximum Use Exemption.

(B) Medically Unlikely Edit.

(C) Medical Usage Evaluation.

(D) Minimum Utilization Enforcement.

(78) A pregnant woman undergoes chorionic villus sampling under ultrasound guidance to diagnose and screen for trisomy disorders. What is the appropriate CPT code?

(A) 76945.

(B) 76944.

(C) 76845.

(D) 76645.

(79) A physician orders a plain X-ray of the shoulder in anteroposterior and lateral views in a patient with suspected shoulder dislocation. What is the CPT code for the procedure?

(A) 73031.

(B) 73030.

(C) 73020.

(D) 73033.

(80) What is the correct CPT code for the use of magnetic resonance imaging guidance to locate parenchymal tissues and monitor their ablation?

(A) 77012.

(B) 77020.

(C) 77022.

(D) 77002.

(81) Which modifier is used to indicate a service provided by a resident under supervision?

(A) -26.

(B) -51.

(C) -76.

(D) -GC.

(82) In ICD-10 coding, what does "CM" stand for?

(A) Clinical modification.

(B) Coding manual.

(C) Condition modifier.

(D) Classification methodology.

(83) Which modifier is used to indicate multiple procedures performed during the same session?

(A) -25.

(B) -51.

(C) -76.

(D) -TC.

(84) What does HCPCS II mostly code?

(A) Diagnosis.

(B) Procedures.

(C) Durable medical equipment (DME).

(D) Surgical interventions.

(85) What does the range of codes 99477-99480 in the CPT codebook refer to?

(A) Adult critical care services.

(B) Initial and subsequent neonatal intensive care services.

(C) Pediatric and neonatal critical care transport.

(D) Intensive cardiac rehabilitation.

(86) Which service is represented by the CPT code 92555?

(A) Speech audiometry threshold.

(B) Comprehensive audiometry threshold evaluation.

(C) Auditory evoked potentials for evoked response audiometry.

(D) Tympanometry.

(87) An 85-year-old established patient is brought in by his son for a physical screening to be enrolled in a group home. The patient has previously been diagnosed with Alzheimer's disease, type 2 diabetes, and grade 1 hypertension. He is compliant with his medications. A comprehensive history and examination are performed, and the medical decision-making is of moderate complexity. Blood work is ordered. Past medical history shows the patient had a left hip replacement 10 years ago. What CPT code should be reported for this patient?

(A) 99397.

(B) 99387.

(C) 99212.

(D) 99213.

(88) What does the CPT code 93458 represent?

(A) Right heart catheterization.

(B) Left heart catheterization including intraprocedural injection(s) for left ventriculography, imaging supervision and interpretation.

(C) Coronary arteriography and left heart catheterization.

(D) Transcatheter therapy, embolic protection only.

(89) What is a type of edit that is seen in NCCI?

(A) PPP.

(B) ATP.

(C) NCI.

(D) MUE.

(90) Mrs. Sanchez presents to Dr. Harold's practice with her son, Chris. She reports that Chris and his sister were jumping on the beds when he fell, and his sister heard a sharp sound. Chris subsequently complained of elbow pain and difficulty using his right arm. Dr. Harold ordered an upper limb X-ray, which showed no fractures or dislocations. Dr. Harold, who had seen Chris for his school physical 14 months prior, documents a detailed examination and decision-making of moderate complexity. He instructs Mrs. Sanchez to visit an orthopedic specialist if Chris has any additional pain or trouble with the use of his arm. What code should be reported for the services offered?

(A) 99214.

(B) 98295.

(C) 99225.

(D) 99203.

(91) Which code range describes services for a 23-day-old patient who is critically ill?

(A) 99291–99292.

(B) 99238–99239.

(C) 99477–99480.

(D) None of the above.

(92) A patient presents for a colonoscopy with possible polyp removal. During the procedure, the surgeon uses the snare technique to remove a polyp in the descending colon. He subsequently removes another polyp in the transverse colon with hot biopsy forceps. What code(s) should be reported by this surgeon?

(A) 45384, 45385–51.

(B) 45384.

(C) 45385.

(D) 45384, 45385–62.

(93) A little girl struggles to see far-away images. Her parents are informed she has myopia. She is fitted for eyeglasses with mono-focal lenses to correct her vision. What is the CPT code for this service?

(A) 92341.

(B) 92342.

(C) 92340.

(D) 92343.

(94) A six-year-old boy is evaluated for language difficulty related to stuttering. The patient is referred for evaluation by a speech-language pathologist. What is the CPT code for the review to be carried out?

(A) 92522.

(B) 92521.

(C) 92524.

(D) 92525.

(95) An eight-year-old boy is brought in for a follow-up visit with the ENT surgeon. He received a cochlear implant a few years ago when he was diagnosed with bilateral profound hearing loss, bordering on deafness. The patient has undergone speech and language therapy. The doctor analyzes the cochlear implant and programs the implant. The boy's parents are counseled on proper care of the implant. What is the CPT code for this encounter?

(A) 92803.

(B) 92603.

(C) 92608.

(D) 92503.

(96) A young girl is noticed to have reduced hearing after treatment for meningitis. Her mother is worried that the girl has become less aware and has poor responses to speech. The girl is brought in for evaluation. The medical provider performs a test where the patient is asked to repeat familiar words that her mother says. What is the CPT code for this?

(A) 92554.

(B) 92555.

(C) 92556.

(D) 92553.

(97) A 62-year-old man presents at a healthcare facility with complaints of severe chest pain after exertion for the last six months. The pain is described as substernal and radiates to his jaw and left shoulder. He has hypertension and hyperlipidemia, for which he takes lisinopril and rosuvastatin. He admits to poor drug and clinic compliance. Cardiac catheterization reveals atherosclerosis of the left coronary artery with narrowed lumen with >85% stenosis. The patient is prepared for balloon stenting into the left coronary artery to expand the vessel. He is discharged for follow-up care with significant relief of symptoms. What CPT code is reported for this single procedure?

(A) 92928.

(B) 92925.

(C) 92927.

(D) 92929.

(98) An interventional radiologist reports a procedure he performed on an older man with suspected unstable angina secondary to myocardial ischemia. The process was carried out via the insertion of a tube through the radial artery. The tube was then threaded into the left side of the heart with dye. Images were collated, and narrowed areas were confirmed in the left anterior descending artery with total occlusion in the distal aspect. The procedure was completed, and the patient was admitted for observation. What is the correct CPT code?

(A) 93455.

(B) 93453.

(C) 93459.

(D) 93458.

(99) What aspect of healthcare is the CPC credential related to?

(A) Clinical pathology compliance.

(B) Certified patient care.

(C) Current procedural terminology coding.

(D) Centralized patient compliance.

(100) What is a key standard emphasized by the AAPC in healthcare coding?

(A) Financial management.

(B) Ethical coding.

(C) Human resources.

(D) Marketing strategies.

## Test 4: Answers and Explanations

(1) (A) SSA.

The Framework for Medical Necessity legislation was based on the Social Security Act (SSA).

(2) (A) Not Elsewhere Classified - Used when a specific code does not exist for a condition and indicates that the information is not available for more specific coding.

It indicates that the information available provides enough detail, but there is not a more specific code available to capture the diagnosis or condition as described. This allows for capturing the details of a condition even when the existing codes do not completely align with the situation.

(3) (B) Cesarean hysterectomy including removal of the uterus at the time of cesarean delivery.

CPT code 59525 is used to report a cesarean hysterectomy, which includes the removal of the uterus at the time of cesarean delivery. This code ensures that the complex procedure is documented and billed.

(4) (A) +59525.

The plus sign signifies an add-on service, which cannot be reported alone.

(5) (C) E89.1.

E11 is used for a confirmed diagnosis of diabetes mellitus. E89.1 is used for a diagnosis of post-pancreatectomy diabetes mellitus. O24.4 is used to code for gestational diabetes mellitus. Y84.2 is unrelated to diabetes. It codes for complications or abnormal reactions to radiation therapy.

(6) (A) Neonatal cerebral ischemia.

ICD-10 code P91.6 denotes Neonatal Cerebral Ischemia. This code is used in medical coding to accurately document cases where a newborn infant experiences a deficiency in blood supply to the brain, which could lead to various degrees of brain damage and requires precise coding for appropriate diagnosis, treatment, and billing purposes.

(7) (B) Superficial.

The anatomical term “superficial” refers to structures closer to the body’s surface or a specific organ. It denotes a position closer to the external layer.

(8) (A) Seropositive rheumatoid arthritis with rheumatoid factor of the unspecified wrist without organ or systems involvement.

This code is used to document cases of rheumatoid arthritis where the condition is seropositive. Rheumatoid factor is an antibody that is present in the blood of individuals with rheumatoid arthritis.

(9) (D) Knee orthosis, suspension sleeve, prefabricated, includes fitting and adjustment.

This code is used to bill for a prefabricated knee orthosis that includes a suspension sleeve. The sleeve is a device used to provide support, stabilization, and alignment for the knee joint. It also helps with pain relief and the healing process after injuries or surgeries.

(10) (A) 94640.

This code is the most appropriate for billing a simple nebulizer treatment, which is a common procedure for administering medication in the form of a mist inhaled into the lungs. Nebulizer treatments are used for patients with conditions such as asthma, COPD, or other respiratory ailments.

(11) (C) Unlisted procedure, diaphragm

This code is used when a specific surgical procedure performed on the diaphragm does not have a predefined CPT code. The "unlisted procedure" codes are critical for medical coding as they provide a way to bill for procedures that are not otherwise classified within the existing CPT code set.

(12) (B) Facilitate global communication in healthcare.

Medical terminology facilitates global communication in healthcare through the use of a standardized language. Healthcare professionals worldwide can use these terms consistently, which transcends language barriers and ensures an accurate understanding of medical information. This contributes to effective collaboration and patient care on an international scale.

(13) (C) E0483.

An airway clearance system is also known as a High Frequency Chest Wall Oscillation (HFCWO) device. This code represents "High frequency chest wall oscillation air-pulse generator system, (includes hoses and vest), each" and is used to document and bill for the provision and use of a device that assists with airway clearance.

(14) (A) Doppler echocardiography color flow velocity mapping.

This code is designated for the additional color flow Doppler service that is performed in conjunction with a primary echocardiography procedure. Color flow Doppler echocardiography is a diagnostic tool that adds color to the Doppler exam, which allows for the visualization of the direction and speed of blood flow through the heart and its valves.

(15) (B) Implantation of a permanent pacemaker with transvenous electrode(s); single chamber, atrial or ventricular.

The procedure includes the introduction of the electrode into the heart, the connection of the electrode to the pacemaker device, and the implantation of the pacemaker device itself, which usually happens subcutaneously in the chest.

(16) (A) K35.80.

Acute appendicitis is a diagnosis within the category of diseases of the gastrointestinal system. It is coded K35.80.

(17) (B) C64.9.

The kidney affected is not specified. The code is under the category of malignant neoplasm, C64.9.

(18) (D) K40.91.

The key word for the diagnosis is hernia, which is a condition listed in category K, specific for recurrent unilateral inguinal hernia. It is coded K40.91.

(19) (D) Leadless pacemaker systems.

This range of codes is used for billing and documentation related to the implantation, interrogation, programming, and removal of leadless pacemaker systems. Leadless pacemakers are a newer type of cardiac pacing device that is implanted directly into the heart without the need for traditional pacing leads. These devices are smaller than conventional pacemakers and are designed to reduce the risk of infections and complications related to leads.

(20) (C) 77.

Modifier 77 is used to report a repeat of a procedure. In this case, the repeat is done by another physician or qualified healthcare professional. If the repeat procedure was done by the same person who performed it the first time, modifier 76 should be used. Modifiers 22 and 25 have other uses unrelated to the question.

(21) (C) 26.

26 is the correct modifier to use to report the professional component of a service that is a combination of both professional and technical components. In this question, the physician will report his service with the modifier 26 to show a technical component not accounted for.

(22) (C) Annually.

The AMA releases yearly updates to the Category I CPT codes.

(23) (D) 15273–58.

The patient had skin graft surgery, which was planned during the initial surgery. The appropriate code is 15273, and the correct modifier for the procedure is 58.

(24) (B) 24685.

The CPT code 24685 is used for the open treatment of an olecranon fracture with internal fixation. This code specifically documents and facilitates billing for the open reduction of an olecranon fracture and internal fixation to stabilize the fracture.

(25) (D) 29881.

CPT code 29881 is used to document and bill arthroscopic procedures that involve the removal of a portion of both the medial and lateral menisci in the knee, along with potential debridement or shaving of articular cartilage.

(26) (C) 27759.

Code 27759 is used to document the open reduction of a tibial shaft fracture and the insertion of an intramedullary nail for stabilization.

(27) (A) L3908.

HCPCS Level II code L3908 code specifies a ready-made orthotic device designed for the wrist, hand, and fingers without articulated joints, and it includes fitting and adjustment services.

(28) (B) L1845.

HCPCS Level II code L1845 represents a custom-fabricated knee orthosis with adjustable knee joints. This includes soft interface material.

(29) (B) To confirm that the healthcare services and procedures billed are reasonable and necessary for the diagnosis or treatment of illness or injury.

This concept is a cornerstone of the healthcare billing process. It ensures that the services provided are appropriate for the specific condition and meet the established standards of medical practice.

(30) (C) I63.9.

Ischemic strokes occur when blood flow to a part of the brain is obstructed, typically by a blood clot, leading to the death of brain cells due to lack of oxygen. The code I63.9 is used when the documentation in the medical record does not specify the area of the brain affected or the cause of the infarction, which makes it a general code for acute ischemic strokes.

(31) (B) S61.201A.

This code is most appropriate for describing a non-specified injury to the right index finger, especially when the injury is an open wound and there's no mention of a foreign body being involved. The code is structured to provide specific details about the injury, including the fact that it's on the right index finger and that it's an open wound, while also indicating it's the initial encounter for treatment.

(32) (B) R40.2110

This code is part of a range that is used to document the level of consciousness in a patient using the Glasgow Coma Scale (GCS), which is a neurological scale that aims to give a reliable, objective way of recording the conscious state of a person for an initial as well as subsequent assessments. A patient who is unconscious would not have their eyes open, but this code is used when the GCS is documented without specifying the time of assessment.

(33) (C) E0465.

The HCPCS Level II code E0465 is used to report the rental of a home ventilator device, which provides respiratory support for patients in their own residence.

(34) (A) A nebulizer with a compressor.

HCPCS Level II code E0570 represents the provision of a nebulizer device that uses compressed air to convert liquid medication into a fine mist for inhalation.

(35) (B) E0650.

The HCPCS Level II code E0650 is used to report the rental or purchase of a pneumatic compression device designed for the treatment of lymphedema.

(36) (B) R56.9.

R56.9, which stands for "Unspecified convulsions," is the most appropriate ICD-10-CM code for a patient diagnosed with a generalized tonic-clonic seizure when there is no mention of epilepsy or a recurrent condition. This code is used to document a single incident of seizure activity without specifying it as part of a broader epileptic disorder.

(37) (B) To indicate that unusual anesthesia was used for a procedure that does not usually require any anesthesia.

This modifier is appended to a procedure code to signify that a procedure, which does not require any form of anesthesia or requires only local anesthesia, was performed under general anesthesia or another form of anesthesia that is not customary for that procedure.

(38) (B) To indicate a service was provided to a newborn patient.

This modifier allows healthcare providers to specify that the care or procedure was performed on a patient who is in the newborn age category, which can have implications for billing and reimbursement, as well as for clinical considerations given the unique needs and vulnerabilities of this patient population.

(39) (B) Type 2 diabetes mellitus without complications.

This code is part of the E11 series that categorizes Type 2 diabetes mellitus, which distinguishes it from other forms of diabetes by its etiology and clinical picture, which is associated with insulin resistance and relative insulin deficiency.

(40) (B) C1888.

Code C1888 specifically designates the procedural details related to the insertion of a stent in the cardiovascular system.

(41) (A) G0422–G0424.

Cardiac rehabilitation services in the HCPCS Level II coding system are usually associated with the code range G0422–G0424. These codes represent various components of comprehensive cardiac rehabilitation programs. This includes initial assessments, exercise sessions, and other services aimed at improving cardiovascular health.

(42) (B) Replacement battery for an implanted pacemaker defibrillator.

The HCPCS (Healthcare Common Procedure Coding System) code K0606 represents a "Replacement battery for implanted pacemaker defibrillator." This code is used in medical billing to denote when a patient requires a new battery for an implanted device that combines the functions of a pacemaker and a defibrillator.

(43) (A) Esophagogastroduodenoscopy (EGD) with removal of foreign body

This procedure involves the use of an endoscope to visually examine the upper part of the gastrointestinal tract, which includes the esophagus, stomach, and the first part of the small intestine (duodenum). When a foreign body is identified during the procedure, this code also includes the removal of that foreign body. This could involve the use of various instruments that can be passed through the endoscope to grasp and retrieve the object.

(44) (D) Esophagogastroduodenoscopy (EGD) with the transoral placement of an intragastric balloon.

This procedure involves the use of an endoscope to guide the placement of a balloon inside the stomach, which is then filled with saline or air. The intragastric balloon is used as a weight loss treatment to help reduce stomach capacity.

(45) (B) Percutaneous skeletal fixation of the posterior pelvic bone.

This code is used for billing and documentation purposes related to the minimally invasive procedure of stabilizing fractures in the posterior portion of the pelvic bone through percutaneous (through the skin) techniques.

(46) (A) Enteral formula, for adults, soy based, lactose-free, with intact nutrients.

This code is specifically designated for billing and documentation purposes related to nutritional support for adults who require enteral feeding. Enteral formulas are used when a person is unable to meet their nutritional needs through oral intake and needs to be fed through a tube directly into their gastrointestinal system.

(47) (B) 51702 is the CPT code for the insertion of a temporary bladder catheter, and N17.0 is the ICD-10-CM code for acute kidney failure.

This code is used in medical billing to document the procedure of placing a temporary catheter into the bladder, which is necessary for patients who are unable to urinate naturally due to various medical conditions or surgical procedures.

(48) (B) Drug- and heavy metal-induced tubulo-interstitial and tubular conditions.

This code is part of the ICD-10-CM range that addresses diseases of the genitourinary system, particularly focusing on the kidney and ureter conditions. Code N14.8 is used to document kidney conditions that are directly caused by the toxic effects of drugs or heavy metals.

(49) (B) 55040-LT is the CPT code for hydrocelectomy of the left testis, and N43.8 is the ICD-10-CM code for other specified hydrocele.

Hydrocelectomy is the surgical removal of a hydrocele, which is a fluid-filled sac around a testicle that results in swelling. This code accurately reflects the procedural aspect of treating a hydrocele by surgical intervention.

(50) (C) C61, N52.35.

The primary diagnosis of this patient is prostate cancer, which is a malignant neoplasm of the prostate. His current complaint of erectile dysfunction is a complication that has occurred due to the radiation therapy used to treat his initial diagnosis. The correct code is C61, N52.35.

(51) (B) N39.0.

ICD-10-CM code N39.0 is for Urinary tract infection, site not specified. This is the most common code used for a general diagnosis of a urinary tract infection (UTI) without specifying the location within the urinary system.

(52) (A) N39.3.

ICD-10-CM code N39.3 is for Stress incontinence (female) (male), which is characterized by the involuntary leakage of urine during activities that increase abdominal pressure, such as coughing or laughing. This code is appropriate for the diagnosis given the description of urine extravasation with the Valsalva maneuver.

(53) (D) Female infertility, unspecified.

This code is used when a woman has been diagnosed with infertility, but the exact cause or origin (such as uterine, ovarian, or tubal) has not been specified or identified. Infertility is defined as the inability to achieve a pregnancy after 12 months or more of regular unprotected sexual intercourse.

(54) (A) Total abdominal hysterectomy, including partial vaginectomy.

This procedure involves the surgical removal of the uterus through an abdominal incision, and it may also include the removal of a part of the vagina (partial vaginectomy) when necessary. The total abdominal hysterectomy is a common gynecological procedure used to treat various conditions such as uterine fibroids, endometriosis, chronic pelvic pain, or uterine cancer.

(55) (A) Communicating hydrocephalus.

Communicating hydrocephalus occurs when the flow of cerebrospinal fluid (CSF) is blocked after it exits the ventricles, which are the spaces in the brain where CSF is produced. This type of hydrocephalus is termed “communicating” because the CSF can still flow between the ventricles, which remain open.

(56) (A) Generalized idiopathic epilepsy and epileptic syndromes, not intractable, without status epilepticus.

This code is used to document a diagnosis of generalized epilepsy, where seizures broadly affect both hemispheres of the brain and are not limited to one specific area.

"Idiopathic" refers to epilepsy with no identifiable cause, which usually suggests a genetic predisposition.

(57) (A) N73.9.

ICD-10-CM code N73.9 is for Female pelvic inflammatory disease, unspecified. This code is used when a diagnosis of pelvic inflammatory disease (PID) is made without specifying the type of PID.

(58) (B) Parkinson's disease.

Parkinson's disease results from the loss of dopamine-producing neurons in the substantia nigra, which is a region of the midbrain, although the exact cause of this neuronal loss is not fully understood. The diagnosis of Parkinson's disease is mainly clinical and based on the presence of its characteristic motor symptoms.

(59) (C) 56420.

CPT code 56420 is for Incision and drainage of Bartholin's gland abscess. This code is appropriate for the procedure described for treating a Bartholin's gland abscess.

(60) (A) Excision of lesion of thyroid, without radical dissection.

This code is applied when a surgeon performs an excision (surgical removal) of a localized lesion within the thyroid gland without undertaking a radical dissection, which implies a more extensive removal of thyroid tissue or surrounding structures.

(61) (C) Enucleation of the eye, without implant; right eye.

The use of modifier RT specifies that the procedure was performed on the right side of the body. For CPT code 65111, it means that the right eye was enucleated without the insertion of an orbital implant to replace the removed eye.

(62) (D) G43.1.

This patient probably has a migraine. This follows with her current clinical symptoms of a unilateral pulsatile headache that is worsened by light or sound triggers. The recent onset of an "off" sensation before the headaches begin is termed an aura. This patient now has a migraine with aura, which has the ICD-10-CM diagnosis code G43.1.

(63) (A) Anesthesia for lower intestinal endoscopic procedures, endoscope introduced distal to duodenum.

This code is used in medical billing to document the administration of anesthesia by a healthcare professional for procedures that involve the use of an endoscope in the lower intestine, such as a colonoscopy or sigmoidoscopy. The specification "endoscope introduced distal to duodenum" indicates that the procedure involves areas of the gastrointestinal tract beyond the duodenum, such as the colon or rectum.

(64) (A) G47.41.

The appropriate diagnosis code for narcolepsy is G47.41.

(65) (A) Anesthesia for upper gastrointestinal endoscopic procedures, endoscope introduced proximal to duodenum.

This code is used in the medical billing process to document the provision of anesthesia services for procedures that involve the use of an endoscope to examine or treat the upper part of the gastrointestinal tract, such as the esophagus, stomach, and the beginning of the small intestine (up to the duodenum). This includes procedures like gastroscopy or esophagogastroduodenoscopy (EGD), where the endoscope does not go beyond the duodenum.

(66) (C) Anesthesia for procedures on the auditory system, not otherwise specified.

This code is used in medical billing to document the provision of anesthesia services for surgical or diagnostic procedures that involve the auditory system (ear and related structures) where the specific type of procedure is not classified under a more specific anesthesia code. The "not otherwise specified" designation indicates that this code serves as a catch-all for auditory system procedures that do not fit more specific descriptions within the anesthesia coding structure.

(67) (D) H90.12.

The correct diagnosis code for unilateral conductive hearing loss with unrestricted hearing on the contralateral side is H90.12.

(68) (C) 66984, modifier 50.

CPT code 66984 is used for Extracapsular cataract removal with insertion of an intraocular lens prosthesis (one stage procedure), phacoemulsification technique. Modifier 50 is used to indicate that the procedure was performed bilaterally.

(69) (A) 65420, modifier LT.

CPT code 65420 is for Excision or transposition of pterygium; without graft. The modifier LT is used to indicate that the procedure was performed on the left side.

(70) (B) Special anesthesia service for a patient of extreme age, younger than 1 year and older than 70.

This code is added to the primary anesthesia code to account for the additional care and monitoring required for these patients due to the increased risks and potential complications associated with administering anesthesia to very young or elderly patients.

(71) (D) 65205, modifier RT; 65235, modifier LT.

Removal of a foreign body in the superficial conjunctiva of the right eye is coded 65205, modifier RT. Removal of the foreign body from the anterior chamber of the left eye is coded 65235, modifier LT.

(72) (B) Ensure patient safety and integrity.

The primary purpose of a compliance program in a healthcare setting is to ensure patient safety and integrity. These programs mitigate risks, prevent fraud, and maintain the highest standards of care. Compliance initiatives encompass regulatory requirements, privacy protections, and ethical conduct, which fosters a culture of transparency and accountability. When patient well-being is prioritized, healthcare compliance programs contribute to the trustworthiness of medical institutions and support quality care and the ethical conduct of healthcare professionals.

(73) (A) 67930, modifier LT.

A suture of the recent wound of the eyelid that involves the lid margin with partial thickness is coded 67930, modifier LT.

(74) (A) 88184.

This code specifically represents flow cytometry; first cell surface, cytoplasmic, or nuclear marker. Additional markers would be coded separately. Flow cytometry is a powerful tool used in many clinical and research applications, including in the fields of immunology, pathology, and genetics.

(75) (B) Identifies repeat procedures by the same physician.

Modifier -76 is used to indicate that a procedure or service was repeated by the same physician or other qualified healthcare professional subsequent to the original service or procedure. It's used when a procedure is repeated on the same day or during the postoperative period and is necessary to distinguish between the services provided.

(76) (B) Hospital discharge day management, 30 minutes or less.

This code specifically pertains to services provided for 30 minutes or less. It includes the time spent at the patient's bedside and on the patient's hospital floor or unit, reviewing the hospital record, discussions with other healthcare professionals, and documentation of the discharge records.

(77) (B) Medically Unlikely Edit.

An MUE (Medically Unlikely Edit) is a Medicare system edit used to control the maximum number of units of service that a provider can report for a single beneficiary on a single date of service for a single HCPCS/CPT code. It is designed to prevent improper payments when services are reported in excessive quantities.

(78) (A) 76945.

Chorionic villus sampling under ultrasound guidance is coded 76945.

(79) (B) 73030.

The appropriate CPT code for an X-ray of the shoulder with two different views is 73030.

(80) (C) 77022.

CPT code 77022 is for magnetic resonance imaging (MRI) guidance for, and monitoring of, parenchymal tissue ablation. This code specifically covers the use of MRI to guide and monitor the ablation of tissues, making it the correct choice for procedures that involve locating parenchymal tissues and monitoring their ablation.

(81) (D) -GC.

The modifier used to indicate a service was provided by a resident under supervision is GC. This modifier signifies that the service was performed by a trainee in a healthcare setting under the direct supervision of an attending or supervising physician.

(82) (A) Clinical modification.

In ICD-10 coding, the "CM" stands for clinical modification. This alphanumeric system is a standardized classification for coding diseases, conditions, and other health-related issues. The inclusion of "CM" emphasizes its clinical relevance and the modifications made for use in the United States healthcare system.

(83) (B) -51.

The modifier used to indicate multiple procedures performed during the same session is 51. This modifier is applied to the secondary and subsequent procedure codes, which signals that multiple distinct services were provided to the patient during a single encounter.

(84) (C) Durable medical equipment (DME)

HCPCS II mainly codes for DME, supplies, drugs, and other non-physician services. It complements CPT codes through the use of a standardized set of codes for services not covered by CPT. HCPCS II includes alphanumeric codes, which facilitate accurate reporting of medical procedures, supplies, and equipment for billing purposes.

(85) (B) Initial and subsequent neonatal intensive care services.

These codes are used to report the intensive care services provided to a newborn who requires constant nursing, intricate medication regimens, frequent monitoring of vital signs, and other life support measures. These services are typically provided in a neonatal intensive care unit.

(86) (A) Speech audiometry threshold.

This code is used to document the procedure where the patient's ability to hear and understand speech is evaluated. The threshold is the softest level of sound that a person can hear and recognize as speech, and determining this level is critical for diagnosing and treating hearing impairments.

(87) (A) 99397.

In the CPT index, preventative medicine codes are from 99381 to 99397. 99397 is used for evaluation and management services provided to an established patient 65 years or older.

(88) (B) Left heart catheterization including intraprocedural injection(s) for left ventriculography, imaging supervision and interpretation.

This code is utilized when a comprehensive diagnostic examination of the left side of the heart is conducted, often including the measurement of pressures and evaluation of the cardiac chambers and associated structures. The inclusion of left ventriculography indicates that contrast is injected to visualize the left ventricular chamber, and the imaging supervision and interpretation component ensures that the procedure and the results are accurately managed and assessed.

(89) (D) MUE.

MUE stands for Medically Unlikely Edits. These are used in the National Correct Coding Initiative (NCCI) to limit the number of times a service can be billed to Medicare on a single day for a single beneficiary, as certain quantities of services provided in a single day may not be medically reasonable or necessary.

(90) (A) 99214.

This patient saw the physician in the outpatient setting. Given that the doctor has seen the patient within the past three years, the MDM level of complexity is documented as moderate. The appropriate code for established patients with moderate MDM in outpatient visits is 99214.

(91) (C) 99477–99480.

Codes 99477–99480 are used for reporting inpatient neonatal and pediatric critical care services. These codes are specific for critically ill infants and young patients, including those who are 23 days old, making them the correct choice for a critically ill 23-day-old patient.

(92) (A) 45384, 45385–51.

When multiple polyps are removed during a colonoscopy using different techniques (snare technique and hot biopsy forceps), both procedures (45384 for removal with hot biopsy forceps and 45385 for removal by snaring) should be reported. The modifier -51 (Multiple Procedures) is used to indicate that more than one procedure was performed during the same session.

(93) (C) 92340.

The service offered is a mono-focal lens fitting for eyeglasses, and the CPT code is 92340.

(94) (B) 92521.

Speech-language pathologists evaluate a patient's speech fluency. This is coded 92521.

(95) (B) 92603.

In this scenario, the provider analyzes and programs a cochlear implant previously placed in an eight-year-old. The provider counsels the parents on proper care of the implant. The appropriate CPT code for the encounter is 92603.

(96) (B) 92555.

CPT code 92555 is for speech audiometry threshold; it involves testing the patient's ability to recognize and repeat words. This is suitable for evaluating a young girl's hearing and speech recognition as described.

(97) (A) 92928.

This patient had angina due to a narrowed lumen of a single major coronary artery. The procedure performed was the inflation of a balloon-tipped catheter into a single major coronary artery to expand the narrowed walls of the vessel and treat stenosis. The CPT code is 92928.

(98) (D) 93458.

CPT code 93458 is used for cardiac catheterization including left heart catheterization, coronary angiograms, and intraprocedural injection(s) for left ventriculography when performed. This code is correct for the procedure described with insertion through the radial artery to the left side of the heart and dye injection for imaging.

(99) (C) Current procedural terminology coding.

The CPC credential is closely tied to current procedural terminology (CPT) coding in healthcare. Awarded by the American Academy of Professional Coders (AAPC), this certification signifies expertise in the accurate translation of medical procedures and services into standardized codes.

(100) (B) Ethical coding.

The AAPC places a strong emphasis on ethical coding as a key standard in healthcare. This involves the accurate and honest representation of medical services provided, which ensures integrity in the billing and reimbursement process.

# Test 5: Questions

(1) Who interprets national health insurance policies into regional policies?

(A) The MAC.

(B) The OIG.

(C) The LCD.

(D) The HMO.

(2) Per HIPAA, which of the following is not a covered entity?

(A) A psychologist.

(B) A healthcare clearinghouse.

(C) An HMO.

(D) A patient.

(3) A patient has white tongue patches and is diagnosed with oral hairy leukoplakia. Blood work is performed, including a test for HIV. Even though the results of the tests are not ready yet, the physician notes that the patient has HIV. The patient smokes marijuana regularly. What is the sequence of these ICD-10 codes?

(A) K13.3, B20, F17.2.

(B) B20, K13.3, F12.2.

(C) Z21, F17.200, 13.3.

(D) K13.3, R75, F17.2.

(4) What is not a category of CPT code as defined by the AMA?

(A) Category I.

(B) Category II.

(C) Category III.

(D) Category IV.

(5) Which of the following is true of disease sequela?

(A) It is noticed at the same time as the onset of the disease.

(B) There is no time limit to when a sequela code can be used.

(C) Three codes are used in sequence for reporting sequela.

(D) The code for the acute phase of a disease can be used together with the late effect code.

(6) A patient presents to the physician's clinic with weight loss, excessive thirst, and increased appetite. He also has polyuria. Blood work shows significantly elevated blood sugar levels. The physician makes a diagnosis of diabetes mellitus. What is the correct code for this diagnosis?

(A) Z79.

(B) E11.

(C) O24.4.

(D) E85.2.

(7) A 22-year-old man is diagnosed with an unclassified bacterial infection that has previously only been seen in large-game animals. What is the appropriate code for this diagnosis?

(A) A15.1.

(B) A28.9.

(C) R22.1.

(D) E89.5.

(8) What is an example of plantar flexion?

(A) The toes are pointed down.

(B) The toes are lifted up.

(C) The knee is bent.

(D) The elbow is extended.

(9) Which anatomical term corresponds to the heel region?

(A) Plantar.

(B) Dorsal.

(C) Palmar.

(D) Calcaneal.

(10) What does "proximal" refer to in anatomical language?

(A) Farther from the point of attachment.

(B) Closer to the point of attachment.

(C) Below or lower.

(D) Above or higher.

(11) What is the term for a movement that decreases the angle between two body parts?

(A) Extension.

(B) Flexion.

(C) Abduction.

(D) Adduction.

(12) In the anatomical position, the palms usually face:

(A) Forward.

(B) Backward.

(C) Toward the midline.

(D) Away from the midline.

(13) What is a movement that brings a body part closer to the body's midline?

(A) Abduction.

(B) Adduction.

(C) Flexion.

(D) Extension.

(14) What is the anatomical term for the back side of the body?

(A) Caudal.

(B) Rostral.

(C) Dorsal.

(D) Ventral.

(15) What is the term for the movement when the head is turned from side to side?

(A) Pronation.

(B) Supination.

(C) Rotation.

(D) Circumduction.

(16) A 65-year-old woman with chronic obstructive pulmonary disease comes into the hospital with a cough and difficulty breathing. Her oxygen saturation is 85% in room air. She receives supplemental oxygen to improve her oxygen saturation to 95%. The attending physician makes an assessment of acute exacerbation of COPD. What is the diagnosis code?

(A) J45.1.

(B) J44.1.

(C) J44.

(D) J44.3.

(17) A 33-year-old woman complains of sudden-onset headache with associated blurry vision and projectile vomiting. There is a family history of polycystic kidney disease, and a magnetic resonance angiography reveals intracerebral hemorrhage. What code does this diagnosis correspond to?

(A) J51.

(B) I61.9.

(C) I61.8.

(D) I61.

(18) What condition does the ICD-10 code I42.0 represent?

(A) Hypertrophic obstructive cardiomyopathy.

(B) Dilated cardiomyopathy.

(C) Restrictive cardiomyopathy.

(D) Arrhythmogenic right ventricular cardiomyopathy.

(19) A gynecologist examines a 30-year-old female with heavy menstrual bleeding, and an abdominal ultrasound scan is requested, which confirms the presence of multiple uterine fibroids. To which ICD-10-CM code does the diagnosis correspond?

(A) D25.0.

(B) D25.

(C) D24.2.

(D) D25.9.

(20) A patient has schizophrenia, but further assessment to classify his condition has yet to be done. What is the diagnosis code?

(A) F20.

(B) F20.3.

(C) F20.9.

(D) F20.23.

(21) How is prostatic cancer coded?

(A) C61.

(B) C60.9.

(C) C63.

(D) C61.9.

(22) Which of the following is incorrect about the HCPCS coding system?

(A) It allows faster billing by providers.

(B) It discourages the use of transportation services.

(C) It reports physician services.

(D) It reports medical supplies outside a physician's office.

(23) A 30-year-old woman presents at the physician's office with complaints of painful unilateral labial swelling and pain when she walks and sits. Following the physician's request, a surgeon reviews and assesses a Bartholin's gland abscess. The patient is scheduled for incision and drainage of the abscess. What are the global days for postoperative care for this procedure?

(A) 0 days.

(B) 10 days.

(C) 30 days.

(D) 90 days.

(24) What does the combination of CPT codes 12002-23 represent?

(A) Simple repair of superficial wounds of scalp, neck, axillae, external genitalia, trunk and/or extremities (including hands and feet); 2.6 cm to 7.5 cm, with added complexity.

(B) Simple repair of superficial wounds of scalp, neck, axillae, external genitalia, trunk and/or extremities (including hands and feet); 2.6 cm to 7.5 cm, with increased procedural services.

(C) Intermediate repair of superficial wounds of scalp, neck, axillae, external genitalia, trunk and/or extremities (including hands and feet); 2.6 cm to 7.5 cm, with increased procedural services.

(D) Intermediate repair of superficial wounds of scalp, neck, axillae, external genitalia, trunk and/or extremities (including hands and feet); 2.6 cm to 7.5 cm, with added complexity.

(25) A patient is scheduled for an interventional procedure in the OR. However, during the surgery, the patient is noticed to have labile vital parameters. This includes blood pressure, pulse rate, and temperature. The surgeon believes there is a significant risk for cardiac arrest intra-op and discontinues the procedure. What is the appropriate modifier for the procedure?

(A) 55.

(B) 53.

(C) 47.

(D) 50.

(26) What condition does the ICD-10 code L25.9 indicate?

(A) Allergic contact dermatitis due to plants, except food.

(B) Unspecified contact dermatitis due to cosmetics.

(C) Unspecified contact dermatitis, unspecified cause.

(D) Irritant contact dermatitis due to detergents.

(27) Which ICD-10 code is used for acne vulgaris?

(A) L70.0.

(B) L73.0.

(C) L76.0.

(D) L80.0.

(28) What is the ICD-10 code for basal cell carcinoma?

(A) C44.9.

(B) D04.9.

(C) L23.9.

(D) L57.0.

(29) What is the ICD-10 code for unspecified malignant melanoma of the skin?

(A) C43.9.

(B) C44.9.

(C) C51.9.

(D) C61.

(30) What is the ICD-10 code for seborrheic dermatitis?

(A) L21.

(B) L23.

(C) L30.

(D) L42.

(31) Which ICD-10 code represents an unspecified disorder of the skin and subcutaneous tissue?

(A) L90.9.

(B) L98.9.

(C) L97.9.

(D) L99.9.

(32) In the ICD-10 coding system, what does the letter "M" in codes for the musculoskeletal system often indicate?

(A) Mental disorders.

(B) Musculoskeletal disorders.

(C) Metabolic disorders.

(D) Malignant neoplasms.

(33) What CPT code is used for a closed treatment of a clavicular fracture without manipulation?

(A) 23500.

(B) 23505.

(C) 23570.

(D) 23615.

(34) Which code represents an injection of a therapeutic substance into the knee joint with ultrasound guidance?

(A) 20610.

(B) 20611.

(C) 20615.

(D) 20616.

(35) What procedure is represented by the CPT code 29823?

(A) Arthroscopy, shoulder, surgical; with removal of loose body or foreign body.

(B) Arthroscopy, shoulder, surgical; debridement, extensive.

(C) Arthroscopy, shoulder, diagnostic, with or without synovial biopsy.

(D) Arthroscopy, knee, surgical; with meniscectomy (medial AND lateral, including any meniscal shaving).

(36) Which CPT code is used for the excision of a tumor of the hand or finger joint with extensive soft tissue removal?

(A) 26116.

(B) 26123.

(C) 26160.

(D) 26170.

(37) What CPT code represents a closed treatment of a hip dislocation without anesthesia or manipulation?

(A) 27250.

(B) 27254.

(C) 27246.

(D) 27280.

(38) An anesthesiologist is paged for an emergency cesarean section. After the CPT code for the anesthesia given during the procedure, what add-on code should be included in the complete medical code reported?

(A) +99100.

(B) +99116.

(C) +99135.

(D) +99140.

(39) What is the ICD-10-CM code for a diaphragmatic hernia?

(A) K44.9.

(B) K40.90.

(C) K46.9.

(D) K31.9.

(40) What is ICD-10-CM code I89.0 used for?

(A) Lymphedema, unspecified.

(B) Phlebitis and thrombophlebitis of unspecified deep vessels of the lower extremity.

(C) Chronic venous insufficiency.

(D) Lymphangitis.

(41) What procedure is represented by the CPT code 31625?

(A) Bronchoscopy, rigid or flexible, with or without fluoroscopic guidance; with bronchial alveolar lavage.

(B) Bronchoscopy, rigid or flexible, including fluoroscopic guidance, when performed; with biopsy, single or multiple sites.

(C) Thoracoscopy, surgical; with diagnostic biopsy(ies) of pleura.

(D) Bronchoscopy, rigid or flexible, with or without fluoroscopic guidance; with transbronchial lung biopsy(s), single lobe.

(42) Which procedure is represented by the CPT code 32554?

(A) Thoracentesis, needle or catheter, aspiration of the pleural space; without imaging guidance.

(B) Thoracentesis, needle or catheter, aspiration of the pleural space; with imaging guidance.

(C) Thoracoscopy, surgical; with pleural biopsy.

(D) Insertion of chest tube, thoracostomy, includes connection to drainage system (e.g., water seal), when performed, open.

(43) What procedure does the CPT code 39400 represent?

(A) Mediastinoscopy, including biopsy by mediastinal incision.

(B) Mediastinoscopy, including biopsy by thoracoscopy.

(C) Mediastinotomy with exploration, drainage, removal of foreign body, or biopsy.

(D) Bronchoscopy, rigid or flexible, including fluoroscopic guidance.

(44) Which ICD-10-CM code is used for angina pectoris?

(A) I20.0.

(B) I25.2.

(C) I48.91.

(D) I50.9.

(45) What is the ICD-10-CM code for unspecified heart failure?

(A) I11.0.

(B) I50.9.

(C) I42.9.

(D) I48.91.

(46) What is the main purpose of an 'X' placeholder in certain ICD-10-CM codes?

(A) To indicate external cause of injury or poisoning.

(B) To provide a placeholder for future code expansion.

(C) To fill in empty characters when a code requires a 7th character.

(D) To designate a new technology or service.

(47) The Medicine section of the CPT code manual is designed for reporting services by:

(A) Surgeons during operations.

(B) Physicians in an office setting.

(C) Providers delivering specialized medical services.

(D) Radiologists conducting imaging procedures.

(48) CPT code range 33530-33536 represents procedures related to:

(A) Vascular shunts.

(B) Cardiac bypass grafting.

(C) Neurological stimulators.

(D) Gastrointestinal endoscopy.

(49) In CPT coding, which modifier is often used to indicate multiple procedures performed during the same session?

(A) -50.

(B) -26.

(C) -51.

(D) -59.

(50) What is the appropriate ICD-10-CM code for irritable bowel syndrome?

(A) K58.9.

(B) K58.0.

(C) K58.1.

(D) K58.2.

(51) Which ICD-10-CM code represents acute gastritis?

(A) K29.0.

(B) K29.1.

(C) K29.2.

(D) K29.9.

(52) B18.2 is the ICD-10 code for:

(A) Acute Hepatitis B without Delta-Agent and without hepatic coma.

(B) Chronic Viral Hepatitis C.

(C) Chronic Viral Hepatitis B without Delta-Agent.

(D) Acute Viral Hepatitis A.

(53) What CPT code is used for a diagnostic esophagogastroduodenoscopy?

(A) 43239.

(B) 43235.

(C) 43250.

(D) 43255.

(54) Which CPT code is appropriate for a colonoscopy with biopsy?

(A) 45380.

(B) 45385.

(C) 45382.

(D) 45387.

(55) What is the CPT code for an upper gastrointestinal endoscopy with dilation?

(A) 43249.

(B) 43239.

(C) 43235.

(D) 43248.

(56) A 60-year-old man presents at his urology appointment for evaluation of his laboratory results. He has had difficulty passing urine for the past eight months, with terminal dribbling and hesitancy. The surgeon informs the patient that his prostate-specific antigen results are markedly elevated and a biopsy is therefore required. The man consents, and the surgeon schedules a punch biopsy. What is the CPT code for this procedure?

(A) 55420.

(B) 53405.

(C) 59700.

(D) 55700.

(57) A 34-year-old man with a completed family has a bilateral vasectomy carried out by his urologist. He is given painkillers after the procedure and discharged to the outpatient clinic to report if he notices any abnormality. What is the CPT code for the procedure that was carried out?

(A) 55250, modifier 50.

(B) 52301, modifier 54.

(C) 55200, modifier 50.

(D) 54202, modifier 51.

(58) A middle-aged woman presents at the hospital for a scheduled surgical laparoscopy with urethral suspension for stress incontinence. The procedure is carried out, and the patient is wheeled into the recovery room. She is eventually discharged with postoperative instructions. What is the CPT code for the surgery?

(A) 51990.

(B) 51450.

(C) 59122.

(D) 51992.

(59) A medical student is instructed to carry out the insertion of a temporary simple indwelling Foley catheter for drainage and monitoring of urine in a 78-year-old woman who just had perineal surgery. The student requests a chaperone, drapes the patient, and requests a catheter insertion tray. The procedure is performed in the operating room, and sterility is maintained. A urine bag is attached to the urethral catheter, and a urine specimen is obtained for microscopy, culture, and sensitivity. What is the CPT code for the procedure carried out by the medical student?

(A) 51702, P9612.

(B) 51784, P9511.

(C) 52705, P9452.

(D) 51702, P515.

(60) A 54-year-old man presents with features suggestive of an obstruction of his lower urinary tract. The surgeon explains the clinical findings and probable diagnosis and schedules the man for further evaluation. On the day of the procedure, the patient is taken to the procedure room, and an injection of dye is performed under radiological supervision with the generation of radiological images, of which the surgeon and surgical assistant take note. After the procedure, the patient is discharged to outpatient follow-up with the interpretation of the retrograde urethrocystography performed. What is the CPT code for the procedure carried out on this patient?

(A) 74450.

(B) 74451.

(C) 74520.

(D) 74520.

(61) A 59-year-old man is brought into the operating room for a scheduled procedure due to symptoms of urethral stricture. Placement of a balloon dilator previously failed, so cystourethroscopy with insertion of a permanent urethral stent is carried out. What is the CPT code reported by the surgeon?

(A) 52248.

(B) 53142.

(C) 52282.

(D) 54120.

(62) A 19-year-old female is brought into the delivery room. She had been in labor at home for over sixteen hours, with arrest of labor for the past four hours. The initial assessment confirms obstructed labor due to cephalopelvic disproportion that resulted in the relative arrest of labor. Fetal heart tone is present. However, there is increased variability and fetal bradycardia. The patient is scheduled for an emergency cesarean delivery. What is the diagnosis code per ICD-10-CM and the current procedural terminology for the scheduled intervention?

(A) O65.5, 59500.

(B) O63.4, 59510.

(C) O65.9, 59514.

(D) O65.4, 59514.

(63) A 25-year-old pregnant woman in labor is monitored by a midwife with a partograph in the delivery room. The chart shows the patient is in a prolonged second stage of labor. What is the ICD-10-CM diagnosis code?

(A) O63.1.

(B) O63.7.

(C) O63.2.

(D) O63.3.

(64) O61.1 is the ICD-10 code for:

(A) Failed attempted termination of pregnancy.

(B) Failed induction of labor.

(C) Failed attempted instrumental delivery.

(D) Complicated delivery by Cesarean section.

(65) O21.1 is the ICD-10 code for:

(A) Mild hyperemesis gravidarum.

(B) Excessive vomiting in pregnancy.

(C) Hyperemesis gravidarum with metabolic disturbance.

(D) Vomiting complicating pregnancy, unspecified.

(66) O21.3 is the ICD-10 code for:

(A) Mild hyperemesis gravidarum.

(B) Excessive vomiting in pregnancy.

(C) Hyperemesis gravidarum with metabolic disturbance.

(D) Late vomiting of pregnancy.

(67) O23.44 is the ICD-10 code for:

(A) Infections of the kidney in pregnancy.

(B) Infections of the bladder in pregnancy.

(C) Infections of the cervix in pregnancy.

(D) Genital tract and urinary tract infections in pregnancy, unspecified.

(68) What is the diagnosis code of primary hyperaldosteronism (Conn's syndrome) per ICD-10-CM?

(A) E26.00.

(B) E26.0.

(C) E26.02.

(D) E26.01.

(69) E26.0 is the ICD-10 code for:

(A) Primary hyperaldosteronism.

(B) Secondary hyperaldosteronism.

(C) Hyperthyroidism.

(D) Hypothyroidism.

(70) I63.3 is the ICD-10 code for:

(A) Cerebral infarction due to thrombosis of cerebral arteries.

(B) Cerebral infarction due to embolism of cerebral arteries.

(C) Cerebral infarction due to unspecified occlusion or stenosis of cerebral arteries.

(D) Stroke, not specified as hemorrhage or infarction.

(71) A seven-year-old boy is transferred to the children's emergency room with a day history of fever, neck pain, and poor feeding. On examination, there is neck stiffness and a positive kerning sign. Temperature is 38.9 C. Heart rate is 106 bpm. Chest is clinically clear. Cerebrospinal fluid is collected via lumbar puncture, and CSF analysis shows an elevated leukocyte count with predominant neutrophilia. A CSF culture is ordered, and the patient is started on intravenous antibiotics at meningitic doses. What is the ICD-10-CM diagnosis code?

(A) G00.

(B) G01.

(C) G04.3.

(D) G00.5.

(72) I67.0 is the ICD-10 code for:

(A) Hypertensive encephalopathy.

(B) Nonpyogenic thrombosis of intracranial venous system.

(C) Cerebral atherosclerosis.

(D) Dissection of cerebral arteries.

(73) A 39-year-old woman visits her neurologist to evaluate recent-onset symptoms. She has noticed progressively worsening tremors and mood problems. Her father died at age 45 from complications that started similarly to hers. She is worried about her prognosis. What ICD-10-CM diagnosis code should be reported for Huntington's disease?

(A) G11.

(B) G09.

(C) G13.

(D) G10.

(74) G06.1 is the ICD-10 code for:

(A) Intracranial abscess.

(B) Intraspinal abscess.

(C) Extradural and subdural abscess.

(D) Brain and spinal abscess, unspecified.

(75) H52.0 is the ICD-10 code for:

(A) Astigmatism.

(B) Myopia.

(C) Hypermetropia.

(D) Presbyopia.

(76) An older man undergoes a visual acuity test after a preliminary assessment of impaired vision that affects both eyes. He has no perception of light in the right eye and a visual acuity of 6/18 in the left eye. What is the appropriate code?

(A) H54.11.

(B) H54.

(C) H54.10.

(D) H53.54.

(77) A 19-year-old boy complains of itching and pain in both ears. He regularly participates in swimming competitions and noticed a yellow discharge from the left ear two days ago. Both ears appear red and swollen, and a purulent discharge is noted from the left ear. He is started on antibiotics and scheduled for a follow-up visit. What is the diagnosis code?

(A) H60.300.

(B) H60.357.

(C) H70.340.

(D) H60.339.

(78) A 26-year-old man presents at a clinic with ringing in the right ear and sharp pain that subsides quickly after instrumentation of the ear to clean wax. Otoscopy confirms a central perforation of the tympanic membrane of the right ear, and the man undergoes a repair of the perforation. The repair is carried out without a mastoidectomy, and the ossicular chain is noted to be intact. What are the ICD-10-CM diagnosis and the CPT code?

(A) H72.01; 69631, modifier RT.

(B) H71.01; 69600, modifier RT.

(C) H62.01; 69631, modifier 77.

(D) H72.01; 68631, modifier 65.

(79) H52.3 is the ICD-10 code for:

(A) Astigmatism.

(B) Myopia.

(C) Hypermetropia.

(D) Presbyopia.

(80) H66.011 is the ICD-10 code for:

(A) Acute suppurative otitis media without spontaneous rupture of the eardrum, right ear.

(B) Acute suppurative otitis media with spontaneous rupture of the eardrum, right ear.

(C) Acute serous otitis media, right ear.

(D) Chronic otitis media, right ear.

(81) What does CPT code 00327 represent?

(A) Anesthesia for procedures on the integumentary system of the head and neck.

(B) Anesthesia for all procedures on the esophagus.

(C) Anesthesia for procedures on the major vessels of the neck.

(D) Anesthesia for procedures involving plastic repair of cleft lip.

(82) A 26-year-old primigravida visits her PCP after labor pains for six hours. There is no history of ruptured membranes or passage of show. She was previously scheduled to receive epidural anesthesia for vaginal delivery. Vaginal examination confirms the latent phase of labor, and the woman subsequently goes into the active phase of labor and delivers a live male neonate with no complications. She receives epidural anesthesia, and pain is well controlled during her labor. What is the correct code to be reported for the form of anesthesia the patient received?

(A) 01968.

(B) 01957.

(C) 01960.

(D) 01967.

(83) A 63-year-old man with suspected prostatic cancer is being prepared for surgical removal of his prostate. The patient consents to a transurethral approach for the removal of the prostate. He undergoes the procedure and receives appropriate anesthesia. The surgery is uneventful, and the patient goes into the recovery room. What is the appropriate code for the anesthesia given during this procedure?

(A) 00914.

(B) 00814.

(C) 00916.

(D) 00915.

(84) A 37-year-old man is referred to an interventional radiologist for continued management of recently diagnosed hepatocellular carcinoma. He is prepared for radioembolization that will use Yttrium-90 to deliver high doses of radioactive materials into the artery that supplies the tumor. This will prevent further spread. He is counseled that the radioactive substance will only target the tumor cells and will not affect the surrounding healthy tissue. What is the correct CPT code that the interventional radiologist should report?

(A) 79455.

(B) 79444.

(C) 79445.

(D) 79443.

(85) A 65-year-old man has been diagnosed with prostatic adenocarcinoma. The tumor is limited to a small part of the prostate, and no evidence of metastasis is found. The patient is counseled on clinical brachytherapy, whereby radioactive implants are inserted near the tumor to stop its growth. The implants are obtained from one to four radioactive sources. What is the appropriate CPT code for the procedure?

(A) 77751.

(B) 77661.

(C) 77701.

(D) 77761.

(86) What does CPT code 77611 represent?

(A) Radiation treatment delivery, single treatment area.

(B) Brachytherapy, complex.

(C) Radiopharmaceutical therapy, therapeutic.

(D) Hemibody irradiation, total body.

(87) As part of a wellness screening, a middle-aged man undergoes a complete abdominal ultrasound scan to view his liver, gallbladder, pancreas, bile ducts, spleen, and abdominal aorta, with real-time image documentation. What is the CPT code for this?

(A) 76701.

(B) 76700.

(C) 76710.

(D) 76711.

(88) A 29-year-old woman is evaluated for infertility. She has a history of secondary amenorrhea that has lasted seven months. Pregnancy tests are negative. She has hirsutism, and her body mass index is 33 kg/m2. A transvaginal ultrasound scan is requested to confirm the diagnosis. What is the CPT code of the requested investigation?

(A) 76820.

(B) 76030.

(C) 76830.

(D) 76820.

(89) A young woman is 28 weeks pregnant with twins. She visits her doctor and asks for an ultrasound for a fetal biophysical profile. What is the CPT code to be reported for this procedure?

(A) 76605, 76810.

(B) 76805, 76610.

(C) 76805, 76800.

(D) 76805, 76810.

(90) What does the acronym "FISH" represent in cytogenetics?

(A) Fluorescent in situ hybridization.

(B) Functional internal system for histology.

(C) Fungal identification through spectroscopy and hybridization.

(D) Flow immunostaining for specific histopathology.

(91) In pathology, what does the name "Hodgkin's lymphoma" honor?

(A) A pioneering microbiologist.

(B) A renowned oncologist.

(C) An influential pathologist.

(D) A famous patient advocate.

(92) What is the meaning of the acronym "ELISA" in laboratory techniques?

(A) Enzyme-linked immunosorbent assay.

(B) Electronically linked imaging and spectroscopy analysis.

(C) Erythrocyte leukocyte identification and screening assay.

(D) Epigenetic laboratory investigation for serum analysis.

(93) What does the eponym "Warthin-Starry stain" refer to in histology?

(A) A technique to identify bacteria.

(B) A stain for connective tissue.

(C) A method for lipid analysis.

(D) A stain for viral inclusions.

(94) In laboratory medicine, what does the acronym "HLA" stand for?

(A) Human leukocyte antigen.

(B) Histopathological laboratory analysis.

(C) High-level automation.

(D) Hematological lymphocyte assessment.

(95) What does the anesthesia CPT code 00792 represent?

(A) Anesthesia for procedures on the esophagus.

(B) Anesthesia for upper abdominal procedures.

(C) Anesthesia for procedures on the lower intestine.

(D) Anesthesia for liver transplant surgery.

(96) What is the appropriate modifier for monitored anesthesia care?

(A) QY.

(B) QS.

(C) QW.

(D) QZ.

(97) A 53-year-old white male was admitted to the hospital to have a splenectomy done after a car accident. The patient was discharged from the hospital after five days. During his hospitalization, he experienced pain and shortness of breath. He was commenced on antibiotic therapy, and he improved. The physician performed a final examination and reviewed the chest X-ray, which revealed possible infiltrates. A CT of the abdomen ruled out any abscess. The man was given oral antibiotics for another 10 days and was told to follow up with his PCP or return to the hospital in case of any pain or bleeding. The physician spent 30 minutes with the patient. What is the appropriate code for this final visit?

(A) 99283.

(B) 99221.

(C) 99231.

(D) 99238.

(98) A physician is notified to go to the hospital floor for medical management of a 56-year-old patient admitted one day ago for aspiration pneumonitis on a background COPD. The physician documents an expanded problem-focused history with no chest pain at present. The woman still has shortness of breath and some swelling in her lower extremities. She was tachypneic yesterday. A focused exam is done, and the lungs reveal coarse crackles in both bases, the right worse than the left. MDM is moderate. The X-ray film and lab results are reviewed, and the patient is continued on intravenous antibiotic treatment and respiratory support. She has improved, and a review by the respiratory team is requested. What CPT code should be reported?

(A) 99221.

(B) 99231.

(C) 99232.

(D) 99223.

(99) An ophthalmologist receives a consult to evaluate a woman with suspected retinopathy secondary to diabetes mellitus. During her first appointment, the woman receives a comprehensive ophthalmological evaluation and fundoscopy. A diagnosis of diabetic retinopathy is confirmed, and a management plan is discussed with the patient. What is the correct CPT code for this service?

(A) 92002.

(B) 92004.

(C) 92001.

(D) 92005.

(100) What does the CPT code 92311 represent?

(A) Contact lens prescription with fitting for both eyes.

(B) Prescription of optical lenses.

(C) Contact lens prescription with fitting for one eye.

(D) Prescription of prosthetic eye.

# Test 5: Answers and Explanations

(1) (A) The MAC.

The medical administrative contractor (MAC) interprets national policies into regional ones. The OIG is mainly concerned with the investigation of healthcare fraud and abuse. The LCD provides guidance on the different services included in a given region and the limitations of these services in their local environments. An HMO is an example of a covered entity designated as a health plan by HIPAA. It is not involved in the national or local interpretation of insurance policies.

(2) (D) A patient.

A patient is not considered a covered entity. HIPAA defines covered institutions as healthcare providers, health plans, and clearinghouses that electronically transmit health information.

(3) (B) B20, K13.3, F12.2.

The correct sequence starts with the primary diagnosis (B20 for HIV disease), followed by conditions that are a consequence of or related to the primary diagnosis (K13.3 for oral hairy leukoplakia, which is associated with HIV), and then other conditions the patient has (F12.2 for cannabis dependence).

(4) (D) Category IV.

Category IV is not a type of CPT code.

(5) (B) There is no time limit to when a sequela code can be used.

There is no time limit to when sequela can occur. Hence, there is no time limit for when the code can be used. This is the only suitable option. Sequelae are late effects of a disease and are seen much later than the onset of the disease. Some occur early (within weeks), and others may be after years. The codes for the acute phase of a disease and sequela cannot be used together as the late effects are seen later, after the acute phase of the disease. Two codes are used, not three.

(6) (B) E11.

For a confirmed diagnosis of diabetes mellitus without a defined type, code E11 is used.

(7) (B) A28.9.

The correct code for this case is A28.9, which is code for unspecified zoonotic bacterial disease. A15.1 codes for tuberculosis of the lungs confirmed by culture. R22.1 codes for pulmonary anthrax. E89.5 codes for postprocedural testicular hypofunction.

(8) (A) The toes are pointed down.

Plantar flexion is the term used to describe the downward action of the toes. “Plantar” is derived from the Latin “planta,” which means sole.

(9) (D) Calcaneal.

The anatomical term for the heel region is the calcaneal region. Derived from the Latin word "calcaneus," it means heel bone.

(10) (B) Closer to the point of attachment.

In anatomical terms, "proximal" refers to a position closer to the point of attachment or the body's center.

(11) (B) Flexion.

Flexion is the anatomical movement that reduces the angle between two body parts. It is common in joints such as knees and elbows. Flexion brings the parts closer together. For instance, when the arm bends at the elbow, this involves flexion.

(12) (A) Forward.

In the anatomical position, the palms face forward. This standard reference point in anatomy helps describe the body's structures consistently. With the body upright, faced forward, arms at the sides, the palms naturally turn toward the front.

(13) (B) Adduction.

The term for a movement that brings a body part closer to the midline is "adduction." This anatomical movement occurs when a limb or body segment moves inward toward the body's central axis.

(14) (C) Dorsal.

The anatomical term for the back side of the body is "dorsal." Dorsal refers to the posterior aspect or the side that faces away from the front.

(15) (C) Rotation.

The anatomical term for the movement of the head from side to side is "rotation." This movement occurs around the axis of the neck and is pivotal for various activities, such as when a person looks over their shoulder.

(16) (B) J44.1.

Chronic obstructive pulmonary disease is listed under the respiratory diseases category and injury index of the ICD-10-CM coding set. The information included reveals an acute exacerbation event listed further within the subcategory. COPD is coded J44.1

(17) (B) I61.9.

Locate the diagnosis under diseases of the circulatory system. Cerebrovascular diseases are in index I60–I69. Nontraumatic intracerebral hemorrhages are located within subcategory I61. Lack of specificity results in a further subcategory, I61.9.

(18) (A) Hypertrophic obstructive cardiomyopathy.

Hypertrophic Obstructive Cardiomyopathy (HOCM) is a condition characterized by abnormal thickening of the heart muscle, and it affects the interventricular septum. This thickening can obstruct blood flow out of the left ventricle and cause various symptoms, such as shortness of breath, chest pain, and palpitations.

(19) (D) D25.9.

Uterine fibroids are benign neoplasms of the uterus with different classifications. The location of these benign growths is not specified. Therefore, the diagnosis of unspecified leiomyoma of the uterus is coded D25.9.

(20) (C) F20.9.

Schizophrenia is a mental disorder classified under the broad category F, with subcategories based on the demonstrated symptoms. The lack of detail of associated symptoms leaves this code as unspecified, F20.9.

(21) (A) C61.

C61 is the primary code for a malignant neoplasm of the prostate, listed under the category of neoplasms. No further subcategory is present in the code set for malignant prostatic lesions.

(22) (B) It discourages the use of transportation services.

This is incorrect. One of the functions of the HCPCS code is to enable reporting and reimbursement for services that are not usually covered by the CPT code set. This may include procedures by healthcare professionals and providers and services, such as medications, transportation, medical devices, and other services needed for functional healthcare service delivery. HCPCS does not discourage the use of transportation services but instead encourages it by making billing and reimbursement easy.

(23) (B) 10 days.

A Bartholin's gland abscess incision and drainage is classified as a minor surgery. In the global package for surgery, for minor procedures/surgeries, the global day is the procedure day for the preoperative period, and the postoperative period is 10 days.

(24) (B) Simple repair of superficial wounds of scalp, neck, axillae, external genitalia, trunk and/or extremities (including hands and feet); 2.6 cm to 7.5 cm, with increased procedural services.

When the code is appended with the modifier -23, it indicates that the procedure required increased procedural services, usually due to factors that make the procedure more complex or time-consuming than usual.

(25) (B) 53.

53 is the appropriate modifier used when a procedure is discontinued at the discretion of the physician or surgeon due to a risk to the patient's well-being.

(26) (C) Unspecified contact dermatitis, unspecified cause.

This code is used when there is insufficient information to assign a more specific code, which indicates a condition of skin inflammation or rash resulting from contact with a substance, but the specific substance or cause is not known.

(27) (A) L70.0.

The ICD-10 code usually used for acne vulgaris is L70.0. Acne vulgaris is identified by comedones, papules, pustules and, occasionally, nodules or cysts. The L70 category in the ICD-10 coding system specifically addresses acne. More detailed codes within this range may be used to indicate the severity, type, and location of acne lesions for accurate medical documentation and billing purposes.

(28) (B) D04.9.

D04.9 is the ICD-10-CM code for basal cell carcinoma, unspecified. It is used to report a diagnosis of basal cell carcinoma when the specific location is not mentioned.

(29) (A) C43.9.

The ICD-10 code for malignant melanoma of the skin with an unspecified site is C43.9. This code is utilized when the specific location of the melanoma is not identified or documented. C43.9 falls within the broader C43 category, which covers malignant melanomas of the skin.

(30) (A) L21.

The ICD-10 code for seborrheic dermatitis is L21. An inflammation of the skin, seborrheic dermatitis is quite prevalent. It is usually identified by the presence of red, itchy, and flaky patches.

(31) (B) L98.9.

The ICD-10 code for an unspecified disorder of the skin and subcutaneous tissue is L98.9. This code is employed when the specific nature or cause of the skin disorder is not provided in medical documentation.

(32) (B) Musculoskeletal disorders.

In the ICD-10 coding system, the "M" serves as the initial character in the alphanumeric code assigned to diseases, conditions, and abnormalities that affect the musculoskeletal system.

(33) (A) 23500.

Code 23500 specifically describes the nonsurgical, closed reduction of a fractured clavicle without the need for manipulation or surgical intervention.

(34) (B) 20611.

Code 20611 is used to document and bill for procedures that involve the injection of therapeutic substances, such as corticosteroids or hyaluronic acid, into the knee joint under ultrasound guidance, with the additional inclusion of arthrography if it is performed during the injection.

(35) (B) Arthroscopy, shoulder, surgical; debridement, extensive.

This procedure involves the surgical removal of extensive amounts of soft tissue and/or bone, which is usually done to treat shoulder conditions where there is significant tissue damage or inflammation. The extensive nature of the debridement distinguishes this procedure from less comprehensive debridement procedures.

(36) (A) 26116.

Code 26116 is specific to surgical procedures that involve the removal of a subcutaneous tumor from the soft tissues in the hand or finger area.

(37) (A) 27250.

Code 27250 is utilized to document and bill for the nonsurgical, closed reduction of a dislocated hip joint without the use of anesthesia or additional manipulative procedures.

(38) (D) +99140.

Code +99140 describes emergency conditions and is found under the qualifying circumstances CPT category in the chapter that covers medicine. The add-on code and a primary anesthesia procedure code are used but only apply when the anesthesia given becomes complex due to an emergency.

(39) (A) K44.9.

Code K44.9 is used to classify herniation of abdominal contents through the diaphragm. This results in potential complications.

(40) (A) Lymphedema, unspecified.

I89.0 is assigned when the cause or location of lymphedema is not further specified.

(41) (B) Bronchoscopy, rigid or flexible, including fluoroscopic guidance, when performed; with biopsy, single or multiple sites.

The code includes the use of fluoroscopic guidance if performed. This procedure allows for direct visualization of the airways and is performed to diagnose and assess lung diseases, infections, or tumors by obtaining tissue samples for histopathological examination.

(42) (A) Thoracentesis, needle or catheter, aspiration of the pleural space; without imaging guidance.

Thoracentesis is a procedure where a needle or catheter is inserted into the pleural space to aspirate fluid for diagnostic or therapeutic purposes. This code represents the procedure when it is done without the aid of imaging technology like ultrasound or CT to guide the needle or catheter placement.

(43) (A) Mediastinoscopy, including biopsy by mediastinal incision.

CPT code 39400 is used for mediastinoscopy, which is a surgical procedure that involves making an incision at the mediastinum (the area between the lungs) and inserting a scope to examine the area and possibly perform a biopsy. This code represents the procedure when a biopsy is taken through a mediastinal incision. Mediastinoscopy is used to diagnose or stage lung cancer, lymphoma, or other diseases in the chest.

(44) (A) I20.0.

Code I20.0 specifically identifies stable angina, a condition characterized by chest pain or discomfort caused by a reduction in blood flow to the heart muscle.

(45) (B) I50.9.

Code I50.9 is utilized when heart failure is diagnosed but not further specified as to type or cause.

(46) (C) To fill in empty characters when a code requires a 7th character.

In ICD-10-CM coding, the 'X' placeholder is used in certain codes that require a 7th character extension to ensure that the code structure remains consistent. The 'X' is placed in the code structure where a specific character is not applicable but a 7th character is required.

(47) (C) Providers delivering specialized medical services.

The Medicine section of the CPT code manual is used to report a wide range of services provided by healthcare professionals, including non-surgical therapeutic, diagnostic, and preventive services. This section encompasses codes for specialized medical services outside of surgery, radiology, and the standard evaluation and management services.

(48) (B) Cardiac bypass grafting.

These codes cover services such as reoperations for cardiac bypass grafting and repairs related to previous cardiac bypass procedures. They are used to accurately report and bill for these complex cardiac procedures.

(49) (C) -51.

In CPT coding, the modifier commonly used to indicate multiple procedures performed during the same session is 51. This modifier is applied when a provider performs multiple distinct procedures during a single encounter.

(50) (A) K58.9.

The appropriate ICD-10-CM code for irritable bowel syndrome is K58.9. This code includes various forms of IBS when specific subtypes are not explicitly identified. IBS refers to a functional gastrointestinal disorder that is marked by abdominal pain, bloating, and alterations in bowel habits.

(51) (A) K29.0.

Code K29.0 is used to document cases of acute inflammation of the gastric mucosa.

(52) (C) Chronic Viral Hepatitis B without Delta-Agent.

This code is used to indicate a diagnosis for healthcare billing and documentation purposes. It specifies that the patient has a chronic form of hepatitis B virus infection without co-infection with the hepatitis D virus, also known as the delta agent.

(53) (B) 43235.

Code 43235 specifically identifies the procedure that visualizes the esophagus, stomach, and duodenum with an endoscope for diagnostic purposes.

(54) (A) 45380.

Code 45380 indicates the complete colonoscopy procedure, which may include the examination and collection of tissue samples for biopsy.

(55) (A) 43249.

Code 43249 represents the procedure that involves the use of an endoscope to visualize the upper gastrointestinal tract. This includes the esophagus, stomach, and duodenum. In addition to visualization, the dilation aspect indicates that therapeutic measures, such as widening of narrowed areas, were performed during the endoscopy.

(56) (D) 55700.

A punch biopsy of the prostate is reported as 55700. No modifiers were reported for this procedure.

(57) (A) 55250, modifier 50.

CPT code 55250 is used for a vasectomy, unilateral or bilateral, including postoperative semen examination(s). Modifier 50 is used to indicate that the procedure was performed on both sides (bilateral).

(58) (A) 51990.

A surgical laparoscopy with urethral suspension for stress incontinence is coded 51990.

(59) (A) 51702, P9612.

The insertion of a temporary simple indwelling Foley catheter for urine drainage in a post-op patient is coded 51702. HCPCS code P9612 is for catheterization for specimen collection in a single patient.

(60) (A) 74450.

CPT code 74450 is used for a radiologic examination, urethra; retrograde, with or without voiding cystourethrography. This code is appropriate for the procedure described, which involves the injection of dye to evaluate the urethra and possibly the bladder, known as retrograde urethrocystography.

(61) (C) 52282.

CPT code 52282 is used for cystourethroscopy with insertion of a permanent urethral stent. This code accurately describes the surgical procedure for urethral stricture when previous dilator placement failed.

(62) (D) O65.4, 59514.

The initial assessment of this patient reveals a diagnosis of obstructed labor due to fetal pelvic disproportion. However, the preliminary nature of this assessment does not specify the cause of this disproportion. Therefore, the subcategory of the diagnosis is reported as unspecified with ICD-10-CM code O65.4. The patient is scheduled for a cesarean delivery, and the CPT code for this emergency intervention is 59514.

(63) (A) O63.1.

The ICD-10-CM diagnosis code for the prolonged second stage of labor is subcategory O63.1.

(64) (B) Failed induction of labor.

This code is important for documenting and communicating this specific obstetric complication.

(65) (B) Excessive vomiting in pregnancy.

This code is used to document cases where the level of vomiting is unusually high and may require medical intervention. It helps with distinguishing this condition from other types of vomiting related to pregnancy, such as mild hyperemesis gravidarum (O21.0) or hyperemesis gravidarum with metabolic disturbance (O21.2).

(66) (D) Late vomiting of pregnancy.

O21.3 specifically represents late vomiting of pregnancy, which occurs typically after the first trimester. This code is used to document cases of vomiting that start later in pregnancy, distinguishing it from early pregnancy vomiting or hyperemesis gravidarum.

(67) (B) Infections of the bladder in pregnancy.

This code is vital for accurate medical documentation, and ensures that healthcare professionals properly recognize and treat bladder infections during pregnancy. It also plays a critical role in healthcare billing, and allows for appropriate reimbursement for services related to the diagnosis and treatment of this condition.

(68) (B) E26.0.

ICD-10-CM diagnosis code E26.0 represents primary hyperaldosteronism, also known as Conn's syndrome. This code is specific for the condition characterized by excessive aldosterone production by the adrenal glands.

(69) (A) Primary hyperaldosteronism.

This condition is characterized by excessive production of the hormone aldosterone by the adrenal glands, leading to hypertension and low potassium levels.

(70) (A) Cerebral infarction due to thrombosis of cerebral arteries.

I63.3 specifically denotes cerebral infarction due to thrombosis of cerebral arteries. This code indicates that the cause of the infarction (tissue death in the brain due to inadequate blood supply) was a thrombus (blood clot) in the cerebral arteries.

(71) (A) G00.

This patient probably has bacterial meningitis, per the CSF analysis findings. The appropriate ICD-10-CM diagnosis code is G00.

(72) (C) Cerebral atherosclerosis.

I67.0 specifically denotes cerebral atherosclerosis, a condition characterized by the buildup of plaques in the arteries of the brain. This can lead to reduced blood flow and potentially cause strokes or transient ischemic attacks. Accurate use of this code is vital for proper diagnosis, treatment planning, and billing for medical services.

(73) (D) G10.

Huntington's disease is a progressive neurological disorder with a poor prognosis. It is characterized by movement disorder and chronic dementia. The disease is inherited in an autosomal dominant fashion, and the ICD-10-CM diagnosis code is G10.

(74) (B) Intraspinal abscess.

G06.1 refers to an intraspinal abscess, an infection characterized by a collection of pus within the spinal canal. This code is used for accurate documentation and billing of medical services related to the diagnosis, treatment, and management of an intraspinal abscess.

(75) (C) Hypermetropia.

H52.0 refers to Hypermetropia, also known as farsightedness or long-sightedness. This condition is characterized by difficulty with focusing on close objects while distant objects can be seen more clearly.

(76) (A) H54.11.

According to the World Health Organization, this patient is diagnosed with blindness in the right eye and low vision in the left eye. The correct code is H54.11.

(77) (D) H60.339.

The diagnosis is swimmer's ear, and the appropriate code for a bilateral presentation is H60.339.

(78) (A) H72.01; 69631, modifier RT.

The appropriate diagnosis code for a central tympanic membrane perforation of only the right ear is H72.01. The subsequent CPT procedure for the repair carried out is 69631, which describes a tympanoplasty without mastoidectomy and ossicular chain reconstruction. The correct modifier is RT.

(79) (A) Astigmatism.

H52.3 refers to Astigmatism, a condition where the cornea or lens of the eye has an irregular shape, causing blurred or distorted vision.

(80) (B) Acute suppurative otitis media with spontaneous rupture of the eardrum, right ear.

H66.011 refers to Acute suppurative otitis media with spontaneous rupture of the eardrum in the right ear. This condition involves an acute infection of the middle ear, and is characterized by the presence of pus and a spontaneous rupture or perforation of the eardrum.

(81) (C) Anesthesia for procedures on the major vessels of the neck.

CPT code 00327 is designated for anesthesia services provided during procedures on the major vessels of the neck.

(82) (D) 01967.

The correct CPT code used to report epidural anesthesia for vaginal delivery, as seen in this case, is 01967.

(83) (A) 00914.

Transurethral prostate removal is a minimally invasive operation. The appropriate code for the anesthesia used in this procedure is 00914.

(84) (C) 79445.

The procedure described in this clinical scenario is the introduction of a liquid that contains radioactive particles into an artery that supplies a tumor. The correct CPT code for this procedure is 79445.

(85) (D) 77761.

Clinical brachytherapy is a form of radiological intervention used for prostate cancer by the application of implants near the tumor from one to four radioactive sources. The appropriate CPT code is 77761.

(86) (B) Brachytherapy, complex.

Brachytherapy is a form of radiation therapy where a radioactive source is placed inside or next to the area requiring treatment. Complex brachytherapy typically involves sophisticated planning and delivery techniques to ensure precise targeting of the radiation dose.

(87) (B) 76700.

The correct CPT code for a complete abdominal ultrasound scan to view the liver, gallbladder, pancreas, bile ducts, spleen, and abdominal aorta, with real-time image documentation, is 76700.

(88) (C) 76830.

The CPT code for a transvaginal ultrasound scan is 76830.

(89) (D) 76805, 76810.

The appropriate CPT code for a transabdominal ultrasound of a single fetus in the second trimester is 76805. For multiple gestation, the add-on code for the second fetus is 76810.

(90) (A) Fluorescent in-situ hybridization.

In cytogenetics, the acronym "FISH" stands for fluorescent in-situ hybridization. This advanced molecular technique allows specific DNA sequences within cells to be visualized and mapped. Through the use of fluorescent probes that bind to target DNA, FISH enables precise identification of genetic abnormalities. This aids in the diagnosis of genetic disorders, cancer, and chromosomal anomalies. FISH helps medical professionals understand vital genomic variations and guides therapeutic interventions in clinical settings.

(91) (C) An influential pathologist.

The name Hodgkin's lymphoma honors the British physician Thomas Hodgkin, an influential pathologist. In the early 19th century, Hodgkin meticulously described a distinct type of lymphatic system cancer characterized by specific cell abnormalities. His groundbreaking work, "On Some Morbid Appearances of the Absorbent Glands and Spleen," published in 1832, laid the foundation for understanding this malignancy. Hodgkin's meticulous observations and contributions to pathology paved the way for further research, classification, and treatment of lymphomas.

(92) (A) Enzyme-linked immunosorbent assay.

In lab techniques, the acronym "ELISA" stands for enzyme-linked immunosorbent assay. This widely used diagnostic method detects the presence of antibodies or antigens in biological samples. ELISA involves binding specific molecules to an enzyme followed by detection of the resultant reaction. The assay's sensitivity and versatility make it pivotal in medical diagnostics. This includes infectious disease testing and allergy detection.

(93) (A) A technique to identify bacteria.

The eponym "Warthin-Starry stain" in histology refers to a specialized staining technique used to identify bacteria, particularly those of the genus Spirochetes. Developed by pathologists Aldred Scott Warthin and Franklin Chester Starry, this stain utilizes silver nitrate to visualize the distinctive spiral-shaped bacteria in tissue sections. The Warthin-Starry stain is particularly valuable in pathogens like Treponema pallidum. This aids in the diagnosis of diseases such as syphilis and other spirochetal infections.

(94) (A) Human leukocyte antigen.

In laboratory medicine, the acronym "HLA" stands for human leukocyte antigen. HLA molecules play a vital role in the immune system when they present antigens to T cells. These genetic markers, found on the surface of cells, are diverse among individuals and influence immune responses and transplantation compatibility. HLA testing is essential for organ and tissue transplantation, as matching HLA types reduces the risk of rejection and enhances the success of transplant procedures in clinical settings.

(95) (C) Anesthesia for procedures on the lower intestine.

This code is used by anesthesiologists and CRNAs to bill for their services when they are involved in procedures such as colonoscopies, lower intestinal resections, or other related surgeries.

(96) (B) QS.

The modifier included when reporting for monitored anesthesia care is QS.

(97) (D) 99238.

Hospital discharge codes are determined based on the time the physician provides discharge-day services, which include evaluation and management. Here, the physician documented 30 minutes, which is reported with 99238.

(98) (C) 99232.

99232 is used to code for subsequent hospital observation or inpatient service with straightforward and moderate medical decision-making.

(99) (B) 92004.

The new patient receives a comprehensive ophthalmological evaluation and diagnostic and treatment program. This is coded 92004.

(100) (C) Contact lens prescription with fitting for one eye.

This code is utilized by eye care professionals to accurately bill for the time and resources involved in evaluating a patient's eye and determining the correct contact lens prescription, including the necessary fitting for one eye.

Made in the USA
Monee, IL
08 October 2026

65145225R00227